New Diagnostic and Therapeutic Aspects of Thrombotic Thrombocytopenic Purpura

New Diagnostic and Therapeutic Aspects of Thrombotic Thrombocytopenic Purpura

Guest Editors

Ilaria Mancini
Andrea Artoni

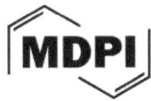

Basel • Beijing • Wuhan • Barcelona • Belgrade • Novi Sad • Cluj • Manchester

Guest Editors

Ilaria Mancini
Università degli Studi di Milano
Milan
Italy

Andrea Artoni
Angelo Bianchi Bonomi Hemophilia
and Thrombosis Center
Milan
Italy

Editorial Office
MDPI AG
Grosspeteranlage 5
4052 Basel, Switzerland

This is a reprint of the Special Issue, published open access by the journal *Journal of Clinical Medicine* (ISSN 2077-0383), freely accessible at: https://www.mdpi.com/journal/jcm/special_issues/242XXPRXN7.

For citation purposes, cite each article independently as indicated on the article page online and as indicated below:

Lastname, A.A.; Lastname, B.B. Article Title. *Journal Name* **Year**, *Volume Number*, Page Range.

ISBN 978-3-7258-2859-3 (Hbk)
ISBN 978-3-7258-2860-9 (PDF)
https://doi.org/10.3390/books978-3-7258-2860-9

© 2025 by the authors. Articles in this book are Open Access and distributed under the Creative Commons Attribution (CC BY) license. The book as a whole is distributed by MDPI under the terms and conditions of the Creative Commons Attribution-NonCommercial-NoDerivs (CC BY-NC-ND) license (https://creativecommons.org/licenses/by-nc-nd/4.0/).

Contents

Stefano Lancellotti, Monica Sacco, Maira Tardugno, Antonietta Ferretti and Raimondo De Cristofaro
Immune and Hereditary Thrombotic Thrombocytopenic Purpura: Can ADAMTS13 Deficiency Alone Explain the Different Clinical Phenotypes?
Reprinted from: *J. Clin. Med.* **2023**, *12*, 3111, https://doi.org/10.3390/jcm12093111 1

Quintijn Bonnez, Kazuya Sakai and Karen Vanhoorelbeke
ADAMTS13 and Non-ADAMTS13 Biomarkers in Immune-Mediated Thrombotic Thrombocytopenic Purpura
Reprinted from: *J. Clin. Med.* **2023**, *12*, 6169, https://doi.org/10.3390/jcm12196169 13

Cristina Dainese, Federica Valeri, Benedetto Bruno and Alessandra Borchiellini
Anti-ADAMTS13 Autoantibodies: From Pathophysiology to Prognostic Impact—A Review for Clinicians
Reprinted from: *J. Clin. Med.* **2023**, *12*, 5630, https://doi.org/10.3390/jcm12175630 25

Raphael Cauchois, Romain Muller, Marie Lagarde, Françoise Dignat-George, Edwige Tellier and Gilles Kaplanski
Is Endothelial Activation a Critical Event in Thrombotic Thrombocytopenic Purpura?
Reprinted from: *J. Clin. Med.* **2023**, *12*, 758, https://doi.org/10.3390/jcm12030758 35

Adrien Joseph, Bérangère S. Joly, Adrien Picod, Agnès Veyradier and Paul Coppo
The Specificities of Thrombotic Thrombocytopenic Purpura at Extreme Ages: A Narrative Review
Reprinted from: *J. Clin. Med.* **2023**, *12*, 3068, https://doi.org/10.3390/jcm12093068 53

Senthil Sukumar, Marshall A. Mazepa and Shruti Chaturvedi
Cardiovascular Disease and Stroke in Immune TTP–Challenges and Opportunities
Reprinted from: *J. Clin. Med.* **2023**, *12*, 5961, https://doi.org/10.3390/jcm12185961 64

Rebecca J. Shaw, Simon T. Abrams, Samuel Badu, Cheng-Hock Toh and Tina Dutt
The Highs and Lows of ADAMTS13 Activity
Reprinted from: *J. Clin. Med.* **2024**, *13*, 5152, https://doi.org/10.3390/jcm13175152 74

Alexandre Soares Ferreira Junior, Morgana Pinheiro Maux Lessa, Samantha Kaplan, Theresa M. Coles, Deirdra R. Terrell and Oluwatoyosi A. Onwuemene
Patient-Reported Outcome Measures in Patients with Thrombotic Thrombocytopenic Purpura: A Systematic Review of the Literature
Reprinted from: *J. Clin. Med.* **2023**, *12*, 5155, https://doi.org/10.3390/jcm12155155 86

Ayesha Butt, Cecily Allen, Adriana Purcell, Satoko Ito and George Goshua
Global Health Resource Utilization and Cost-Effectiveness of Therapeutics and Diagnostics in Immune Thrombotic Thrombocytopenic Purpura (TTP)
Reprinted from: *J. Clin. Med.* **2023**, *12*, 4887, https://doi.org/10.3390/jcm12154887 101

Kazuya Sakai and Masanori Matsumoto
Clinical Manifestations, Current and Future Therapy, and Long-Term Outcomes in Congenital Thrombotic Thrombocytopenic Purpura
Reprinted from: *J. Clin. Med.* **2023**, *12*, 3365, https://doi.org/10.3390/jcm12103365 115

Leslie Skeith, Kelle Hurd, Shruti Chaturvedi, Lorraine Chow, Joshua Nicholas, Adrienne Lee, et al.
Hypercoagulability and Inflammatory Markers in a Case of Congenital Thrombotic Thrombocytopenic Purpura Complicated by Fetal Demise
Reprinted from: *J. Clin. Med.* **2022**, *11*, 7115, https://doi.org/10.3390/jcm11237115 . . . . **127**

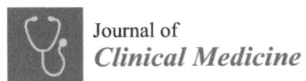

Review

Immune and Hereditary Thrombotic Thrombocytopenic Purpura: Can ADAMTS13 Deficiency Alone Explain the Different Clinical Phenotypes?

Stefano Lancellotti [1,†], Monica Sacco [2,†], Maira Tardugno [2], Antonietta Ferretti [2] and Raimondo De Cristofaro [1,2,*]

1 Servizio Malattie Emorragiche e Trombotiche, Fondazione Policlinico Universitario "A. Gemelli" IRCCS, 00168 Roma, Italy; stefano.lancellotti@policlinicogemelli.it
2 Dipartimento di Medicina e Chirurgia Traslazionale, Facoltà di Medicina e Chirurgia "Agostino Gemelli", Università Cattolica S. Cuore, 00168 Roma, Italy; monicasacco.89@gmail.com (M.S.); maira.tardugno@gmail.com (M.T.)
* Correspondence: raimondo.decristofaro@unicatt.it; Tel.: +39-0630156329; Fax: +39-0630155915
† These authors contributed equally to this work.

Abstract: Thrombotic thrombocytopenic purpura (TTP) is a thrombotic microangiopathy caused by a hereditary or immune-mediated deficiency of the enzyme ADAMTS13 (a disintegrin and metalloproteinase with a thrombospondin type 1 motif, member 13). TTPs are caused by the following pathophysiological mechanisms: (1) the presence of inhibitory autoantibodies against ADAMTS13; and (2) hereditary mutations of the *ADAMTS13* gene, which is present on chromosome 9. In both syndromes, TTP results from a severe deficiency of ADAMTS13, which is responsible for the impaired proteolytic processing of high-molecular-weight von Willebrand factor (HMW-VWF) multimers, which avidly interact with platelets and subendothelial collagen and promote tissue and multiorgan ischemia. Although the acute presentation of the occurring symptoms in acquired and hereditary TTPs is similar (microangiopathic hemolytic anemia, thrombocytopenia, and variable ischemic end-organ injury), their intensity, incidence, and precipitating factors are different, although, in both forms, a severe ADAMTS13 deficiency characterizes their physiopathology. This review is aimed at exploring the possible factors responsible for the different clinical and pathological features occurring in hereditary and immune-mediated TTPs.

Keywords: pathophysiology of iTTP; autoantibodies to ADAMTS-13; thrombotic microangiopathy

1. Introduction

Thrombotic microangiopathies (TMAs) are a heterogeneous group of syndromes associated with the generation of disseminated microthrombi responsible for a clinical triad composed of microangiopathic hemolytic anemia (MAHA), thrombocytopenia, and variable ischemic end-organ injury [1]. Such syndromes, although stemming from different pathophysiological mechanisms, present with a similar clinical phenotype. The main diagnostic aspects of different TMAs are summarized in Table 1, which includes the most recent clinical form associated with coronavirus disease-19 (COVID-19), whose pathogenesis is still under investigation [2]. The latter, although it would resemble the pathophysiology of complement-mediated TMAs, shows genetic and functional evidence of complement dysregulation. Thrombotic thrombocytopenic purpura (TTP) is caused by a hereditary (cTTP) or immune-mediated (iTTP) deficiency of the enzyme ADAMTS13 (a disintegrin and metalloproteinase with a thrombospondin type 1 motif, member 13) [3,4] and is one of the best characterized TMAs [5–8]. After the initial discovery of the main culprit for TTPs, further understanding of the underlying pathophysiology of TTP has led to significant advancements in the diagnosis [9–12] and clinical management of these patients [13–15], as well as increasing interest in issues related to TTP survivorship. Although the acute clinical phenomena occurring in iTTP and cTTP are similar (MAHA, thrombocytopenia, and variable ischemic end-organ injury), their intensity, incidence, and precipitating factors are different, despite the fact that in both forms, a severe ADAMTS13 deficiency characterizes their physiopathology.

Table 1. Diagnostic features of different thrombotic microangiopathies (TMAs).

Clinical Form	Diagnostic Features
Thrombotic Thrombocytopenic Purpura (TTP)	ADAMTS13 deficiency
Infection-associated TMA	Shiga-toxin, Streptococcus pneumonia, Campylobacter jejuni, Cytomegalovirus, Human immunodeficiency virus, Parvovirus B19, Epstein–Barr virus, BK virus, Influenza
Complement-mediated hemolytic uremic syndrome (HUS)	Dysregulation of complement factors and their inhibitors
Secondary TMAs	Cancer, Transplantation, Antiphospholipid antibody Systemic lupus erythematosus syndrome, Scleroderma, Vasculitis/glomerulonephritis
Disseminated intravascular coagulation	Sepsis, cancer
Drug-induced TMA	Calcineurin or mTOR inhibitors, Quinine, Interferon Vascular endothelial growth factor or proteasome inhibitors Estrogen/progesterone, Gemcitabine/mitomycin C, Cocaine
Malignant hypertension-induced TMA	Extreme levels of blood pressure, severe headache, papilledema
Pregnancy-associated TMA	HELLP (hemolysis, elevated liver enzymes, and low platelets) syndrome, HUS, TTP
Metabolism-associated TMA	Cobalamin responsive methylmalonic acidemia, mutation of Diacylglycerolkinase epsilon
COVID-19 associated TMA	SARS-COV2 infection, evidence of microangiopathy

The present review is aimed at exploring the possible factors responsible for the different clinical and pathological features of TTP.

2. TTP Pathophysiology

TTPs are caused by different pathophysiological mechanisms, which include the following: (1) the presence of inhibitory autoantibodies against ADAMTS13; and (2) hereditary mutations of the *ADAMTS13* gene, which is present on chromosome 9q34 [4]. In both syndromes, TTP results from a severe deficiency of ADAMTS13, which is responsible for the impaired proteolytic processing of high-molecular-weight von Willebrand factor (HMW-VWF) multimers that, under shear stress of >30 dyn/cm^2, are stretched and form long strings that are able to avidly interact with platelets and subendothelial collagen. Moreover, the longer the VWF multimer, the higher its sensitivity to shear stress [16]. In fact, the tensile force F(j) to the inside of any sphere pair j in a chain with N dimers, such as in a VWF multimer, is the sum of the forces on all the outer dimer pairs. The total tensile force, F(j), is calculated as follows [17]:

$$F(j) \approx \sum_{i=j}^{N} f[ix(d+2a)] \approx \frac{(N+j)(N+1-j)}{2} f(d+2a) \quad (1)$$

where f(i) is the normal force between two spheres that are a certain distance (x) apart. From Equation (1), a is the radius of the sphere; the normal force on a monomer in the center of a multimer is approximately proportional to N^2 (i.e., when j = 1), whereas the force on a monomer at the end of a multimer is proportional to N (i.e., when j = N). This is why the prothrombotic potential of VWF multimers occurs in the microcirculation. Here, hemodynamic principles indicate the presence of the highest shear stress in the entire circulatory tree that can induce a drastic conformational change and stretch the VWF multimers that interact and aggregate a great number of blood platelets with the resulting ischemic effects.

3. Immune TTP (iTTP)

Most patients with iTTP have detectable anti-ADAMTS13 autoantibodies that may have inhibitory or non-inhibitory features [18–21]. The former block the proteolysis of HMW-VWF, whereas ADAMTS13 clearance from the circulatory tree is accelerated by non-inhibitory antibodies [18]. The latter were found to target several domains of ADAMTS13. The spacer domain of the metalloprotease represents a hotspot for interacting antibodies. In fact, antibodies against the spacer domain are present in the majority of iTTP patients, inhibiting the enzyme's activity [22–25]. The mechanisms of action of non-inhibitory antibodies, also defined as "clearing" antibodies, are not fully clarified. For instance, Thomas M.R. and colleagues found non-inhibitory antibodies in 15 out of 43 patients during an acute iTTP episode [21]. Moreover, the ADAMTS13 antigen levels were found to be very low in the early phase of acute iTTP, and the patients falling in the lowest quartile of the ADAMTS13 antigen level showed the highest mortality rate [21]. ADAMTS13, which would usually circulate in a "closed" globular conformation, was found in an "open" conformation, both during acute iTTP episodes and phases of clinical remission with subnormal ADAMTS13 levels [26]. In studies by Roose and colleagues, autoantibodies against ADAMTS13 have been described to induce a conformational transition of the ADAMTS13 molecules from a native "closed" state to an "open" state [11,26], causing the exposure of cryptic epitopes in the spacer region. Furthermore, different autoantibodies directed against the distal carboxy terminal of ADAMTS13, where CUB domains are present, modulate its susceptibility to inhibitory antibodies [27]. The complete list of the negative activities exerted by these autoantibodies in the pathophysiology of iTTP is yet to be fully characterized. The detailed and specific mechanisms leading to the loss of tolerance for ADAMTS13 in iTTP are still far from being identified. Similar to any autoimmune disorder, environmental factors such as female sex, ethnicity/race, or obesity may represent risk factors for iTTP [28–31]. Some human leukocyte antigen (HLA) haplotypes seem to be associated with iTTP occurrence. A higher prevalence of Class II locus DRB1*11 and DQB1*03 alleles was found in Caucasian patients. At variance, the HLA-DRB1*04 haplotype showed a protective effect in this population [32–35], while in African patients, the frequency of this haplotype is markedly reduced. This haplotype pattern could explain the 8-fold higher incidence of iTTP among black people in the United States [29,30]. In another study, the HLA-DRB1*11 or HLADRB1*04 alleles did not show a protective or predisposing effect on iTTP in a cohort of Japanese patients [36]. By contrast, HLA-DRB1*08:03, HLA-DRB3/4/5*blank, HLA-DQA1*01:03, and HLA-DQB*06:01 have been suggested as possible risk factors [36]. ADAMTS13 deficiency is a necessary but not always sufficient element to trigger an iTTP relapse [37–39]. Hence, it is likely that other synergic mechanisms may provide a "second hit", responsible for iTTP initiation [40]. In this respect, the activation of the alternative pathway of the complement system may act as a facilitating mechanism to induce an acute phase of iTTP [41–43], where ULVWF multimers can be involved in the activation of the alternative complement pathway [44]. It has to be noted that the complement factors, VWF multimers, and the ADAMTS13 level of patients in remission of iTTP were shown to be entangled [42]. High levels of HMW multimers were in fact associated with increased levels of biomarkers of complement activation, such as sC5b-9, C3a, and C5a [42]. The latter were demonstrated to be less efficient regulatory elements to inhibit the activation of the alternative complement pathway. A specific interaction between C3b and the A2 domain of VWFs was demonstrated [45]. These findings are in line with published data showing high-affinity binding between VWF and C3b in surface plasmon resonance experiments and colocalization of C3/C3b with ULVWF on histamine-stimulated HUVECs [46,47]. Upon a trigger event that activates or injures the endothelial cells, ULVWF multimers are secreted from Weibel–Palade bodies on the endothelial cells' surfaces, and the binding of C3b may amplify the alternative complement pathway cascade by forming a C3 convertase complex. In normal subjects, ADAMTS13 cleaves the ULVWF multimers from the cell surface and prevents the activation of the alternative complement pathway, maintaining homeostasis. Normal VWF multimers act as cofactors for complement factor I, an inhibitor of complement activation via the cleavage of complement C3b [48]. Zheng and colleagues demonstrated in a murine model that ADAMTS13 deficiency and the dysregulated complement pathway have synergistic effects [49]. KO mice with $Adamts13$ ($Adamts13^{-/-}$) or loss-of-function heterozygous mutant complement factor H (cfh) mutations ($cfh^{W/R}$) did not develop spontaneous TTP. By contrast, animals with both $Adamts13^{-/-}$ and $cfh^{W/R}$ developed a TTP. Of note, the homozygous $cfh^{R/R}$ form only developed a TTP independently from $Adamts13^{-/-}$ [49]. The interplay between ADAMTS13 activity and complement activation was also shown in human iTTPs, where the mortality rate correlates with complement dysregulation [43]. How complement dysregulation during the acute phase of disease could provide better prognostic elements concerning disease recrudescence, relapse, and mortality predictions remains to be established.

4. Clinical Symptoms of First Episodes and Relapse Incidence of iTTP

The classical symptoms of a first episode of iTTP are represented by variable neurological symptoms (from headache to seizures and coma), severe thrombocytopenia, MAHA with schistocytes, and different degrees of multiorgan failure (heart, kidney, gastrointestinal system) [8]. TTP is a rare disease that mainly affects young people and requires urgent treatment. Despite adequate treatment, 10% of patients will die from this disease, and up to 50% of patients will have recurrent episodes [28]. A recent study was performed in Spain with the application of the French TMA Reference Center Score and the mortality in TTP Score in 20 patients suffering from de novo and relapsed episodes of iTTP [50]. The median age of these patients was 46 (IQR 39–56). Of interest, among exacerbation and relapse episodes, thirteen (45%) were relapses of a previously diagnosed TTP, 14% corresponded to second episodes, 14% to third episodes, 7% to fourth episodes, and 10% to fifth episodes or beyond. The median time elapsed from the previous episode to relapse was ≈36 months (IQR 9–82 months). Thirteen episodes (45%) were associated with potential triggers. The most frequent triggers were infections/antibiotic use (52%), surgery (16%), the onset of an autoimmune disease (16%), pregnancy (8%), and cocaine use (8%). A real-world analysis of a large US health records database found high mortality and morbidity in patients with iTTP, despite treatments with plasma exchange and immunosuppression [51]. The relapse rate observed in this study was 11% over a shorter follow-up period of 4 years [51], whereas the exacerbations (within 1 month since the diagnosis and onset of therapy) were equal to 17% [51]. The observed mortality rate of 14% among patients with one or more iTTP episodes is consistent with the 8–20% reported in the literature for patients treated with plasma exchange and immunosuppression [51].

Hence, from these findings, a high incidence of exacerbation and relapse episodes emerged from these real-world data for iTTP patients. Thus, once iTTP is triggered, the prevalence and incidence of disease relapse are significantly higher than analog phenomena in hereditary TTP (see below). These observations deserve adequate hypotheses about possible differences in the pathophysiology of the two forms, which share the same ADAMTS13 deficiency.

5. Clinical Symptoms of First Episodes and Relapse Incidence of Hereditary TTP

Hereditary TTP is considered a rare syndrome, as most estimates suggest an overall prevalence of $<1/1 \times 10^6$. However, a greater prevalence has been observed in the Central Norway Health Region, where the estimated prevalence of the p.R1060W mutation is 16.7 cases per million people [52]. More than 200 ADAMTS13 mutations have been identified in all of the ADAMTS13 protein domains [53–55]. Of note, some missense ADAMTS13 single-nucleotide polymorphisms have also been identified, which, in some cases, are in strong linkage disequilibrium with specific ADAMTS13 mutations, influencing their molecular effects [56–58]. The clinical manifestations of hereditary TTP (also referred to as the Upshaw–Schulman syndrome) are typical of other TMA forms and comprise thrombocytopenia, MAHA, and multiorgan failure. Although patients with hereditary TTP are at increased risk for typical manifestations of microvascular thrombosis throughout their lives, two periods appear to be associated with high risks. These periods are represented by neonatal life and pregnancy/puerperium. In the former case, characterized by jaundice, anemia, and severe thrombocytopenia, the syndrome may also be fatal and diagnosed only post-mortem, as reported [59]. Beside pregnancy/puerperium and neonatal life, other clinical settings, such as infections and alcohol abuse, may be characterized by hereditary TTP episodes. In a recent study based on data from 87 patients followed in the Hereditary TTP Registry (clinicaltrials.gov #NCT01257269), a wide variety of incidence and severity of clinical manifestations of this syndrome have been reported [60]. Hereditary TTP exacerbations can mimic iTTP but may be less acute in onset, and renal failure is more common. The laboratory parameters may only be slightly perturbed or even normal. It is possible that cTTP patients can present neurologic symptoms with essentially normal platelet counts. Likewise, one of the most frequent symptoms is headache, which may occur without significant thrombocytopenia or any organ failure. It is not uncommon that cTTP patients, even with ADAMTS13 levels of 1–3%, are completely asymptomatic. Globally, the data provided by the above registry showed that the annual incidence of acute episodes is equal to 0.41 (95% CI, 0.30–0.56) for patients without regular plasma treatments. Moreover, an annual low incidence rate of acute episodes of ≤ 0.5 was recorded in 67.3% of patients with an ADAMTS13 activity of <1% [60]. Notably, many patients that are homozygous for the c.4143_4144drupA mutation have an ADAMTS13 activity of <1% but widely varying clinical courses [61]. Based on the above findings, an interesting question may emerge, which is as follows: Why is the comparably severe deficiency of ADAMTS13 observed in both iTTP and cTTP associated with a much higher incidence of exacerbations and relapse episodes in the former? In the next section, we will discuss the potential reason for this apparent discrepancy, remarking on the possible direct involvement of the anti-ADAMTS13 antibodies on the severity and prevalence of thrombotic complications in iTTP.

6. The Role of Anti-ADAMTS13 Antibodies in the Pathological Complications of iTTP

All of the IgG subclasses of anti-ADAMTS13 antibodies were detected in patients with iTTP, with the IgG(4) isotype followed by IgG(1) and IgA antibodies dominating the anti-ADAMTS13 immune response [62]. IgG(1) seems to be the dominant subclass during the first acute episode, whereas IgG(4) would be dominant during or following a relapse [63]. The IgG(1) subclass is a potent inducer of inflammation, as it can effectively bind to Fcγ receptors and activate the classical pathway of the complement system. At variance, IgG(4) tends to be anti-inflammatory, as it is not able to activate the complement system via the classical pathway and binds to Fcγ receptors with low affinity [64]. Hence, the levels of IgG(4) could be efficiently monitored for the identification of patients at risk of disease relapse. In a recent and elegant study, anti-ADAMTS13 IgG and their F(ab)′2 fragments, purified from 62 iTTP patients but not free from heme and nucleosomes, showed a specific effect on endothelial cells (ECs), in which the autoantibodies elicited in vitro the Ca^{2+}-mediated activation of endothelial cells [65]. However, it should be noted that some authors found that free heme and nucleosomes may induce degranulation of

WPBs through TLR4 ligation [66]. Likewise, free heme can facilitate the activation of the complement pathway on the surface of endothelial cells, empowering the dysregulation of this compartment and rendering it prone to thrombotic phenomena [67,68]. Plasma from TTP patients was demonstrated to induce endothelial cell apoptosis and platelet activation [69]. The possible involvement of endothelial cell dysregulation in the thrombotic phenomena of TTP is a debated topic. It is still unclear whether the endothelial activation detected through measurements of endothelial biomarkers is the cause or a consequence of the disease. Increased levels of endothelial microvesicles in TTP patients during the acute phase of the disease were previously documented, whereas during the remission period, the endothelial microparticles strongly decreased [70]. Of interest, TTP plasmas induce procoagulant endothelial microvesicle generation from cultured brain and renal microvascular endothelium [70]. Likewise, an elevated level of circulating endothelial cells was described in a prospective multicentric study in France during the acute phase of TTP, which was normalized during remission [71]. However, further studies are needed to validate in vivo the hypothesis concerning the activation of endothelial cells by anti-ADAMTS13 antibodies. It should be noted, however, that the activation and possible apoptosis of endothelial cells by the purified anti-ADAMTS13 antibodies in vitro caused a rapid VWF release and P-selectin exposure on human dermal microvascular endothelial cell (HMVEC-d) surfaces, associated with angiopoietin-2 and endothelin-1 secretions from the Weibel–Palade bodies [72]. Notably, calcium (Ca^{2+}) blockades with the calcium chelator MAPTAM (1,2-bis-5-methylaminophenoxylethane-NNN'-tetraacetoxymethyl acetate) significantly decreased the VWF release [72]. The authors of this study did not report the molecular mechanisms through which the anti-ADAMTS13 antibodies can induce Ca^{2+} liberation inside endothelial cells. Ca^{2+} signaling in ECs plays a key role in the release of several biochemical mediators, such as NO, prostacyclin (PGI_2), platelet activating factor (PAF), VWF, tissue plasminogen activator (tPA), and tissue factor pathway inhibitor (TFPI). Ca^{2+} signaling in ECs involves an initial increase in the intracellular free $[Ca^{2+}]$ ($[Ca^{2+}]_i$). The rise in $[Ca^{2+}]_i$ takes place via second messenger-mediated processes, which, in turn, trigger the release from intracellular Ca^{2+} stores in the endoplasmic reticulum (ER), and this is followed by Ca^{2+} entry from the extracellular space. This mechanism of Ca^{2+} entry can involve ER Ca^{2+} depletion but also directly receptor-activated Ca^{2+} entry. Of interest, the influx of Ca^{2+} into ECs occurs via some channels that are not gated by voltage. Among these, several polymodal transient receptor potential cation/canonical channels (TRPCs) have been shown to mediate the endothelial Ca^{2+} influx in ECs [73]. Seven TRPC isoforms (TRPC1 to 7) have been described in mammalian species, which have been classified into the following four subfamilies on the basis of their structural homologies and functional similarities: TRPC1, TRPC2, TRPC4/5, and TRPC3/6/7 [74]. TRPC5 expression has been found in many cell types with inherited mechanosensitive Ca^{2+} influx, including ECs [75]. TRPC5 channels have been involved in different physiological and pathophysiological processes, including endothelial functions and vascular smooth muscles [75]. TRPC5 participates in endothelial cell injury and dysfunction, migration and proliferation of vascular smooth muscle cells, cardiac hypertrophy, and lipid deposition. Moreover, a pharmacological block of the TRPC5 channels can inhibit atherosclerotic plaque progression, improve renal function, play a synergistic role in improving the prognosis of CVD patients, and, importantly, prevent depression and anxiety [75], the latter being a common symptom of the long-term effects of iTTP [76]. Thus, TRPC inhibitors may represent an intriguing target for the pharmacological control of cardiovascular morbidity and mortality in iTTP. A vast class of TRPC inhibitors has been synthesized, comprising pyrazoles, 2-aminoquinolines (among these compounds, ML204 is a potent inhibitor of TRPC5), phenylethylimidazoles, piperazine/piperidine analogues, naphthalene sulfonamides, N-phenylanthranilic acid, polyphenols, and 2-aminothiazoles [65]. However, due to the tissue-specificity of TRPC expression, the possibility of obtaining a selective and positive effect on endothelial cells is still far from being reached. However, independently from this possible pharmacological intervention, the direct effect of anti-ADAMTS13 antibodies on endothelial cells cannot be ignored any longer in the pursuit of better therapeutic controls for the severe cardiovascular complications of iTTP.

7. Effects on Therapies of the Different Pathogenetic Effectors of cTTP and iTTP

The different pathogenetic effectors and varying clinical phenotypes described above in cTTP and iTTP determine the different therapeutic approaches for their treatments. Plasma infusion may be administered in both clinical forms, but it is predominantly used in cTTP while waiting for the final approval of recombinant ADAMTS13 by regulatory agencies [77]. By contrast, plasma exchange is mandatory for iTTP to eliminate the anti-ADAMTS13 antibodies and, at the same time, provide sufficient amounts of ADAMTS13. However, plasmapheresis may be administered, even to patients with relapses of the refractory forms of cTTP, to deliver sufficient amounts of ADAMTS13 and avoid volume overload. As for caplacizumab, this drug is approved for the treatment of iTTP and is given daily after plasmapheresis plus 30 days following remission. However, off-label use of caplacizumab has been previously reported in a cTTP case with severe multiorgan thrombotic microangiopathy and was associated with a positive outcome [78]. The substantial difference concerns the immunosuppressive therapy (high doses of corticosteroids, cyclophosphamide, rituximab, etc.) that is administered in iTTP only, while theoretically, in severe cTTP cases with complete ADAMTS13 deficiency, the formation of inhibitory antibodies against the metalloprotease could derive from the treatment with plasma.

8. Conclusions

In conclusion, the understanding of the immunological basis of iTTP, which accounts for the majority of TTP cases, has progressively increased in the last few years. Plenty of previous studies investigated the contribution of antibodies against different ADAMTS13 domains to the inhibitory potential in plasma and revealed how these autoantibodies may cause both accelerated clearance with depletion of the metalloprotease and inhibition of its activity (Figure 1A). However, recent studies have also noted a direct activity of the various IgG subclasses on the activation of endothelial cells and platelets responsible for the pathological phenomena of iTTP (Figure 1B). Hence, the application in the future of more specific drugs able to control even the direct cellular effects of the TTP-associated autoantibodies, besides the immunological response, will provide an additional strategy for disease control, together with the fundamental therapeutic tools represented by plasma exchange, immunosuppressors, and caplacizumab.

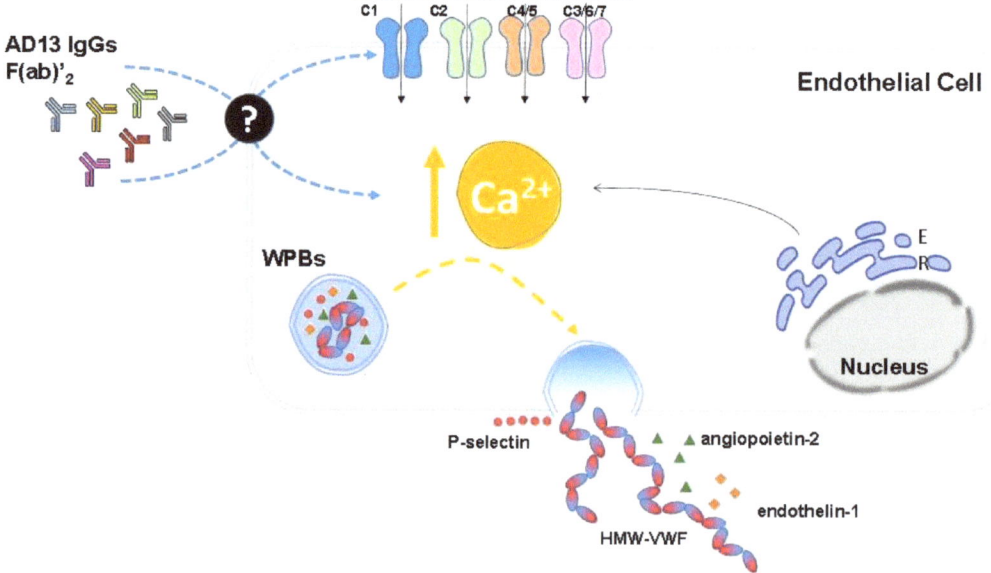

Figure 1. Scheme of the canonical (**A**) and putative (**B**) mechanisms responsible for the thrombotic phenomena in iTTP and cTTP, occurring at the endothelial level. In the putative mechanism shown in (**B**), endothelial activation occurs through stimulation of the Ca^{2+} entry and signaling responsible for the secretion of Weibel–Palade bodies and other biochemical mediators able to activate platelets.

Funding: This research was funded by Fondazione Policlinico Universitario Agostino Gemelli IRCCs, grant "Ricerca corrente 2022".

Institutional Review Board Statement: Not applicable.

Informed Consent Statement: Not applicable.

Acknowledgments: Financial support from Fondazione Policlinico Universitario "Gemelli" IRCCS (Ricerca corrente 2022) is gratefully acknowledged.

Conflicts of Interest: The authors declare no conflict of interest.

References

1. Moake, J. Thrombotic microangiopathies: Multimers, metalloprotease, and beyond. *Clin. Transl. Sci.* **2009**, *2*, 366–373. [CrossRef] [PubMed]
2. Malgaj Vrecko, M.; Ales Rigler, A.; Veceric-Haler, Z. Coronavirus Disease 2019-Associated Thrombotic Microangiopathy: Literature Review. *Int. J. Mol. Sci.* **2022**, *23*, 11307. [CrossRef]
3. Zheng, X.; Chung, D.; Takayama, T.K.; Majerus, E.M.; Sadler, J.E.; Fujikawa, K. Structure of von Willebrand factor-cleaving protease (ADAMTS13), a metalloprotease involved in thrombotic thrombocytopenic purpura. *J. Biol. Chem.* **2001**, *276*, 41059–41063. [CrossRef] [PubMed]
4. Levy, G.G.; Nichols, W.C.; Lian, E.C.; Foroud, T.; McClintick, J.N.; McGee, B.M.; Yang, A.Y.; Siemieniak, D.R.; Stark, K.R.; Gruppo, R.; et al. Mutations in a member of the ADAMTS gene family cause thrombotic thrombocytopenic purpura. *Nature* **2001**, *413*, 488–494. [CrossRef] [PubMed]
5. Furlan, M.; Robles, R.; Galbusera, M.; Remuzzi, G.; Kyrle, P.A.; Brenner, B.; Krause, M.; Scharrer, I.; Aumann, V.; Mittler, U.; et al. von Willebrand factor-cleaving protease in thrombotic thrombocytopenic purpura and the hemolytic-uremic syndrome. *N. Engl. J. Med.* **1998**, *339*, 1578–1584. [CrossRef]
6. Tsai, H.M.; Lian, E.C. Antibodies to von Willebrand factor-cleaving protease in acute thrombotic thrombocytopenic purpura. *N. Engl. J. Med.* **1998**, *339*, 1585–1594. [CrossRef]
7. Chung, D.W.; Fujikawa, K. Processing of von Willebrand factor by ADAMTS-13. *Biochemistry* **2002**, *41*, 11065–11070. [CrossRef]
8. George, J.N. Clinical practice. Thrombotic thrombocytopenic purpura. *N. Engl. J. Med.* **2006**, *354*, 1927–1935. [CrossRef]
9. Roose, E.; Vidarsson, G.; Kangro, K.; Verhagen, O.; Mancini, I.; Desender, L.; Pareyn, I.; Vandeputte, N.; Vandenbulcke, A.; Vendramin, C.; et al. Anti-ADAMTS13 Autoantibodies against Cryptic Epitopes in Immune-Mediated Thrombotic Thrombocytopenic Purpura. *Thromb. Haemost.* **2018**, *118*, 1729–1742. [CrossRef]
10. Roose, E.; Veyradier, A.; Vanhoorelbeke, K. Insights into ADAMTS13 structure: Impact on thrombotic thrombocytopenic purpura diagnosis and management. *Curr. Opin. Hematol.* **2020**, *27*, 320–326. [CrossRef]
11. Roose, E.; Schelpe, A.S.; Tellier, E.; Sinkovits, G.; Joly, B.S.; Dekimpe, C.; Kaplanski, G.; Le Besnerais, M.; Mancini, I.; Falter, T.; et al. Open ADAMTS13, induced by antibodies, is a biomarker for subclinical immune-mediated thrombotic thrombocytopenic purpura. *Blood* **2020**, *136*, 353–361. [CrossRef]
12. Scully, M. Inhibitory anti-ADAMTS 13 antibodies: Measurement and clinical application. *Blood Rev.* **2010**, *24*, 11–16. [CrossRef] [PubMed]
13. Froissart, A.; Buffet, M.; Veyradier, A.; Poullin, P.; Provot, F.; Malot, S.; Schwarzinger, M.; Galicier, L.; Vanhille, P.; Vernant, J.P.; et al. Efficacy and safety of first-line rituximab in severe, acquired thrombotic thrombocytopenic purpura with a suboptimal response to plasma exchange. Experience of the French Thrombotic Microangiopathies Reference Center. *Crit. Care Med.* **2012**, *40*, 104–111. [CrossRef] [PubMed]
14. Peyvandi, F.; Callewaert, F. Caplacizumab for Acquired Thrombotic Thrombocytopenic Purpura. *N. Engl. J. Med.* **2016**, *374*, 2497–2498. [CrossRef]
15. Scully, M.; Cataland, S.R.; Peyvandi, F.; Coppo, P.; Knobl, P.; Kremer Hovinga, J.A.; Metjian, A.; de la Rubia, J.; Pavenski, K.; Callewaert, F.; et al. Caplacizumab Treatment for Acquired Thrombotic Thrombocytopenic Purpura. *N. Engl. J. Med.* **2019**, *380*, 335–346. [CrossRef] [PubMed]
16. Lancellotti, S.; Sacco, M.; Basso, M.; De Cristofaro, R. Mechanochemistry of von Willebrand factor. *Biomol. Concepts* **2019**, *10*, 194–208. [CrossRef]
17. Shankaran, H.; Neelamegham, S. Hydrodynamic forces applied on intercellular bonds, soluble molecules, and cell-surface receptors. *Biophys. J.* **2004**, *86*, 576–588. [CrossRef] [PubMed]
18. Scheiflinger, F.; Knobl, P.; Trattner, B.; Plaimauer, B.; Mohr, G.; Dockal, M.; Dorner, F.; Rieger, M. Nonneutralizing IgM and IgG antibodies to von Willebrand factor-cleaving protease (ADAMTS-13) in a patient with thrombotic thrombocytopenic purpura. *Blood* **2003**, *102*, 3241–3243. [CrossRef]
19. Shelat, S.G.; Smith, P.; Ai, J.; Zheng, X.L. Inhibitory autoantibodies against ADAMTS-13 in patients with thrombotic thrombocytopenic purpura bind ADAMTS-13 protease and may accelerate its clearance in vivo. *J. Thromb. Haemost.* **2006**, *4*, 1707–1717. [CrossRef] [PubMed]

20. Rieger, M.; Mannucci, P.M.; Kremer Hovinga, J.A.; Herzog, A.; Gerstenbauer, G.; Konetschny, C.; Zimmermann, K.; Scharrer, I.; Peyvandi, F.; Galbusera, M.; et al. ADAMTS13 autoantibodies in patients with thrombotic microangiopathies and other immunomediated diseases. *Blood* **2005**, *106*, 1262–1267. [CrossRef]
21. Thomas, M.R.; de Groot, R.; Scully, M.A.; Crawley, J.T. Pathogenicity of Anti-ADAMTS13 Autoantibodies in Acquired Thrombotic Thrombocytopenic Purpura. *EBioMedicine* **2015**, *2*, 942–952. [CrossRef] [PubMed]
22. Soejima, K.; Matsumoto, M.; Kokame, K.; Yagi, H.; Ishizashi, H.; Maeda, H.; Nozaki, C.; Miyata, T.; Fujimura, Y.; Nakagaki, T. ADAMTS-13 cysteine-rich/spacer domains are functionally essential for von Willebrand factor cleavage. *Blood* **2003**, *102*, 3232–3237. [CrossRef] [PubMed]
23. Luken, B.M.; Turenhout, E.A.; Hulstein, J.J.; Van Mourik, J.A.; Fijnheer, R.; Voorberg, J. The spacer domain of ADAMTS13 contains a major binding site for antibodies in patients with thrombotic thrombocytopenic purpura. *Thromb. Haemost.* **2005**, *93*, 267–274. [CrossRef]
24. Luken, B.M.; Turenhout, E.A.; Kaijen, P.H.; Greuter, M.J.; Pos, W.; van Mourik, J.A.; Fijnheer, R.; Voorberg, J. Amino acid regions 572-579 and 657-666 of the spacer domain of ADAMTS13 provide a common antigenic core required for binding of antibodies in patients with acquired TTP. *Thromb. Haemost.* **2006**, *96*, 295–301. [CrossRef] [PubMed]
25. Velasquez Pereira, L.C.; Roose, E.; Graca, N.A.G.; Sinkovits, G.; Kangro, K.; Joly, B.S.; Tellier, E.; Kaplanski, G.; Falter, T.; Von Auer, C.; et al. Immunogenic hotspots in the spacer domain of ADAMTS13 in immune-mediated thrombotic thrombocytopenic purpura. *J. Thromb. Haemost.* **2021**, *19*, 478–488. [CrossRef] [PubMed]
26. Roose, E.; Schelpe, A.S.; Joly, B.S.; Peetermans, M.; Verhamme, P.; Voorberg, J.; Greinacher, A.; Deckmyn, H.; De Meyer, S.F.; Coppo, P.; et al. An open conformation of ADAMTS-13 is a hallmark of acute acquired thrombotic thrombocytopenic purpura. *J. Thromb. Haemost.* **2018**, *16*, 378–388. [CrossRef]
27. Halkidis, K.; Siegel, D.L.; Zheng, X.L. A human monoclonal antibody against the distal carboxyl terminus of ADAMTS-13 modulates its susceptibility to an inhibitor in thrombotic thrombocytopenic purpura. *J. Thromb. Haemost.* **2021**, *19*, 1888–1895. [CrossRef]
28. Mariotte, E.; Azoulay, E.; Galicier, L.; Rondeau, E.; Zouiti, F.; Boisseau, P.; Poullin, P.; de Maistre, E.; Provot, F.; Delmas, Y.; et al. Epidemiology and pathophysiology of adulthood-onset thrombotic microangiopathy with severe ADAMTS13 deficiency (thrombotic thrombocytopenic purpura): A cross-sectional analysis of the French national registry for thrombotic microangiopathy. *Lancet Haematol.* **2016**, *3*, e237–e245. [CrossRef]
29. Reese, J.A.; Muthurajah, D.S.; Kremer Hovinga, J.A.; Vesely, S.K.; Terrell, D.R.; George, J.N. Children and adults with thrombotic thrombocytopenic purpura associated with severe, acquired Adamts13 deficiency: Comparison of incidence, demographic and clinical features. *Pediatr. Blood Cancer* **2013**, *60*, 1676–1682. [CrossRef]
30. Martino, S.; Jamme, M.; Deligny, C.; Busson, M.; Loiseau, P.; Azoulay, E.; Galicier, L.; Pene, F.; Provot, F.; Dossier, A.; et al. Thrombotic Thrombocytopenic Purpura in Black People: Impact of Ethnicity on Survival and Genetic Risk Factors. *PLoS ONE* **2016**, *11*, e0156679. [CrossRef]
31. Hrdinova, J.; D'Angelo, S.; Graca, N.A.G.; Ercig, B.; Vanhoorelbeke, K.; Veyradier, A.; Voorberg, J.; Coppo, P. Dissecting the pathophysiology of immune thrombotic thrombocytopenic purpura: Interplay between genes and environmental triggers. *Haematologica* **2018**, *103*, 1099–1109. [CrossRef]
32. Coppo, P.; Busson, M.; Veyradier, A.; Wynckel, A.; Poullin, P.; Azoulay, E.; Galicier, L.; Loiseau, P.; French Reference Centre For Thrombotic, M. HLA-DRB1*11: A strong risk factor for acquired severe ADAMTS13 deficiency-related idiopathic thrombotic thrombocytopenic purpura in Caucasians. *J. Thromb. Haemost.* **2010**, *8*, 856–859. [CrossRef]
33. Scully, M.; Brown, J.; Patel, R.; McDonald, V.; Brown, C.J.; Machin, S. Human leukocyte antigen association in idiopathic thrombotic thrombocytopenic purpura: Evidence for an immunogenetic link. *J. Thromb. Haemost.* **2010**, *8*, 257–262. [CrossRef] [PubMed]
34. Mancini, I.; Giacomini, E.; Pontiggia, S.; Artoni, A.; Ferrari, B.; Pappalardo, E.; Gualtierotti, R.; Trisolini, S.M.; Capria, S.; Facchini, L.; et al. The HLA Variant rs6903608 Is Associated with Disease Onset and Relapse of Immune-Mediated Thrombotic Thrombocytopenic Purpura in Caucasians. *J. Clin. Med.* **2020**, *9*, 3379. [CrossRef] [PubMed]
35. John, M.L.; Hitzler, W.; Scharrer, I. The role of human leukocyte antigens as predisposing and/or protective factors in patients with idiopathic thrombotic thrombocytopenic purpura. *Ann. Hematol.* **2012**, *91*, 507–510. [CrossRef] [PubMed]
36. Sakai, K.; Kuwana, M.; Tanaka, H.; Hosomichi, K.; Hasegawa, A.; Uyama, H.; Nishio, K.; Omae, T.; Hishizawa, M.; Matsui, M.; et al. HLA loci predisposing to immune TTP in Japanese: Potential role of the shared ADAMTS13 peptide bound to different HLA-DR. *Blood* **2020**, *135*, 2413–2419. [CrossRef]
37. Jin, M.; Casper, T.C.; Cataland, S.R.; Kennedy, M.S.; Lin, S.; Li, Y.J.; Wu, H.M. Relationship between ADAMTS13 activity in clinical remission and the risk of TTP relapse. *Br. J. Haematol.* **2008**, *141*, 651–658. [CrossRef]
38. Peyvandi, F.; Lavoretano, S.; Palla, R.; Feys, H.B.; Vanhoorelbeke, K.; Battaglioli, T.; Valsecchi, C.; Canciani, M.T.; Fabris, F.; Zver, S.; et al. ADAMTS13 and anti-ADAMTS13 antibodies as markers for recurrence of acquired thrombotic thrombocytopenic purpura during remission. *Haematologica* **2008**, *93*, 232–239. [CrossRef]
39. Page, E.E.; Kremer Hovinga, J.A.; Terrell, D.R.; Vesely, S.K.; George, J.N. Clinical importance of ADAMTS13 activity during remission in patients with acquired thrombotic thrombocytopenic purpura. *Blood* **2016**, *128*, 2175–2178. [CrossRef]
40. Miyata, T.; Fan, X. A second hit for TMA. *Blood* **2012**, *120*, 1152–1154. [CrossRef]

41. Reti, M.; Farkas, P.; Csuka, D.; Razso, K.; Schlammadinger, A.; Udvardy, M.L.; Madach, K.; Domjan, G.; Bereczki, C.; Reusz, G.S.; et al. Complement activation in thrombotic thrombocytopenic purpura. *J. Thromb. Haemost.* **2012**, *10*, 791–798. [CrossRef] [PubMed]
42. Wu, H.; Jay, L.; Lin, S.; Han, C.; Yang, S.; Cataland, S.R.; Masias, C. Interrelationship between ADAMTS13 activity, von Willebrand factor, and complement activation in remission from immune-mediated trhrombotic thrombocytopenic purpura. *Br. J. Haematol.* **2020**, *189*, e18–e20. [CrossRef] [PubMed]
43. Wu, T.C.; Yang, S.; Haven, S.; Holers, V.M.; Lundberg, A.S.; Wu, H.; Cataland, S.R. Complement activation and mortality during an acute episode of thrombotic thrombocytopenic purpura. *J. Thromb. Haemost.* **2013**, *11*, 1925–1927. [CrossRef] [PubMed]
44. Turner, N.; Sartain, S.; Moake, J. Ultralarge von Willebrand factor-induced platelet clumping and activation of the alternative complement pathway in thrombotic thrombocytopenic purpura and the hemolytic-uremic syndromes. *Hematol. Oncol. Clin. N. Am.* **2015**, *29*, 509–524. [CrossRef] [PubMed]
45. Bettoni, S.; Galbusera, M.; Gastoldi, S.; Donadelli, R.; Tentori, C.; Sparta, G.; Bresin, E.; Mele, C.; Alberti, M.; Tortajada, A.; et al. Interaction between Multimeric von Willebrand Factor and Complement: A Fresh Look to the Pathophysiology of Microvascular Thrombosis. *J. Immunol.* **2017**, *199*, 1021–1040. [CrossRef]
46. Turner, N.A.; Moake, J. Assembly and activation of alternative complement components on endothelial cell-anchored ultra-large von Willebrand factor links complement and hemostasis-thrombosis. *PLoS ONE* **2013**, *8*, e59372. [CrossRef]
47. Feng, S.; Liang, X.; Cruz, M.A.; Vu, H.; Zhou, Z.; Pemmaraju, N.; Dong, J.F.; Kroll, M.H.; Afshar-Kharghan, V. The interaction between factor H and Von Willebrand factor. *PLoS ONE* **2013**, *8*, e73715. [CrossRef]
48. Feng, S.; Liang, X.; Kroll, M.H.; Chung, D.W.; Afshar-Kharghan, V. von Willebrand factor is a cofactor in complement regulation. *Blood* **2015**, *125*, 1034–1037. [CrossRef]
49. Zheng, L.; Zhang, D.; Cao, W.; Song, W.C.; Zheng, X.L. Synergistic effects of ADAMTS13 deficiency and complement activation in pathogenesis of thrombotic microangiopathy. *Blood* **2019**, *134*, 1095–1105. [CrossRef]
50. Domingo-Gonzalez, A.; Regalado-Artamendi, I.; Martin-Rojas, R.M.; Perez-Rus, G.; Perez-Corral, A.; Diez-Martin, J.L.; Pascual-Izquierdo, C. Application of the French TMA Reference Center Score and the mortality in TTP Score in de novo and relapsed episodes of acquired thrombotic thrombocytopenic purpura at a tertiary care facility in Spain. *J. Clin. Apher.* **2021**, *36*, 420–428. [CrossRef]
51. Adeyemi, A.; Razakariasa, F.; Chiorean, A.; de Passos Sousa, R. Epidemiology, treatment patterns, clinical outcomes, and disease burden among patients with immune-mediated thrombotic thrombocytopenic purpura in the United States. *Res. Pract. Thromb. Haemost.* **2022**, *6*, e12802. [CrossRef]
52. von Krogh, A.S.; Quist-Paulsen, P.; Waage, A.; Langseth, O.O.; Thorstensen, K.; Brudevold, R.; Tjonnfjord, G.E.; Largiader, C.R.; Lammle, B.; Kremer Hovinga, J.A. High prevalence of hereditary thrombotic thrombocytopenic purpura in central Norway: From clinical observation to evidence. *J. Thromb. Haemost.* **2016**, *14*, 73–82. [CrossRef] [PubMed]
53. van Dorland, H.A.; Taleghani, M.M.; Sakai, K.; Friedman, K.D.; George, J.N.; Hrachovinova, I.; Knobl, P.N.; von Krogh, A.S.; Schneppenheim, R.; Aebi-Huber, I.; et al. The International Hereditary Thrombotic Thrombocytopenic Purpura Registry: Key findings at enrollment until 2017. *Haematologica* **2019**, *104*, 2107–2115. [CrossRef]
54. Lancellotti, S.; Peyvandi, F.; Pagliari, M.T.; Cairo, A.; Abdel-Azeim, S.; Chermak, E.; Lazzareschi, I.; Mastrangelo, S.; Cavallo, L.; Oliva, R.; et al. The D173G mutation in ADAMTS-13 causes a severe form of congenital thrombotic thrombocytopenic purpura. A clinical, biochemical and in silico study. *Thromb. Haemost.* **2016**, *115*, 51–62. [CrossRef]
55. Alwan, F.; Vendramin, C.; Liesner, R.; Clark, A.; Lester, W.; Dutt, T.; Thomas, W.; Gooding, R.; Biss, T.; Watson, H.G.; et al. Characterization and treatment of congenital thrombotic thrombocytopenic purpura. *Blood* **2019**, *133*, 1644–1651. [CrossRef] [PubMed]
56. Kokame, K.; Matsumoto, M.; Soejima, K.; Yagi, H.; Ishizashi, H.; Funato, M.; Tamai, H.; Konno, M.; Kamide, K.; Kawano, Y.; et al. Mutations and common polymorphisms in ADAMTS13 gene responsible for von Willebrand factor-cleaving protease activity. *Proc. Natl. Acad. Sci. USA* **2002**, *99*, 11902–11907. [CrossRef]
57. Plaimauer, B.; Fuhrmann, J.; Mohr, G.; Wernhart, W.; Bruno, K.; Ferrari, S.; Konetschny, C.; Antoine, G.; Rieger, M.; Scheiflinger, F. Modulation of ADAMTS13 secretion and specific activity by a combination of common amino acid polymorphisms and a missense mutation. *Blood* **2006**, *107*, 118–125. [CrossRef]
58. Akiyama, M.; Kokame, K.; Miyata, T. ADAMTS13 P475S polymorphism causes a lowered enzymatic activity and urea lability in vitro. *J. Thromb. Haemost.* **2008**, *6*, 1830–1832. [CrossRef] [PubMed]
59. Hager, H.B.; Andersen, M.T. A neonate presenting with jaundice, anemia, and thrombocytopenia. *Blood* **2018**, *131*, 1627. [CrossRef] [PubMed]
60. Tarasco, E.; Butikofer, L.; Friedman, K.D.; George, J.N.; Hrachovinova, I.; Knobl, P.N.; Matsumoto, M.; von Krogh, A.S.; Aebi-Huber, I.; Cermakova, Z.; et al. Annual incidence and severity of acute episodes in hereditary thrombotic thrombocytopenic purpura. *Blood* **2021**, *137*, 3563–3575. [CrossRef] [PubMed]
61. Sukumar, S.; Lammle, B.; Cataland, S.R. Thrombotic Thrombocytopenic Purpura: Pathophysiology, Diagnosis, and Management. *J. Clin. Med.* **2021**, *10*, 536. [CrossRef] [PubMed]
62. Ferrari, S.; Mudde, G.C.; Rieger, M.; Veyradier, A.; Kremer Hovinga, J.A.; Scheiflinger, F. IgG subclass distribution of anti-ADAMTS13 antibodies in patients with acquired thrombotic thrombocytopenic purpura. *J. Thromb. Haemost.* **2009**, *7*, 1703–1710. [CrossRef] [PubMed]

63. Sinkovits, G.; Szilagyi, A.; Farkas, P.; Inotai, D.; Szilvasi, A.; Tordai, A.; Razso, K.; Reti, M.; Prohaszka, Z. Concentration and Subclass Distribution of Anti-ADAMTS13 IgG Autoantibodies in Different Stages of Acquired Idiopathic Thrombotic Thrombocytopenic Purpura. *Front. Immunol.* **2018**, *9*, 1646. [CrossRef]
64. Bruhns, P.; Iannascoli, B.; England, P.; Mancardi, D.A.; Fernandez, N.; Jorieux, S.; Daeron, M. Specificity and affinity of human Fcgamma receptors and their polymorphic variants for human IgG subclasses. *Blood* **2009**, *113*, 3716–3725. [CrossRef]
65. Tellier, E.; Widemann, A.; Cauchois, R.; Faccini, J.; Lagarde, M.; Brun, M.; Robert, P.; Robert, S.; Bachelier, R.; Poullin, P.; et al. Immune thrombotic thrombocytopenic purpura plasmas induce calcium- and IgG-dependent endothelial activation: Correlations with disease severity. *Haematologica* **2023**, *108*, 1127–1140. [CrossRef] [PubMed]
66. Merle, N.S.; Paule, R.; Leon, J.; Daugan, M.; Robe-Rybkine, T.; Poillerat, V.; Torset, C.; Fremeaux-Bacchi, V.; Dimitrov, J.D.; Roumenina, L.T. P-selectin drives complement attack on endothelium during intravascular hemolysis in TLR-4/heme-dependent manner. *Proc. Natl. Acad. Sci. USA* **2019**, *116*, 6280–6285. [CrossRef]
67. Frimat, M.; Tabarin, F.; Dimitrov, J.D.; Poitou, C.; Halbwachs-Mecarelli, L.; Fremeaux-Bacchi, V.; Roumenina, L.T. Complement activation by heme as a secondary hit for atypical hemolytic uremic syndrome. *Blood* **2013**, *122*, 282–292. [CrossRef]
68. Cauchois, R.; Muller, R.; Lagarde, M.; Dignat-George, F.; Tellier, E.; Kaplanski, G. Is Endothelial Activation a Critical Event in Thrombotic Thrombocytopenic Purpura? *J. Clin. Med.* **2023**, *12*, 758. [CrossRef]
69. Wu, X.W.; Li, Q.Z.; Lian, E.C. Plasma from a patient with thrombotic thrombocytopenic purpura induces endothelial cell apoptosis and platelet aggregation. *Thromb. Res.* **1999**, *93*, 79–87. [CrossRef]
70. Jimenez, J.J.; Jy, W.; Mauro, L.M.; Horstman, L.L.; Ahn, Y.S. Elevated endothelial microparticles in thrombotic thrombocytopenic purpura: Findings from brain and renal microvascular cell culture and patients with active disease. *Br. J. Haematol.* **2001**, *112*, 81–90. [CrossRef]
71. Widemann, A.; Pasero, C.; Arnaud, L.; Poullin, P.; Loundou, A.D.; Choukroun, G.; Sanderson, F.; Lacroix, R.; Sabatier, F.; Coppo, P.; et al. Circulating endothelial cells and progenitors as prognostic factors during autoimmune thrombotic thrombocytopenic purpura: Results of a prospective multicenter French study. *J. Thromb. Haemost.* **2014**, *12*, 1601–1609. [CrossRef] [PubMed]
72. Feys, H.B.; Roodt, J.; Vandeputte, N.; Pareyn, I.; Lamprecht, S.; van Rensburg, W.J.; Anderson, P.J.; Budde, U.; Louw, V.J.; Badenhorst, P.N.; et al. Thrombotic thrombocytopenic purpura directly linked with ADAMTS13 inhibition in the baboon (*Papio ursinus*). *Blood* **2010**, *116*, 2005–2010. [CrossRef] [PubMed]
73. Thakore, P.; Earley, S. Transient Receptor Potential Channels and Endothelial Cell Calcium Signaling. *Compr. Physiol.* **2019**, *9*, 1249–1277. [CrossRef]
74. Birnbaumer, L. The TRPC class of ion channels: A critical review of their roles in slow, sustained increases in intracellular Ca^{2+} concentrations. *Annu. Rev. Pharmacol. Toxicol.* **2009**, *49*, 395–426. [CrossRef] [PubMed]
75. Yip, H.; Chan, W.Y.; Leung, P.C.; Kwan, H.Y.; Liu, C.; Huang, Y.; Michel, V.; Yew, D.T.; Yao, X. Expression of TRPC homologs in endothelial cells and smooth muscle layers of human arteries. *Histochem. Cell Biol.* **2004**, *122*, 553–561. [CrossRef]
76. Graciaa, S.; Adeagbo, S.; Fong, G.; Rollins, M.; McElfresh, P.; Zerra, P.E.; Bennett, C.; Josephson, C.D.; Briones, M.; Fasano, R.M.; et al. Clinical features and neurological outcomes in pediatric immune-mediated thrombotic thrombocytopenic purpura: A report from a large pediatric hematology center. *Pediatr. Blood Cancer* **2022**, *69*, e29992. [CrossRef]
77. Scully, M.; Knobl, P.; Kentouche, K.; Rice, L.; Windyga, J.; Schneppenheim, R.; Kremer Hovinga, J.A.; Kajiwara, M.; Fujimura, Y.; Maggiore, C.; et al. Recombinant ADAMTS-13: First-in-human pharmacokinetics and safety in congenital thrombotic thrombocytopenic purpura. *Blood* **2017**, *130*, 2055–2063. [CrossRef]
78. Boothby, A.; Mazepa, M. Caplacizumab for congenital thrombotic thrombocytopenic purpura. *Am. J. Hematol.* **2022**, *97*, E420–E421. [CrossRef]

Disclaimer/Publisher's Note: The statements, opinions and data contained in all publications are solely those of the individual author(s) and contributor(s) and not of MDPI and/or the editor(s). MDPI and/or the editor(s) disclaim responsibility for any injury to people or property resulting from any ideas, methods, instructions or products referred to in the content.

Review

ADAMTS13 and Non-ADAMTS13 Biomarkers in Immune-Mediated Thrombotic Thrombocytopenic Purpura

Quintijn Bonnez [1], Kazuya Sakai [1,2] and Karen Vanhoorelbeke [1,*]

[1] Department of Chemistry, KU Leuven Campus Kulak Kortrijk, 8500 Kortrijk, Belgium
[2] Department of Blood Transfusion Medicine, Nara Medical University, Kashihara 634-8522, Japan
* Correspondence: karen.vanhoorelbeke@kuleuven.be; Tel.: +32-5624-6061

Abstract: Immune-mediated thrombotic thrombocytopenic purpura (iTTP) is a rare medical emergency for which a correct and early diagnosis is essential. As a severe deficiency in A Disintegrin And Metalloproteinase with ThromboSpondin type 1 repeats, member 13 (ADAMTS13) is the underlying pathophysiology, diagnostic strategies require timely monitoring of ADAMTS13 parameters to differentiate TTP from alternative thrombotic microangiopathies (TMAs) and to guide initial patient management. Assays for conventional ADAMTS13 testing focus on the enzyme activity and presence of (inhibitory) anti-ADAMTS13 antibodies to discriminate immune-mediated TTP (iTTP) from congenital TTP and guide patient management. However, diagnosis of iTTP remains challenging when patients present borderline ADAMTS13 activity. Therefore, additional biomarkers would be helpful to support correct clinical judgment. Over the last few years, the evaluation of ADAMTS13 conformation has proven to be a valuable tool to confirm the diagnosis of acute iTTP when ADAMST13 activity is between 10 and 20%. Screening of ADAMTS13 conformation during long-term patient follow-up suggests it is a surrogate marker for undetectable antibodies. Moreover, some non-ADAMTS13 parameters gained notable interest in predicting disease outcome, proposing meticulous follow-up of iTTP patients. This review summarizes non-ADAMTS13 biomarkers for which inclusion in routine clinical testing could largely benefit differential diagnosis and follow-up of iTTP patients.

Keywords: immune-mediated thrombotic thrombocytopenic purpura; differential diagnosis; ADAMTS13 testing; ADAMTS13 activity; ADAMTS13 conformation; ADAMTS13 antigen; non-ADAMTS13 biomarkers

1. TTP: Pathophysiology, Diagnosis, Therapy and Follow-Up

1.1. Pathophysiology

Thrombotic thrombocytopenic purpura (TTP) is a rare disease with an incidence estimated at around four cases per million, caused by a severe deficiency of the enzyme ADAMTS13 (A Disintegrin And Metalloproteinase with ThromboSpondin type 1 repeats, member 13), and is recognized as thrombotic microangiopathy (TMA) that is characterized by severe thrombocytopenia, hemolytic anemia, and ischemic organ failure [1,2]. The substrate of ADAMTS13 is the multimerc protein von Willebrand factor (VWF). VWF is synthesized in endothelial cells and megakaryocytes, where it is stored as ultra-large prothrombotic multimers in Weibel Palade bodies and α-granules respectively. Release of the ultra-large (UL) VWF multimers results in unfolding of the VWF molecule and exposure of the ADAMTS13 cleavage site and platelet binding sites. Subsequent cleavage of UL-VWF results in smaller VWF multimers that are not prothrombotic and hence do not spontaneously bind platelets. Therefore, ADAMTS13 deficiency in TTP patients results in systemic microvascular thrombi formation, leading to platelet consumption and ischemic organ damage [3,4]. About 5% of the TTP patients suffer from the congenital form of the disease, while 95% have the acquired form of TTP. Of those, up to 90% of the TTP cases are classified as immune-mediated TTP (iTTP), resulting from the acquired production of anti-ADAMTS13 autoantibodies [5,6] while the remaining patients suffer from TTP of unknown cause (uTTP) [7,8].

1.2. Diagnosis

Historically, a clinical pentad has been used for the clinical diagnosis of TTP by screening for fever, thrombocytopenia, hemolytic anemia, and renal and neurologic dysfunction [9]. It was shown that patients with all five symptoms, only seen in 40% of cases, have poorer outcomes than those without [9]. Based on the current consensus and guidelines, TTP is clinically diagnosed by the presence of severe thrombocytopenia (<30×10^9/L) and microangiopathic hemolytic anemia with highly elevated lactate dehydrogenase (LDH) and indirect bilirubin [10–12]. Since these signs and symptoms overlap with those of other microangiopathies, confirmation of severely reduced ADAMTS13 activity (<10%) is crucial to confirm the diagnosis of TTP. Current diagnostic assays to determine ADAMTS13 activity are based on the use of a VWF fragment, which has an exposed ADAMTS13 cleavage site. Indeed, full-length VWF adopts a folded conformation with a cryptic ADAMTS13 cleavage site and can only be used in vitro under static conditions as an ADAMTS13 substrate when it is denatured [13]. Frequently used ADAMTS13 assays include the fluorescence resonance energy transfer (FRET)-VWF73 assay and the chromogenic ADAMTS13 activity ELISA, both using an artificial 73 amino acid residue-long VWF A2 peptide (VWF73) that contains the exposed ADAMTS13 cleavage site. In the FRET-VWF73 assay, an increased fluorescence is generated when the substrate is cleaved by plasma ADAMTS13 [14]. In the chromogenic ADAMTS13 activity ELISA, the anti-N10 monoclonal antibody recognizes the digested VWF73 fragment when cleaved by ADAMTS13 [15]. Of note, the use of EDTA-treated plasma should be avoided since EDTA retrieves divalent cations from the ADAMTS13 metalloprotease domain, rendering ADAMTS13 inactive [16]. To discriminate iTTP from cTTP, the presence of autoantibodies is studied using either an anti-ADAMTS13 IgG detection ELISA or a Bethesda assay [17]. In a few iTTP cases, autoantibodies are undetectable, which is explained by the presence of immune complex formation [18].

1.3. Therapy

Standard iTTP therapy combines therapeutic plasma exchange (TPE) and corticosteroids and has significantly reduced mortality in acute-phase iTTP below 10–20% [19,20]. Recently, targeted therapies can be administered, including anti-CD20 monoclonal antibody (rituximab) [21–23] and anti-VWF A1 nanobody (caplacizumab) [24,25], and these therapies enable successful treatment of iTTP patients in the acute phase. However, prophylactic treatment options to prevent iTTP relapse during remission remain urgent since 20–50% of patients experience at least one clinical relapse [26–29]. Standard cTTP therapy includes plasma infusions until TTP-related symptoms have resolved and platelet counts have normalized. Prophylactic plasma infusions are given in the remission phase to prevent the recurrence of cTTP [2,8].

1.4. Follow-Up

During remission, treating physicians typically provide monthly follow-up for the first three months, three-monthly follow-up for the first year, and six-monthly or yearly follow-up when stable [30]. Platelet counts, LDH levels, ADAMTS13 activity, and inhibitory and non-inhibitory ADAMTS13 antibodies should be carefully followed during each visit to anticipate an ADAMTS13 or clinical relapse in the super early stage and to treat the patients accordingly. Nonetheless, accurately identifying patients at risk of relapse in iTTP remains a significant challenge due to the absence of reliable biomarkers. However, numerous studies have focused on assessing the prognostic potential of various biomarkers in order to enhance the prediction of relapse. In the next section, these different biomarkers and their role in predicting an iTTP relapse will be discussed.

2. ADAMTS13 Antigen, Autoantibodies and Conformation to Advance Diagnosis and Follow-Up

2.1. ADAMTS13 Activity, Antigen and Autoantibodies

2.1.1. Low ADAMTS13 Activity and/or Presence of Anti-ADAMTS13 IgG and Their Link with Relapse

When iTTP patients suffer from clinical relapse, ADAMTS13 tests reveal severely deficient ADAMTS13 activity and positive anti-ADAMTS13 IgG as laboratory findings. Persistent or recurrent deficiency of ADAMTS13 activity during follow-up of survivors of acute iTTP is an established risk factor for disease recurrence [27,31]. Accordingly, many groups have discussed the importance of monitoring ADAMTS13 activity and anti-ADAMTS13 IgG titers in the follow-up. Ferrari et al. reported a prospective cohort study that enrolled 35 iTTP patients during an 18-month follow-up [26]. Occurring on one or two occasions (19%) throughout the follow-up period, elevated levels of inhibitory anti-ADAMTS13 IgG upon initial presentation were linked to the continuous absence of detectable ADAMTS13 activity during remission. Among 13 survivors with undetectable ADAMTS13 activity in remission, six experienced a relapse. Hence, depleted ADAMTS13 activity with detectable autoantibodies was indicative of forthcoming relapses within an 18-month timeframe [26]. Peyvandi et al. also confirmed these findings in a retrospective iTTP cohort; severe deficiency of ADAMTS13 activity and positive anti-ADAMTS13 antibodies were more identified in patients with recurrent iTTP relapses than those without relapses [27]. In addition, the likelihood of relapse was 3.6 times higher when patients had both severe ADAMTS13 deficiency and anti-ADAMTS13 antibodies [27]. Using a logistic regression model, Jin et al. assessed the relationship between ADAMTS13 activity level and the probability of iTTP relapse in 157 serial samples from 24 patients [31]. The authors revealed that lower ADAMTS13 activity and younger age were significantly linked to a higher risk of relapse three months after sample withdrawal, whereas ADAMTS13 antibody IgG levels were not predictive of iTTP relapses [31]. Schieppati et al. revealed in a multi-institutional study that the correlation between ADAMTS13 activity being $\leq 20\%$ and a significant anti-ADAMTS13 titer during remission, along with a duration of at least 13 days for the initial treatment's response, were autonomous prognostic indicators for the recurrence of the disease [32].

As for ADAMTS13 parameters in acute phase, Sui et al. described that while plasma levels of ADAMTS13 activity, antigen, and anti-ADAMTS13 IgG on admission could not predict exacerbation or recurrence in patients with iTTP, persistently low plasma ADAMTS13 activity below 10 U/dL (HR, 4.4; $p < 0.005$) or high anti-ADAMTS13 IgG (HR, 3.1; $p < 0.016$) 3 to 7 days after the initiation of TPE was associated with a higher risk for exacerbation or recurrence [33].

In conclusion, persistently depleted ADAMTS13 activity accompanied by positive ADAMTS13 autoantibodies in the middle of the acute phase and during remission causes earlier iTTP relapse.

2.1.2. Low ADAMTS13 Antigen and High Anti-ADAMTS13 IgG and Their Link with Disease Outcome and Prognosis

To date, the ADAMTS13 antigen is not routinely evaluated in clinical practice. In healthy individuals, normal ADAMTS13 antigen levels are found to range between 0.5 and 1.8 µg/mL [34–37]. Although iTTP patients sporadically display ADAMTS13 antigen within the normal range, almost all patients present with severely deficient antigen levels during acute phase iTTP [34–36]. ADAMTS13 antigen depletion at presentation is statistically associated with disease severity, as significantly lower presenting antigen levels are detected in patients with fatal disease outcomes, and a five-fold higher mortality rate is associated with ADAMTS13 antigen levels in the lowest quartile [34,35]. Therefore, ADAMTS13 antigen levels could serve as a prognostic factor to predict disease outcome. Follow-up of ADAMTS13 antigen during treatment could also provide helpful information to guide patient management, as higher antigen levels at clinical response suggest patients should sustain remission [36]. Intriguingly, iTTP patients displaying no inhibitory antibodies were found to have significantly lower ADAMTS13 antigen levels at first presentation [34]. However, when inhibitory antibodies are detected, lower antigen levels are observed in patients with autoantibodies against both N- and C-terminal ADAMTS13 domains compared to patients with only N-terminal antibodies [34].

Despite the polyclonal immune response in iTTP, dominant immunoprofiles suggest that nearly all patients display antibodies targeted against immunogenic hotspots mainly located in the ADAMTS13 Spacer (S) and Cysteine-rich (C) domains (hereafter referred to as anti-CS antibodies) [34,38–42]. However, the domain specificity of presenting anti-ADAMTS13 antibodies does not differ between surviving and deceased iTTP patients. Moreover, disease severity, prognosis, or patient management to enable remission could not be linked to antibody domain specificity nor to the three most dominant patient immunoprofiles [34,39,42]. Aberrantly high antibody titers, typically found when multiple domains are targeted by anti-ADAMTS13 antibodies [42], are displayed in over 90% of presenting patients, even though elevated titers could often only be measured at the later stages of relapse episodes [35]. Interestingly, patients with antibody titers in the highest quartile showed a three-fold increased mortality rate when compared to those in the lowest quartile. Additionally, elevated troponin levels, a lowered Glasgow Coma Scale (GCS) score, and a larger number of plasma exchange sessions were associated with patients in the highest quartile [35]. Therefore, both ADAMTS13 antibody (i.e., titers of the highest quartile) and antigen (i.e., titers of the lowest quartile) are reported to adversely affect TTP outcome by means of elevated mortality rates as well as raised cardiac and neurological involvement [34,35,42].

2.2. Open ADAMTS13 Conformation and Its Link with Diagnosis and Follow-Up

As previously described, the diagnosis of iTTP is always confirmed when the laboratory parameters show an ADAMTS13 activity below 10% and the presence of anti-ADAMTS13 antibodies [2,10,42]. However, diagnosis remains challenging when borderline ADAMTS13 activity levels fluctuate between 10–20%, as alternative thrombotic microangiopathies could be differentially diagnosed [11,42]. To correctly diagnose such iTTP patients, clinical attention is attracted towards a novel biomarker: an open ADAMTS13 conformation, as conformationally altered self-antigens are also observed in other autoimmune diseases [42–47]. Indeed, our group showed that an open ADAMTS13 conformation is a specific biomarker for acute iTTP as well as for subclinical iTTP [43,44]. In acute iTTP patients, the ADAMTS13 conformation is open, whereas the evaluation of healthy individuals, sepsis patients, and hemolytic uremic syndrome (HUS) patients all showed a closed conformation [43]. This suggests successful differentiation of acute iTTP patients from patients with alternative TMAs such as HUS, which could thereby largely benefit the diagnosis of iTTP patients that present ADAMTS13 activity ranging from 10 to 20%. Long-term follow-up of individual iTTP patients revealed that nearly all remission patients with ADAMTS13 activity below 50% had an ADAMTS13 with an open ADAMTS13 conformation, demonstrating that open ADAMTS13 is not only a biomarker for acute iTTP but also for subclinical disease. Intriguingly, ADAMTS13 conformation was closed in over 60% of remission patients with >50% ADAMTS13 activity, indicating that open ADAMTS13 might predict relapse in these patients [44].

We showed that iTTP patient anti-ADAMTS13 antibodies induce an open ADAMTS13 conformation. Indeed, purified iTTP patient IgG and, more specifically, purified anti-CS antibodies induced an open ADAMTS13 conformation [47]. This finding linked the open ADAMTS13 conformation with the most dominant immunoprofile (i.e., presence of only anti-CS antibodies) described in both Caucasian and Japanese iTTP patient cohorts [34,39,42,47]. On the other hand, purification of patient anti-CUB antibodies, present in over 50% of patients [39,42], revealed that only some of these anti-CUB fractions could induce an open ADAMTS13 conformation. This observation might explain how ADAMTS13 could adopt an open conformation in iTTP patients without detectable anti-CS antibodies [47]. The role of anti-ADAMTS13 antibodies in opening ADAMTS13 is in line with the observation that in acquired TTP of unknown pathophysiology (uTTP), a closed ADAMTS13 conformation is typically presented by such patients (>85%), and no anti-ADAMTS13 antibodies are detected [48]. The role of anti-ADAMTS13 antibodies in opening ADAMTS13 was also confirmed by the observed changes in ADAMTS13 conformations when preemptive rituximab administration was used. Patients responsive to rituximab treatment (i.e., >50% ADAMTS13 activity recovery) systematically recovered a closed ADAMTS13 conformation; however, a borderline open conformation was also reported in some patients [44,49]. Alternatively, an open ADAMTS13 conformation was sustained in patients poorly responding to preemptive rituximab, as no ADAMTS13 activity restoration or anti-ADAMTS13 antibody titer reduction occurred [49].

Finally, although ADAMTS13 activity was decreased in the remission patients with an activity <50%, anti-ADAMTS13 antibodies were often undetectable [44,49,50]. Since we showed that iTTP patient anti-ADAMTS13 antibodies induce an open ADAMTS13 conformation, open ADAMTS13 could be a surrogate marker for the presence of anti-ADAMTS13 antibodies when these antibodies are undetectable in the plasma of these patients. As ELISA-assays used to detect anti-ADAMTS13 antibodies in patient plasma typically only identify free antibodies, undetectable antibody levels can be explained by their presence in immune complexes. On the other hand, very low levels of free antibodies might be undetectable in the current ELISAs [18,44,51,52].

To date, the reference assay to evaluate ADAMTS13 conformation is the 1C4 open/closed ELISA developed in our group, in which a cryptic epitope in the Spacer domain of open ADAMTS13 is specifically recognized [42–44,47]. Novel diagnostic tests to evaluate ADAMTS13 conformation that are fast, automated, and easy-to-use could be beneficial to promote iTTP diagnosis and ameliorate patient follow-up and management.

3. Non-ADAMTS13 Parameters

3.1. Troponin-T/I and Glasgow Coma Score and Their Link with Acute iTTP Death

Cardiac troponin-T and -I (cTnT and cTnI) are biomarkers commonly used for detecting myocardial injury and the differential diagnosis of acute coronary syndrome [53,54]. Patients with acute decompensated heart failure with positive cardiac troponin tests had lower systolic blood pressure on admission, a lower ejection fraction, and higher in-hospital mortality than those with negative tests [55]. In addition, patients with a positive troponin are 2.55 times more likely to die than those not positive for troponin (95% confidence interval, 2.24 to 2.89; $p < 0.001$ by the Wald test) [55]. Although induction of plasma exchange has dramatically improved the survival rate in acute iTTP, the 30-day mortality rate remains 10–20% [19,20]. Acute cardiac events in iTTP are myocardial infarction, congestive heart failure, fatal arrhythmias, and cardiogenic shock, leading to fatal outcomes in the acute phase [56]. A Japanese retrospective study revealed that 26 out of 32 patients experienced sudden death, mostly following radical hypotension and bradycardia. The median follow-up time after admission was 5.0 days, and nine patients underwent autopsy and had cardiac microvascular thrombi in arterioles [57]. The UK group reported a retrospective study on cardiac involvement in acute iTTP. A positive cTnT test was identified in 54% of patients, and half had cardiac symptoms [58]. Intriguingly, an elevated anti-ADAMTS13 IgG titer was associated with positive cTnT above 0.25 ng/mL (normal range 0–0.01 ng/mL), and both parameters predicted mortality and acute morbidity in acute iTTP [58]. Moreover, cTnI in iTTP was also assessed by the French TMA reference center [59]. An increased cTnI above 0.1 ng/mL was seen in 78 out of 133 non-selected patients, of whom 46 had no clinical cardiac involvement. A cTnI level of >0.25 ng/mL was determined as an independent predictive factor in death and refractoriness (odds ratio 2.87 and 3.03, respectively) [59]. Based on these studies, elevated cTnT/cTnI on admission would predict poor clinical outcomes, probably because patients with higher cTnT/cTnI substantially suffer from a cardiac injury due to microthrombi [58,59]. However, it should be noted that not all patients with positive cTnT/cTnI develop cardiac involvement in the acute phase [58,59].

The GCS is a clinical scale used to reliably measure a person's level of consciousness after a brain injury. Its score is based on eye opening (ocular response, 1–4), verbal (oral response, 1–5), and motor responses (motoric response, 1–6). The combined score, which ranges from 3 to 15, reflects consciousness. Generally, brain injury is classified as Severe, GCS $\leq$ 8; Moderate, GCS 9–12; or Minor, GCS $\geq$ 13 [60]. Alwan et al. reported that 24% of iTTP patients had a reduced GCS, defined as a GCS score of 14 or below, at presentation, with a ninefold increase in mortality (20% vs. 2.2% for normal GCS at presentation, $p < 0.0001$) [35]. In this study, while cardiac involvement was also identified as a risk for mortality, there was no synergistic effect on the mortality rate of a combined decreased GCS and elevated cardiac troponin compared with the mortality for a single abnormal prognostic factor [35,61]. A further prospective investigation is required to conclude if a novel anti-VWF A1 nanobody, caplacizumab, could improve patients with positive cTnT/cTnI and/or impaired GCS.

3.2. Markers of Endothelial Activation and Inflammation

Endothelial cell (EC) activation and inflammation have been linked to the pathophysiology of iTTP [62–66]. Hence, proteins secreted from endothelial cells and/or circulating endothelial cells (CECs) or proteins secreted from leukocytes during acute iTTP and in remission might be interesting biomarkers to predict disease outcome and relapse. In this section, proteins and cells that have been studied as possible biomarkers for disease outcome will be discussed.

Although VWF antigen is increased during the acute phase upon EC activation, high VWF antigen levels were not predictive of disease outcome or relapse [27,67]. In contrast, decreased high molecular weight (HMW) VWF multimers were associated with the presence and severity of neurological symptoms in acute phase iTTP, while no association was found between HMW VWF and relapse in the French retrospective cohort study [68]. In the Mainz prospective cohort study, a newly defined fraction of HMW compared to LMW VWF multimers (VWF MM ratio) was shown to be higher in patient plasma samples obtained a few days to several weeks before a relapse compared to patients remaining in remission [69]. Whether changes in HMW VWF multimers during remission predict relapse remains to be determined. Moreover, soluble P-selectin (sP-selectin) concentration is elevated in the acute phase upon EC activation; however, increased sP-selectin concentrations were not associated with neurological symptoms nor with disease severity [66].

Another protein secreted upon EC activation is big endothelin-1 (Big ET-1). Big ET-1 is a 38-amino acid polypeptide and the precursor of ET-1, a potent vasoconstrictor. The half-life of ET-1 is less than one minute, while Big ET-1 is more slowly cleared. Big ET-1 is synthesized in vascular ECs, where it has been identified in Weibel Palade bodies. It was shown that plasma levels of Big ET-1 are significantly elevated upon admission and during clinical response/remission [65]. Elevated levels of plasma Big ET-1 upon admission were linked to acute renal insufficiency and higher in-hospital mortality rates. Furthermore, persistently elevated plasma levels of Big ET-1 during clinical response/remission are associated with exacerbations of iTTP. Whether plasma levels of Big ET-1 were associated with the risk of relapse was not investigated [65]. A possible role of Big ET-1 in the pathophysiology of iTTP is not known.

Finally, CECs, which are stressed endothelial cells that become detached from the endothelial membrane and indicate endothelial damage, were elevated during acute phase iTTP. This increase was linked to the presence of initial neurological symptoms and demonstrated a correlation with the patient's clinical outcome. Whether an increase in CECs predicts relapse remains to be determined [66].

Syndecan-1 (Sdc-1) and soluble thrombomodulin (sTM) are the main components of the endothelial glycocalyx, a layer of membrane-bound macromolecules anchored to the luminal surface of the vascular endothelium. In specific pathologic conditions, such as acute inflammation and ischemia-reperfusion injury [70–72], leukocyte-derived proteases, metalloproteinases, and heparinases cleave the ectodomains of Sdc-1 and TM. Upon admission, individuals with acute iTTP exhibit significantly higher plasma levels of Sdc-1 and/or sTM, and these levels remain elevated during clinical response/remission. Increased plasma levels of Sdc-1 and/or sTM on admission are linked to mortality in patients experiencing acute iTTP. A concurrent rise in plasma Sdc-1 and sTM during clinical response/remission is associated with a higher recurrence rate of acute iTTP [64].

Granular, azurophilic neutrophil content, such as S100A8/A9, human neutrophil peptides 1–3 (HNP1–3), and neutrophil extracellular traps (NETs), are released upon inflammation or neutrophil activation [62]. Moreover, neutrophils, as a NET component, as well as different cell processes such as necrosis and apoptosis, cause the release of cell-free DNA (cfDNA). And as NETs consist of neutrophil proteases and histone/DNA complexes, increased levels of these plasma markers (i.e., cfDNA, S100A8/A9, and histone/DNA complexes) are reported in acute iTTP patients. Notably, elevated levels of these plasma markers at admission are associated with in-hospital patient mortality [62]. Interestingly, HNP1-3 is described to bind the VWF A2 domain, which could thereby inhibit multimeric VWF cleavage by ADAMTS13. Intriguingly, HNP1–3 share a RRY peptide motif with the immunogenic ADAMTS13 spacer domain, which might suggest that HNPs could enhance pathogenic autoantibody production [73].

Markers of endothelial and leukocyte activation are increased in acute iTTP, and some of these are associated with neurological symptoms or patient outcomes. However, larger prospective studies are needed to prove their usefulness in predicting disease outcome and relapse.

4. Conclusions

This review summarizes essential biomarkers to differentially diagnose iTTP from alternative TMAs and allow subdiagnosis of various iTTP forms (Figure 1). Clinical evaluation of ADAMTS13 parameters (activity, antibody, conformation, and antigen) is essential to specifically diagnose iTTP, with an open ADAMTS13 conformation serving as a sensitive tool to confirm iTTP when ADAMTS13 activity ranges between 10 and 20%, even when anti-ADAMTS13 antibodies remain undetectable. ADAMTS13 antigen levels as well as some non-ADAMTS13 parameters could be assessed to predict iTTP disease severity and mortality. To date, the role of each ADAMTS13 parameter for clinical diagnosis and prognosis of iTTP patients has been thoroughly evaluated, whereas the role of various non-ADAMTS13 biomarkers remains indefinite. Accurate and easily available tests are prerequisites, and additional clinical studies are needed to clarify the potential role of each of these non-ADAMTS13 parameters in iTTP diagnosis and prognosis. Therefore, the inclusion of automated, easy-to-use assays for these novel biomarkers in routine clinical testing might largely benefit on-demand diagnosis and follow-up of iTTP patients while providing essential insights into disease progression and allowing rapid switching of treatment administration.

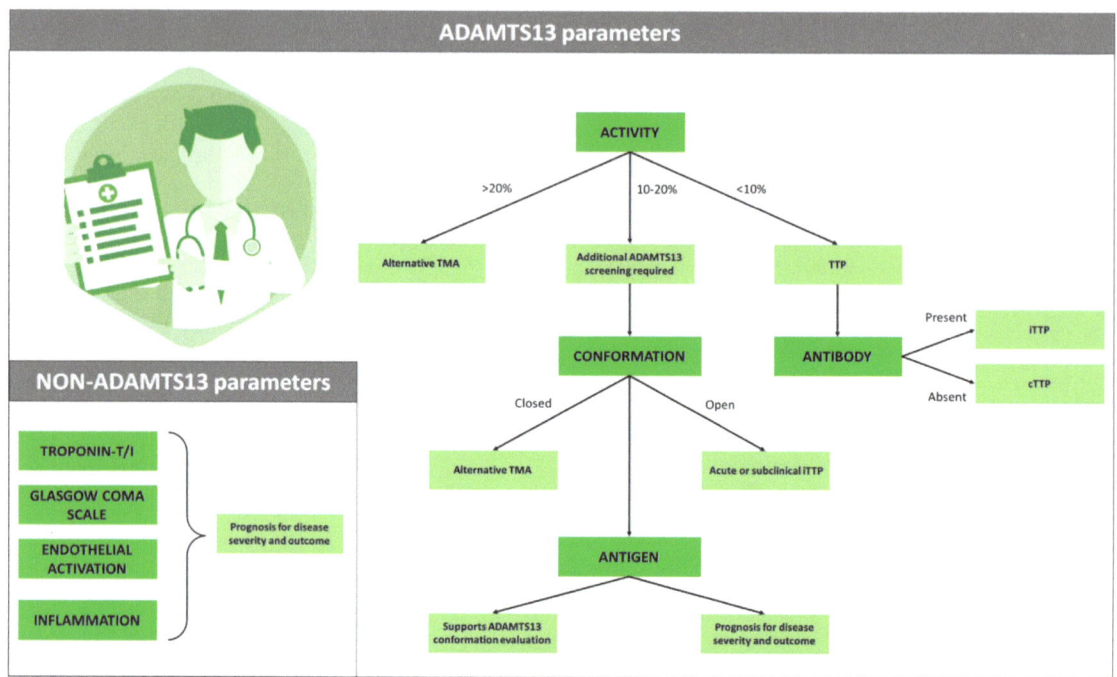

Figure 1. (Non)-ADAMTS13 diagnostic parameters for iTTP. To diagnose TTP, evaluation of different ADAMTS13 parameters is paramount. ADAMTS13 activity levels below 10% of normal activity specifically discriminate TTP from alternative TMAs. Diagnosis remains challenging when an activity between 10 and 20% is presented, requiring additional ADAMTS13 testing to correctly recognize TTP. The presence of anti-ADAMTS13 antibodies suggests the subdiagnosis of iTTP, whereas its absence could indicate cTTP. Within this 10–20% activity range, the ADAMTS13 conformation, relying on ADAMTS13 antigen evaluation, provides crucial information to properly (sub)diagnose TTP disease. Anyway, its contribution to conformation determination, the ADAMTS13 antigen is described as a prognostic factor for disease severity and clinical outcome. Non-ADAMTS13 parameters (troponin levels, GCS, endothelin-1, histone/DNA complexes, and syndecan-1) lack specificity to diagnose TTP, despite being described as valuable tools to predict disease outcome and guide patient management. TMA, thrombotic microangiopathy; ADAMTS13 (A Disintegrin And Metalloproteinase with ThromboSpondin type 1 Repeats, Member 13); TTP, thrombotic thrombocytopenic purpura; iTTP, immune-mediated TTP; cTTP, congenital TTP.

Author Contributions: Q.B., K.S. and K.V. were involved in the conceptualization, writing, reviewing, and editing of the manuscript. All authors have read and agreed to the published version of the manuscript.

Funding: This work was supported by the "Fonds voor Wetenschappelijk Onderzoek—Toegepast Biomedisch onderzoek met een primair Maatschappelijke finaliteit" (FWO-TBM) (T002918N), FWO G090120N, and the Answering T.T.P. Thrombotic Thrombocytopenic Purpura Foundation awarded to K.V.

Conflicts of Interest: The authors declare no conflict of interest.

References

1. Sadler, J.E. Pathophysiology of thrombotic thrombocytopenic purpura. *Blood* **2017**, *130*, 1181–1188. [CrossRef] [PubMed]
2. Kremer Hovinga, J.A.; Coppo, P.; Lämmle, B.; Moake, J.L.; Miyata, T.; Vanhoorelbeke, K. Thrombotic thrombocytopenic purpura. *Nat. Rev. Dis. Primers* **2017**, *3*, 1–17. [CrossRef]

3. South, K.; Lane, D.A. ADAMTS-13 and von Willebrand factor: A dynamic duo. *J. Thromb. Haemost.* **2018**, *16*, 6–18. [CrossRef]
4. Sarig, G. ADAMTS-13 in the Diagnosis and Management of Thrombotic Microangiopathies. *Rambam Maimonides Med. J.* **2014**, *5*, e0026. [CrossRef]
5. Furlan, M.; Robles, R.; Solenthaler, M.; Lämmle, B. Acquired Deficiency of von Willebrand Factor-Cleaving Protease in a Patient With Thrombotic Thrombocytopenic Purpura. *Blood* **1998**, *91*, 2839–2846. [CrossRef] [PubMed]
6. Tsai, H.M.; Lian, E.C.Y. Antibodies to von Willebrand factor-cleaving protease in acute thrombotic thrombocytopenic purpura. *N. Engl. J. Med.* **1998**, *339*, 1585–1594. [CrossRef] [PubMed]
7. Mariotte, E.; Azoulay, E.; Galicier, L.; Rondeau, E.; Zouiti, F.; Boisseau, P.; Poullin, P.; de Maistre, E.; Provôt, F.; Delmas, Y.; et al. Epidemiology and pathophysiology of adulthood-onset thrombotic microangiopathy with severe ADAMTS13 deficiency (thrombotic thrombocytopenic purpura): A cross-sectional analysis of the French national registry for thrombotic microangiopathy. *Lancet Haematol.* **2016**, *3*, e237–e245. [CrossRef] [PubMed]
8. Joly, B.S.; Paul Coppo, A.V. Thrombotic thrombocytopenic purpura. *Blood* **2017**, *129*, 2836–2846. [CrossRef]
9. Amorosi, E.; Ultmann, J. Thrombotic thrombocytopenic purpura. *Medicine* **1966**, *45*, 139–160. [CrossRef]
10. Scully, M.; Hunt, B.J.; Benjamin, S.; Liesner, R.; Rose, P.; Peyvandi, F.; Cheung, B.; Machin, S.J.; British Committee for Standards in Haematology. Guidelines on the diagnosis and management of thrombotic thrombocytopenic purpura and other thrombotic microangiopathies. *Br. J. Haematol.* **2012**, *158*, 323–335. [CrossRef]
11. Zheng, X.L.; Vesely, S.K.; Cataland, S.R.; Coppo, P.; Geldziler, B.; Iorio, A.; Matsumoto, M.; Mustafa, R.A.; Pai, M.; Rock, G.; et al. ISTH guidelines for the diagnosis of thrombotic thrombocytopenic purpura. *J. Thromb. Haemost.* **2020**, *18*, 2486–2495. [CrossRef]
12. Matsumoto, M.; Miyakawa, Y.; Kokame, K.; Ueda, Y.; Wada, H.; Higasa, S.; Higasa, S.; Moriki, T.; Yagi, H.; Miyata, T.; et al. Diagnostic and treatment guidelines for thrombotic thrombocytopenic purpura (TTP) in Japan 2023. *Int. J. Hematol.* **2023**, *106*, 3–15. [CrossRef]
13. Furlan, M.; Robles, R.; Galbusera, M.; Remuzzi, G.; Kyrle, P.A.; Brenner, B.; Krause, M.; Scharrer, I.; Aumann, V.; Mittler, U.; et al. von Willebrand factor-cleaving protease in thrombotic thrombocytopenic purpura and the hemolytic-uremic syndrome. *N. Engl. J. Med.* **1998**, *339*, 1578–1584. [CrossRef]
14. Kokame, K.; Nobe, Y.; Kokubo, Y.; Okayama, A.; Miyata, T. FRETS-VWF73, a first fluorogenic substrate for ADAMTS13 assay. *Br. J. Haematol.* **2005**, *129*, 93–100. [CrossRef]
15. Kato, S.; Matsumoto, M.; Matsuyama, T.; Isonishi, A.; Hiura, H.; Fujimura, Y. Novel monoclonal antibody-based enzyme immunoassay for determining plasma levels of ADAMTS13 activity. *Transfusion* **2006**, *46*, 1444–1452. [CrossRef]
16. Liu, L.; Choi, H.; Bernardo, A.; Bergeron, A.L.; Nolasco, L.; Ruan, C.; Moake, J.L.; Dong, J.F. Platelet-derived VWF-cleaving metalloprotease ADAMTS-13. *J. Thromb. Haemost.* **2005**, *3*, 2536–2544. [CrossRef] [PubMed]
17. Vendramin, C.; Thomas, M.; Westwood, J.P.; Scully, M. Bethesda Assay for Detecting Inhibitory Anti-ADAMTS13 Antibodies in Immune-Mediated Thrombotic Thrombocytopenic Purpura. *TH Open* **2018**, *2*, e329–e333. [CrossRef] [PubMed]
18. Lotta, L.A.; Valsecchi, C.; Pontiggia, S.; Mancini, I.; Cannavò, A.; Artoni, A.; Mikovic, D.; Meloni, G.; Peyvandi, F. Measurement and prevalence of circulating ADAMTS13-specific immune complexes in autoimmune thrombotic thrombocytopenic purpura. *J. Thromb. Haemost.* **2014**, *12*, 329–336. [CrossRef] [PubMed]
19. Rock, G.A.; Shumak, K.H.; Buskard, N.A.; Blanchette, V.S.; Kelton, J.G.; Nair, R.C.; Spasoff, R.A. Comparison of plasma exchange with plasma infusion in the treatment of thrombotic thrombocytopenic purpura. Canadian Apheresis Study Group. *N. Engl. J. Med.* **1991**, *325*, 393–397. [CrossRef] [PubMed]
20. Bell, W.R.; Braine, H.G.; Ness, P.M.; Kickler, T.S. Improved survival in thrombotic thrombocytopenic purpura-hemolytic uremic syndrome. Clinical experience in 108 patients. *N. Engl. J. Med.* **1991**, *325*, 398–403. [CrossRef]
21. Scully, M.; McDonald, V.; Cavenagh, J.; Hunt, B.J.; Longair, I.; Cohen, H.; Machin, S.J. A phase 2 study of the safety and efficacy of rituximab with plasma exchange in acute acquired thrombotic thrombocytopenic purpura. *Blood* **2011**, *118*, 1746–1753. [CrossRef] [PubMed]
22. Sun, L.; Mack, J.; Li, A.; Ryu, J.; Upadhyay, V.A.; Uhl, L.; Kaufman, R.M.; Stowell, C.P.; Dzik, W.S.; Makar, R.S.; et al. Predictors of relapse and efficacy of rituximab in immune thrombotic thrombocytopenic purpura. *Blood Adv.* **2019**, *3*, 1512–1518. [CrossRef] [PubMed]
23. Kubo, M.; Sakai, K.; Yoshii, Y.; Hayakawa, M.; Matsumoto, M. Rituximab prolongs the time to relapse in patients with immune thrombotic thrombocytopenic purpura: Analysis of off-label use in Japan. *Int. J. Hematol.* **2020**, *112*, 764–772. [CrossRef] [PubMed]
24. Peyvandi, F.; Scully, M.; Kremer Hovinga, J.A.; Cataland, S.; Knöbl, P.; Wu, H.; Artoni, A.; Westwood, J.P.; Mansouri Taleghani, M.; Jilma, B.; et al. Caplacizumab for Acquired Thrombotic Thrombocytopenic Purpura. *N. Engl. J. Med.* **2016**, *374*, 511–522. [CrossRef]
25. Scully, M.; Cataland, S.R.; Peyvandi, F.; Coppo, P.; Knöbl, P.; Kremer Hovinga, J.A.; Metjian, A.; de la Rubia, J.; Pavenski, K.; Callewaert, F.; et al. Caplacizumab Treatment for Acquired Thrombotic Thrombocytopenic Purpura. *N. Engl. J. Med.* **2019**, *380*, 335–346. [CrossRef] [PubMed]
26. Ferrari, S.; Scheiflinger, F.; Rieger, M.; Mudde, G.; Wolf, M.; Coppo, P.; Girma, J.P.; Azoulay, E.; Brun-Buisson, C.; Fakhouri, F.; et al. Prognostic value of anti-ADAMTS 13 antibody features (Ig isotype, titer, and inhibitory effect) in a cohort of 35 adult French patients undergoing a first episode of thrombotic microangiopathy with undetectable ADAMTS 13 activity. *Blood* **2007**, *109*, 2815–2822. [CrossRef]

27. Peyvandi, F.; Lavoretano, S.; Palla, R.; Feys, H.B.; Vanhoorelbeke, K.; Battaglioli, T.; Valsecchi, C.; Canciani, M.T.; Fabris, F.; Zver, S.; et al. ADAMTS13 and anti-ADAMTS13 antibodies as markers for recurrence of acquired thrombotic thrombocytopenic purpura during remission. *Haematologica* **2008**, *93*, 232–239. [CrossRef]
28. Falter, T.; Herold, S.; Weyer-Elberich, V.; Scheiner, C.; Schmitt, V.; von Auer, C.; Messmer, X.; Wild, P.; Lackner, K.J.; Lämmle, B.; et al. Relapse Rate in Survivors of Acute Autoimmune Thrombotic Thrombocytopenic Purpura Treated with or without Rituximab. *Thromb. Haemost.* **2018**, *118*, 1743–1751. [CrossRef]
29. Coppo, P.; Cuker, A.; George, J.N. Thrombotic thrombocytopenic purpura: Toward targeted therapy and precision medicine. *Res. Pract. Thromb. Haemost.* **2018**, *3*, 26–37. [CrossRef]
30. Zheng, X.L.; Vesely, S.K.; Cataland, S.R.; Coppo, P.; Geldziler, B.; Iorio, A.; Matsumoto, M.; Mustafa, R.A.; Pai, M.; Rock, G.; et al. Good practice statements (GPS) for the clinical care of patients with thrombotic thrombocytopenic purpura. *J. Thromb. Haemost.* **2020**, *18*, 2503–2512. [CrossRef]
31. Jin, M.; Casper, T.C.; Cataland, S.R.; Kennedy, M.S.; Lin, S.; Li, Y.J.; Wu, H.M. Relationship between ADAMTS13 activity in clinical remission and the risk of TTP relapse. *Br. J. Haematol.* **2008**, *141*, 651–658. [CrossRef]
32. Schieppati, F.; Russo, L.; Marchetti, M.; Barcella, L.; Cefis, M.; Gomez-Rosas, P.; Caldara, G.; Carpenedo, M.; D'Adda, M.; Rambaldi, A.; et al. Low levels of ADAMTS-13 with high anti-ADAMTS-13 antibodies during remission of immune-mediated thrombotic thrombocytopenic purpura highly predict for disease relapse: A multi-institutional study. *Am. J. Hematol.* **2020**, *95*, 953–959. [CrossRef]
33. Sui, J.; Cao, W.; Halkidis, K.; Abdelgawwad, M.S.; Kocher, N.K.; Guillory, B.; Williams, L.A.; Gangaraju, R.; Marques, M.B.; Zheng, X.L. Longitudinal assessments of plasma ADAMTS13 biomarkers predict recurrence of immune thrombotic thrombocytopenic purpura. *Blood Adv.* **2019**, *3*, 4177–4186. [CrossRef] [PubMed]
34. Thomas, M.R.; de Groot, R.; Scully, M.A.; Crawley, J.T.B. Pathogenicity of Anti-ADAMTS13 Autoantibodies in Acquired Thrombotic Thrombocytopenic Purpura. *EBioMedicine* **2015**, *2*, 942–952. [CrossRef]
35. Alwan, F.; Vendramin, C.; Vanhoorelbeke, K.; Langley, K.; McDonald, V.; Austin, S.; Clark, A.; Lester, W.; Gooding, R.; Biss, T.; et al. Presenting ADAMTS13 antibody and antigen levels predict prognosis in immune-mediated thrombotic thrombocytopenic purpura. *Blood* **2017**, *130*, 466–471. [CrossRef] [PubMed]
36. Yang, S.; Jin, M.; Lin, S.; Cataland, S.; Wu, H. ADAMTS13 activity and antigen during therapy and follow-up of patients with idiopathic thrombotic thrombocytopenic purpura: Correlation with clinical outcome. *Haematologica* **2011**, *96*, 1521–1527. [CrossRef] [PubMed]
37. Rieger, M.; Ferrari, S.; Kremer Hovinga, J.A.; Konetschny, C.; Herzog, A.; Koller, L.; Weber, A.; Remuzzi, G.; Dockal, M.; Plaimauer, B.; et al. Relation between ADAMTS13 activity and ADAMTS13 antigen levels in healthy donors and patients with thrombotic microangiopathies (TMA). *Thromb. Haemost.* **2006**, *95*, 212–220.
38. Kangro, K.; Roose, E.; Schelpe, A.S.; Tellier, E.; Kaplanski, G.; Voorberg, J.; De Meyer, S.F.; Männik, A.; Vanhoorelbeke, K. Generation and validation of small ADAMTS13 fragments for epitope mapping of anti-ADAMTS13 autoantibodies in immune-mediated thrombotic thrombocytopenic purpura. *Res. Pract. Thromb. Haemost.* **2020**, *4*, 918–930. [CrossRef]
39. Kangro, K.; Roose, E.; Joly, B.S.; Sinkovits, G.; Falter, T.; von Auer, C.; Rossmann, H.; Reti, M.; Voorberg, J.; Prohászka, Z.; et al. Anti-ADAMTS13 autoantibody profiling in patients with immune-mediated thrombotic thrombocytopenic purpura. *Blood Adv.* **2021**, *5*, 3427–3435. [CrossRef]
40. Velásquez Pereira, L.C.; Roose, E.; Graça, N.A.G.; Sinkovits, G.; Kangro, K.; Joly, B.S.; Tellier, E.; Kaplanski, G.; Falter, T.; Von Auer, C.; et al. Immunogenic hotspots in the spacer domain of ADAMTS13 in immune-mediated thrombotic thrombocytopenic purpura. *J. Thromb. Haemost.* **2021**, *19*, 478–488. [CrossRef]
41. Luken, B.M.; Turenhout, E.A.; Kaijen, P.H.; Greuter, M.J.; Pos, W.; van Mourik, J.A.; Fijnheer, R.; Voorberg, J. Amino acid regions 572–579 and 657–666 of the spacer domain of ADAMTS13 provide a common antigenic core required for binding of antibodies in patients with acquired TTP. *Thromb. Haemost.* **2006**, *96*, 295–301. [CrossRef] [PubMed]
42. Sakai, K.; Matsumoto, M.; De Waele, L.; Dekimpe, C.; Hamada, E.; Kubo, M.; Tersteeg, C.; De Meyer, S.F.; Vanhoorelbeke, K. ADAMTS13 conformation and immunoprofiles in Japanese patients with immune-mediated thrombotic thrombocytopenic purpura. *Blood Adv.* **2022**, *7*, 131–140. [CrossRef] [PubMed]
43. Roose, E.; Schelpe, A.S.; Joly, B.S.; Peetermans, M.; Verhamme, P.; Voorberg, J.; Greinacher, A.; Deckmyn, H.; De Meyer, S.F.; Coppo, P.; et al. An open conformation of ADAMTS-13 is a hallmark of acute acquired thrombotic thrombocytopenic purpura. *J. Thromb. Haemost.* **2018**, *16*, 378–388. [CrossRef] [PubMed]
44. Roose, E.; Schelpe, A.S.; Tellier, E.; Sinkovits, G.; Joly, B.S.; Dekimpe, C.; Kaplanski, G.; Le Besnerais, M.; Mancini, I.; Falter, T.; et al. Open ADAMTS13, induced by antibodies, is a biomarker for subclinical immune-mediated thrombotic thrombocytopenic purpura. *Blood* **2020**, *136*, 353–361. [CrossRef] [PubMed]
45. Brandt, S.; Krauel, K.; Gottschalk, K.E.; Renné, T.; Helm, C.A.; Greinacher, A.; Block, S. Characterisation of the conformational changes in platelet factor 4 induced by polyanions: Towards in vitro prediction of antigenicity. *J. Thromb. Haemost.* **2014**, *112*, 53–64. [CrossRef] [PubMed]
46. De Laat, B.; van Berkel, M.; Urbanus, R.T.; Siregar, B.; de Groot, P.G.; Gebbink, M.F.; Maas, C. Immune Responses against Domain I of 2-Glycoprotein I Are Driven by Conformational Changes Domain I of 2-Glycoprotein I Harbors a Cryptic Immunogenic Epitope. *Arthritis Rheum.* **2011**, *63*, 3960–3968. [CrossRef]

47. De Waele, L.; Curie, A.; Kangro, K.; Tellier, E.; Kaplanski, G.; Männik, A.; Tersteeg, C.; Joly, B.S.; Coppo, P.; Veyradier, A.; et al. Anti-cysteine/spacer antibodies that open ADAMTS13 are a common feature in iTTP. *Blood Adv.* **2021**, *5*, 4480–4484. [CrossRef]
48. Joly, B.S.; Roose, E.; Coppo, P.; Vanhoorelbeke, K.; Veyradier, A. ADAMTS13 conformation is closed in non-immune acquired thrombotic thrombocytopenic purpura of unidentified pathophysiology. *Haematologica* **2023**, *108*, 638–644. [CrossRef]
49. Jestin, M.; Benhamou, Y.; Schelpe, A.S.; Roose, E.; Provôt, F.; Galicier, L.; Hié, M.; Presne, C.; Poullin, P.; Wynckel, A.; et al. Preemptive rituximab prevents long-term relapses in immune-mediated thrombotic thrombocytopenic purpura. *Blood* **2018**, *132*, 2143–2153. [CrossRef]
50. Doyle, A.J.; Stubbs, M.J.; Dutt, T.; Lester, W.; Thomas, W.; van Veen, J.; Hermans, J.; Cranfield, T.; Hill, Q.A.; Clark, A.; et al. Long-term risk of relapse in immune-mediated thrombotic thrombocytopenic purpura and the role of anti-CD20 therapy. *Blood* **2023**, *141*, 285–294. [CrossRef]
51. Ferrari, S.; Palavra, K.; Gruber, B.; Kremer Hovinga, J.A.; Knöbl, P.; Caron, C.; Cromwell, C.; Aledort, L.; Plaimauer, B.; Turecek, P.L.; et al. Persistence of circulating ADAMTS13-specific immune complexes in patients with acquired thrombotic thrombocytopenic purpura. *Haematologica* **2014**, *99*, 779–787. [CrossRef]
52. Mancini, I.; Ferrari, B.; Valsecchi, C.; Pontiggia, S.; Fornili, M.; Biganzoli, E.; Peyvandi, F. ADAMTS13-specific circulating immune complexes as potential predictors of relapse in patients with acquired thrombotic thrombocytopenic purpura. *Eur. J. Intern. Med.* **2017**, *39*, 79–83. [CrossRef]
53. Adams, J.E.; Bodor, G.S.; Davila-Roman, V.G.; Delmez, J.A.; Apple, F.S.; Ladenson, J.H.; Jaffe, A.S. Cardiac troponin I. A marker with high specificity for cardiac injury. *Circulation* **1993**, *88*, 101–106. [CrossRef]
54. Ohman, E.M.; Armstrong, P.W.; Christenson, R.H.; Granger, C.B.; Katus, H.A.; Hamm, C.W.; O'Hanesian, M.A.; Wagner, G.S.; Kleiman, N.S.; Harrell, F.E.; et al. Cardiac troponin T levels for risk stratification in acute myocardial ischemia. GUSTO IIA Investigators. *N. Engl. J. Med.* **1996**, *335*, 1333–1342. [CrossRef] [PubMed]
55. Peacock, W.F.; De Marco, T.; Fonarow, G.C.; Diercks, D.; Wynne, J.; Apple, F.S.; Wu, A.H.B. Cardiac troponin and outcome in acute heart failure. *N. Engl. J. Med.* **2008**, *358*, 2117–2126. [CrossRef]
56. Patschan, D.; Witzke, O.; Dührsen, U.; Erbel, R.; Philipp, T.; Herget-Rosenthal, S. Acute myocardial infarction in thrombotic microangiopathies—Clinical characteristics, risk factors and outcome. *Nephrol. Dial. Transplant.* **2006**, *21*, 1549–1554. [CrossRef] [PubMed]
57. Kayashima, M.; Sakai, K.; Harada, K.; Kanetake, J.; Kubo, M.; Hamada, E.; Hayakawa, M.; Hatakeyama, K.; Matsumoto, M. Strong association between insufficient plasma exchange and fatal outcomes in Japanese patients with immune-mediated thrombotic thrombocytopenic purpura. *Int. J. Hematol.* **2021**, *114*, 415–423. [CrossRef]
58. Hughes, C.; McEwan, J.R.; Longair, I.; Hughes, S.; Cohen, H.; Machin, S.; Scully, M. Cardiac involvement in acute thrombotic thrombocytopenic purpura: Association with troponin T and IgG antibodies to ADAMTS 13. *J. Thromb. Haemost.* **2009**, *7*, 529–536. [CrossRef] [PubMed]
59. Benhamou, Y.; Boelle, P.Y.; Baudin, B.; Ederhy, S.; Gras, J.; Galicier, L.; Azoulay, E.; Provôt, F.; Maury, E.; Pène, F.; et al. Cardiac troponin-i on diagnosis predicts early death and refractoriness in acquired thrombotic thrombocytopenic purpura. experience of the french thrombotic microangiopathies reference center. *J. Thromb. Haemost.* **2015**, *13*, 293–302. [CrossRef]
60. Rowley, G.; Fielding, K. Reliability and accuracy of the Glasgow Coma Scale with experienced and inexperienced users. *Lancet* **1991**, *337*, 535–538. [CrossRef]
61. Staley, E.M.; Cao, W.; Pham, H.P.; Kim, C.H.; Kocher, N.K.; Zheng, L.; Gangaraju, R.; Lorenz, R.G.; Williams, L.A.; Marques, M.B.; et al. Clinical factors and biomarkers predict outcome in patients with immune-mediated thrombotic thrombocytopenic purpura. *Haematologica* **2019**, *104*, 166–175. [CrossRef] [PubMed]
62. Sui, J.; Lu, R.; Halkidis, K.; Kocher, N.K.; Cao, W.; Marques, M.B.; Zheng, X.L. Plasma levels of S100A8/A9, histone/DNA complexes, and cell-free DNA predict adverse outcomes of immune thrombotic thrombocytopenic purpura. *J. Thromb. Haemost.* **2021**, *19*, 370–379. [CrossRef] [PubMed]
63. Fuchs, T.A.; Kremer Hovinga, J.A.; Schatzberg, D.; Wagner, D.D.; Lämmle, B. Circulating DNA and myeloperoxidase indicate disease activity in patients with thrombotic microangiopathies. *Blood* **2012**, *120*, 1157–1164. [CrossRef] [PubMed]
64. Lu, R.; Sui, J.; Zheng, X.L. Elevated plasma levels of syndecan-1 and soluble thrombomodulin predict adverse outcomes in thrombotic thrombocytopenic purpura. *Blood Adv.* **2020**, *4*, 5378–5388. [CrossRef] [PubMed]
65. Lu, R.; Zheng, X.L. Plasma Levels of Big Endothelin-1 Are Associated with Renal Insufficiency and In-Hospital Mortality of Immune Thrombotic Thrombocytopenic Purpura. *Thromb. Haemost.* **2022**, *122*, 344–352. [CrossRef]
66. Widemann, A.; Pasero, C.; Arnaud, L.; Poullin, P.; Loundou, A.D.; Choukroun, G.; Sanderson, F.; Lacroix, R.; Sabatier, F.; Coppo, P.; et al. Circulating endothelial cells and progenitors as prognostic factors during autoimmune thrombotic thrombocytopenic purpura: Results of a prospective multicenter French study. *J. Thromb. Haemost.* **2014**, *12*, 1601–1609. [CrossRef]
67. Veyradier, A.; Obert, B.; Houllier, A.; Meyer, D.; Girma, J.P. Specific von Willebrand factor-cleaving protease in thrombotic microangiopathies: A study of 111 cases. *Blood* **2001**, *98*, 1765–1772. [CrossRef]
68. Béranger, N.; Benghezal, S.; Savigny, S.; Capdenat, S.; Joly, B.S.; Coppo, P.; Stepanian, A.; Veyradier, A. Loss of von Willebrand factor high-molecular-weight multimers at acute phase is associated with detectable anti-ADAMTS13 IgG and neurological symptoms in acquired thrombotic thrombocytopenic purpura. *Thromb. Res.* **2019**, *181*, 29–35. [CrossRef]

69. Falter, T.; Rossmann, H.; de Waele, L.; Dekimpe, C.; von Auer, C.; Müller-Calleja, N.; Häuser, F.; Degreif, A.; Marandiuc, D.; Messmer, X.; et al. A novel von Willebrand factor multimer ratio as marker of disease activity in thrombotic thrombocytopenic purpura. *Blood Adv.* **2023**, *7*, 5091–5102. [CrossRef]
70. Gonzalez Rodriguez, E.; Cardenas, J.C.; Cox, C.S.; Kitagawa, R.S.; Stensballe, J.; Holcomb, J.B.; Johansson, P.I.; Wade, C.E. Traumatic brain injury is associated with increased syndecan-1 shedding in severely injured patients. *Scand. J. Trauma. Resusc. Emerg. Med.* **2018**, *26*, 102. [CrossRef]
71. Pruessmeyer, J.; Martin, C.; Hess, F.M.; Schwarz, N.; Schmidt, S.; Kogel, T.; Ikeda, A.; Oikawa, K.; Takikawa, Y.; Masuda, T. A Disintegrin and metalloproteinase 17 (ADAM17) mediates inflammation-induced shedding of syndecan-1 and -4 by lung epithelial cells. *J. Biol. Chem.* **2010**, *285*, 137–144. [CrossRef] [PubMed]
72. Mulivor, A.W.; Lipowsky, H.H. Inflammation- and ischemia-induced shedding of venular glycocalyx. *Am. J. Physiol. Heart Circ. Physiol.* **2004**, *286*, H1672–H1680. [CrossRef] [PubMed]
73. Pillai, V.G.; Bao, J.; Zander, C.B.; McDaniel, J.K.; Chetty, P.S.; Seeholzer, S.H.; Bdeir, K.; Cines, D.B.; Zheng, X.L. Human neutrophil peptides inhibit cleavage of von Willebrand factor by ADAMTS13: A potential link of inflammation to TTP. *Blood* **2016**, *128*, 110–119. [CrossRef] [PubMed]

Disclaimer/Publisher's Note: The statements, opinions and data contained in all publications are solely those of the individual author(s) and contributor(s) and not of MDPI and/or the editor(s). MDPI and/or the editor(s) disclaim responsibility for any injury to people or property resulting from any ideas, methods, instructions or products referred to in the content.

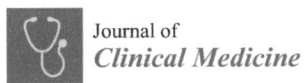 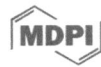

Review

Anti-ADAMTS13 Autoantibodies: From Pathophysiology to Prognostic Impact—A Review for Clinicians

Cristina Dainese [1,2,*], Federica Valeri [1,2], Benedetto Bruno [2,3] and Alessandra Borchiellini [1,2]

1. Regional Centre for Hemorrhagic and Thrombotic Diseases, AOU Città Della Salute e Della Scienza, 10126 Turin, Italy; fvaleri@cittadellasalute.to.it (F.V.); aborchiellini@cittadellasalute.to.it (A.B.)
2. Division of Hematology, AOU Città Della Salute e Della Scienza and University of Turin, 10124 Turin, Italy; benedetto.bruno@unito.it
3. Department of Molecular Biotechnology and Health Sciences, University of Turin, 10124 Turin, Italy
* Correspondence: cdainese@cittadellasalute.to.it; Tel.: +39-0116335329 (ext. 4418)

Abstract: Thrombotic thrombocytopenic purpura (TTP) is a fatal disease in which platelet-rich microthrombi cause end-organ ischemia and damage. TTP is caused by markedly reduced ADAMTS13 (a disintegrin and metalloproteinase with a thrombospondin type 1 motif, member 13) activity. ADAMTS13 autoantibodies (autoAbs) are the major cause of immune TTP (iTTP), determining ADAMTS13 deficiency. The pathophysiology of such autoAbs as well as their prognostic role are continuous objects of scientific studies in iTTP fields. This review aims to provide clinicians with the basic information and updates on autoAbs' structure and function, how they are typically detected in the laboratory and their prognostic implications. This information could be useful in clinical practice and contribute to future research implementations on this specific topic.

Keywords: thrombotic thrombocytopenic purpura; Moskowitz syndrome; ADAMTS13 autoantibodies; ADAMTS13 inhibitors

Citation: Dainese, C.; Valeri, F.; Bruno, B.; Borchiellini, A. Anti-ADAMTS13 Autoantibodies: From Pathophysiology to Prognostic Impact—A Review for Clinicians. *J. Clin. Med.* **2023**, *12*, 5630. https://doi.org/10.3390/jcm12175630

Academic Editors: Ilaria Mancini and Andrea Artoni

Received: 30 June 2023
Revised: 26 July 2023
Accepted: 27 July 2023
Published: 29 August 2023

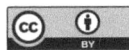

Copyright: © 2023 by the authors. Licensee MDPI, Basel, Switzerland. This article is an open access article distributed under the terms and conditions of the Creative Commons Attribution (CC BY) license (https://creativecommons.org/licenses/by/4.0/).

1. Introduction

Thrombotic thrombocytopenic purpura (TTP) is a rare hematological disorder caused by a deficiency in the enzymatic function of a member of the disintegrin and metalloprotease with thrombospondin-type motifs family, an enzyme called ADAMTS13, which is synthesized primarily in the liver and, in limited quantities, by vascular endothelial cells, megakaryocytes, platelets, glomerular podocytes and glial cells. ADAMTS13 binds soluble von Willebrand Factor (VWF) and interacts with endothelium-anchored Ultra-Large VWF Multimers (ULVWFMs), resulting in the cleavage of ULVWFM strings or bundles to regulate their interaction with platelets, thus preventing the formation of blood clots in normal circulation. In patients with immune TTP (iTTP), ADAMTS13 activity is significantly reduced due to the binding of anti-ADAMTS13 autoantibodies (autoAbs) to the metalloprotease. Consequently, ULVWFMs remain uncleaved in circulation, forming platelet-rich thrombi in the microvessels under conditions of high shear stress [1]. The mechanisms by which these autoAbs inhibit ADAMTS13 enzymatic function are not fully understood, and in recent years many scientific efforts have been made to improve our knowledge on this specific topic.

2. Anti-ADAMTS13 Autoantibodies Pathophysiology: Production, Structure and Function

As in other autoimmune disorders, iTTP is characterized by a loss of tolerance resulting in a shift to autoimmunity [2]. Antigens derived from ADAMTS13 molecules, processed by dendritic cells, activate cross-reactive naïve CD4+ T cells, which, in turn, differentiate into autoreactive effector CD4+ T cells [3,4]. Autoreactive B cells recirculate into the germinal center (GC) of secondary lymph nodes, stimulated by antigens and auto reactive T helper cells and differentiate into autoAb-producing plasma cells or long-lived memory B cells [5]. Shin and colleagues performed an analysis of B cell subsets and circulating follicular T helper (cfTh) cell changes in iTTP [2]. A decreased number of post-GC memory B cells, an increased number of plasma blasts and a reduction of cfTh compared to healthy controls were found in the acute phase of iTTP. Furthermore, the authors of that study described an association between higher plasma blasts and higher ADAMTS13 autoAbs levels, with a trend toward reduced ADAMTS13 antigen levels. The same group also demonstrated that, in asymptomatic patients that underwent an ADAMTS13 relapse prior to preemptive therapy with rituximab (RTX), a significantly increased naïve B cell population, a global decrease in all memory subsets and a trend toward increased plasma blasts were present.

The autoimmune response against ADAMTS13 is polyclonal and heterogeneous [6,7]. A study demonstrated that ADAMTS13 autoAbs are primarily composed of immunoglobulin G (IgG), approximately 90% of which are of the IgG4 subtype [8]. In the cases presenting with detectable IgG4 autoAbs, IgG4 were found alone in 33% of the cases and with other IgG subtypes in 67%. The second most frequent subtype detected was IgG1 (52%), followed by IgG2 (50%) and IgG3 (33%). None of these subtypes were detected alone. Only 10–20% of the patients presented with autoAbs of IgA and IgM classes [8].

Several scientific groups are working to better understand which epitope/epitopes of ADAMTS13 these autoAbs recognize and bind to. Figure 1 proposes a simplified version of the ADAMTS13 structure. The physiologic functions of most of the domains are unknown. The inhibition or depletion of ADAMTS13 activity may be attributable to various mechanisms, depending on the epitope bound by the autoAbs [9]. ADAMTS13 circulates in a folded conformation through an S-CUB interaction, which is disrupted upon binding to its substrate, VWF or to opening antibodies, which allosterically activate ADAMTS13. Thus, the open conformation of ADAMTS13 induced by autoAbs is considered a hallmark of iTTP [10–12].

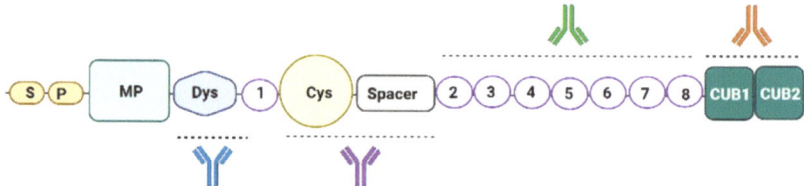

Figure 1. ADAMTS13 enzyme structure and major autoAbs binding sites. ADAMTS13 is a multidomain metalloprotease consisting of a signal peptide domain (S), a short propeptide domain (P), a metalloprotease (M) domain, a disintegrin-like (Dis) domain, a first thrombospondin type 1 (TSP1) repeat, a cysteine-rich (Cys) domain and a Spacer domain. It has seven additional thrombospondin type 1 repeats (TSP2-8) and two CUB domains (CUB1-2) [13]. Major epitope binding sites are the Cys-Spacer domain, the CUBs domain (see main text), the Dys domain and the TSP fragments and domains.

Several authors have demonstrated that a major binding site for autoAbs in iTTP is the cysteine-rich/Spacer (CS) domain [14–17]. Klaus and colleagues, by inducing the expression of a series of ADAMTS13 domains in E. coli, evaluated the reactivity of purified recombinant fragments with ADAMTS13 autoAbs from 25 patients with iTTP in vitro [18]. All the plasma samples contained autoAbs directed against the CS domain. AutoAbs reacting exclusively with the CS domain were found in 12% of plasmas, underscoring the importance of this region for the functional activity of ADAMTS13. In 64% of the plasma samples, autoAbs reacted with the two CUB domains, with the TSP-1 repeat compound fragment and the TSP-1 domain in 56%. Less frequently, autoAbs reacted with TSP1 repeats 2 to 8 (28%). Unexpectedly, autoAbs reacting with the propeptide region were found in 20% of the plasmas samples. These results indicate that, even though ADAMTS13 autoAbs react with multiple protease domains, the CS domain is consistently involved in antibody reactivity. Also, Osertag and colleagues cloned ADAMTS13 autoAbs using phage display and characterized them with respect to genetic origin, inhibition of ADAMTS13 activity and epitope specificity. It was noted that both autoAbs directed against the amino-terminal domains and those requiring the ADAMTS13 CS domains for binding inhibited proteolytic activity, while those solely targeting carboxy-terminal domains were non-inhibitory [19]. A different group isolated ADAMTS13 autoAbs sequences from the peripheral blood mononuclear cells of iTTP patients. Three IgG ADAMTS13 autoAbs were cloned (TTP73–1 and TR8C11 binding to the CS domains, ELH2–1 recognizing the T2–T3 domains). Interestingly, none of the autoAbs had inhibitory activity and all three antibodies recognized cryptic epitopes, in accordance with the hypothesis that the conformation of ADAMTS13 is open during acute iTTP [12]. Thomas and colleagues also found that almost 97% of iTTP episodes had IgG recognizing ADAMTS13 N-terminal domains and S domain. In the same study, functional analyses were performed on IgG from 43 patients and revealed that inhibitory IgG was limited to anti-S domain autoAbs [20]. AutoAbs with no detectable inhibitory action were found in 35% of patients, while 74% of patients had autoAbs with inhibitory function that was insufficient to account for the severe deficiency state, suggesting a possible alternative pathogenic mechanism. A multicenter European study determined anti-ADAMTS13 immunoprofiles based on the presence or absence of anti-M, anti-Dys, anti-CS, anti-T2-T5, anti-T6-T8 and anti-CUB1-2 autoAbs in a large cohort of both acute and remission iTTP plasma and serum samples (365 samples from 213 iTTP patients) [21]. Three main profiles were identified: only anti-CS autoAbs (profile 1); anti-CS and anti-CUB1-2 AutoAbs (profile 2); and anti-Dys, anti-CS, anti-T2-T5, anti-T6-T8 and anti-CUB1-2 autoAbs (profile 3). In both acute and remission phases, profile 1 was the dominant immunoprofile, suggesting that anti-CS autoAbs are the first to reappear or are the ones that persist during remission, while the other domain-specific autoAbs mainly appear in the acute phase. A similar analysis was performed on a Japanese iTTP cohort: more than 70% of patients had anti-CS autoAbs, in agreement with the Caucasian cohorts, but the Japanese cohort only showed one dominant immunoprofile, profile 1, with only autoAbs against the CS domain [22].

Increasing knowledge on autoAb immunoprofiles might support the improvement of targeted therapies for better iTTP patient management. For example, if a patient has only anti-S autoantibodies, an rADAMTS13 variant, mutated in the S domain, could be used to escape the binding of anti-S autoAbs [23,24].

How do ADAMST13 autoAbs work? ADAMTS13 deficiency may manifest with reduced activity and/or a reduction in circulating antigen depending on the autoAbs mechanism. Thus, the autoAbs response to ADAMTS13 includes neutralizing and/or non-neutralizing antibodies. Neutralizing autoAbs block the proteolytic activity of ADAMTS13 towards VWF, primarily reducing the enzymatic function of the molecule, while non-neutralizing autoAbs may contribute to increasing ADAMTS13 clearance or interfere with ADAMTS13 interaction with cells or other plasma proteins. As previously reported, anti-CS domain autoAbs mainly inhibit the function of ADAMTS13 by targeting the S domain, which plays a key role in VWF binding [25]. Thus, the inhibition of ADAMTS13's function has long been thought to be the major cause of ADAMTS13 deficiency in iTTP. However, many iTTP plasma samples do not contain inhibitory ADAMTS13 autoAbs and, on the other hand, ADAMTS13 antigen levels can be severely decreased even in the presence of inhibitory ADAMTS13 autoAbs. Hence, some authors have suggested that ADAMTS13 clearance rather than ADAMTS13 inhibition could be the major pathogenic cause of ADAMTS13 deficiency in iTTP [20]. A possible enhanced clearance pathway could be the formation of ADAMTS13 antigen–antibody immune complexes (ICs), described in acute iTTP and during remission [26–28]. The clearance of IgG containing ICs occurs primarily in the liver, through both Fc receptor-dependent and receptor-independent mechanisms [29–33]. Complement also plays an important role in the elimination of IC, with C3b binding keeping ICs soluble [30]. Erythrocytes bind these opsonized ICs in the circulation via C3b receptors and expose them to tissue macrophages for elimination [31].

Recently, Underwood and colleagues demonstrated the enhanced rate of ADAMTS13 clearance and how this appears to be the major mechanism of reduced ADAMTS13 activity during plasma exchange (PEX) [34]. The authors observed that, at presentation, the vast majority of patients included in the study had ADAMTS13 antigen levels of <10%, suggesting a major contribution of ADAMTS13 clearance to the deficiency state. After the first PEX, both ADAMTS13 antigen and activity levels increased similarly, while the ADAMTS13 autoAb titer decreased in all patients, revealing ADAMTS13 inhibition to be a modest modifier of ADAMTS13 function. Analysis of ADAMTS13 antigen levels between consecutive PEX treatments revealed that the rate of ADAMTS13 clearance in more than half of patients analyzed was 4- to 10-fold faster than the estimated normal rate of clearance, again supporting the hypothesis that ADAMTS13 clearance mediated by autoAbs plays a major role in iTTP. The real picture is probably much more complicated, and it is possible that more mechanisms could act simultaneously in inducing ADAMTS13 deficiency, just as it is possible that different mechanisms could be activated in the acute phase and in case of recurrence.

In summary, the development of ADAMTS13 autoAbs is the result of an immune imbalance involving B cells, cTfh cells and plasmablasts, leading to a polyclonal autoimmune response. Most ADAMTS13 autoAbs belong to the IgG family and recognize the CS domain of the ADAMTS13 molecule. One matter of debate is the main function of autoAbs, neutralizing or non-neutralizing, in the enhancement of ADAMTS13 clearance. Increasing knowledge about the structure, function and specific epitope recognition of ADAMTS13 autoAbs not only helps to better understand iTTP pathophysiology but, as seen here, could have important clinical-therapeutic implications in the future, especially with the advent of new molecules.

3. Anti-ADAMTS13 Autoantibodies Detection

A test of ADAMTS13 activity is required to confirm TTP diagnosis. Then, in order to differentiate iTTP from congenital TTP (cTTP), the identification of ADAMTS13 autoAbs is mandatory. Diagnostic samples for ADAMTS13 activity and autoAbs testing should be collected prior to treatment [35]. Severe deficiency is defined as ADAMTS13 activity < 10 IU/dL (or <10% of normal values) [36,37]. Rare cases of iTTP with normal ADAMTS13 activity have been reported. This is attributed to the disassociation of neutralizing autoAbs from ADAMTS13 in vitro, allowing the recovery of activity in vitro [38]. False-negative autoAbs testing can occur with low-antibody titers or if autoAbs are highly bound in antigen–antibody complexes. This may be diagnostically misleading, masking the underlying immune mechanism of the disorder; it is thus crucial to differentiate iTTP from cTTP [39].

Bethesda assays are used to detect and titer neutralizing autoAbs. Test plasma is heat-treated to inactivate any ADAMTS13 still present, leaving autoAbs in the plasma intact. One volume of heat-treated plasma is added to one volume of normal pooled plasma (NPP), the source of ADAMTS13 in the assay. A separate control mixture is prepared, comprising equal volumes of NPP and buffer; in this way, both tubes begin the procedure with identical levels of ADAMTS13. Then, both tubes are incubated for 30 to 120 min, depending on the protocol, to permit the formation of antigen–antibody complexes. The ADAMTS13 activity of the test and control mixtures is then measured in a functional assay and the residual ADAMTS13 activity of the test sample is calculated as a percentage of that of the control sample subjected to identical incubation conditions. One Bethesda unit (BU) is an inhibitor titer that decreases the residual activity to 50% of the expected value. Performing a dilution series allows for titer determination. Rather than wait for the result on just the 1 + 1 dilution, it is common to perform the assay on a range of dilutions in the first instance, then correcting for the dilution factor [40]. Some authors suggest that an incubation period of at least 2 h and not immediate incubation is the required time for detecting inhibitory anti-ADAMTS13 antibodies [41]. It is important to note that the Bethesda-like detection of ADAMTS13 inhibitors also shows variability, dependent on the analytical technique.

The tests commonly referred to as ADAMTS13 autoAbs tests utilize enzyme-linked immunosorbent assay (ELISA) [35]. ELISA identifies all autoAbs, regardless of neutralizing or non-neutralizing activities. For this reason, IgG ELISA is more sensitive for iTTP, but less specific, since non-neutralizing autoAbs have been reported in a small percentage of healthy individuals and patients with other autoimmune disorders (e.g., systemic lupus erythematosus (SLE) or antiphospholipid antibody syndrome (APS)) [42–44]. For this assay, the microplate walls are supplied coated with rADAMTS13 to capture autoAbs. The first step of the assay is the addition of calibration and control plasmas containing ADAMTS13 autoAbs, as well as diluted test plasmas potentially containing ADAMTS13 autoAbs. After incubation, residual plasma is washed off, and an anti-human IgG antibody conjugated to the enzyme horseradish peroxidase (HRP) is added. The amount that binds is proportional to the amount of anti-ADAMTS13 antibody captured by the rADAMTS13. After incubation, excess conjugate is washed off, and a colorless HRP substrate, $3,3',5,5'$-tetramethylbenzidine (e.g., TMB or OPD), is added that reacts with HRP to generate a blue-colored product. After incubation, the reaction is stopped with sulfuric acid to stabilize color development, generating a clear yellow color due to TMB oxidation. Color intensity is proportional to bound conjugate and, hence, to the ADAMTS13 autoAbs level. Different ELISA set-ups are used in clinical and research laboratories, which vary in the presentation of rADAMTS13 and the type of detection autoAbs [40]. One commonly used ELISA assay is available from Technoclone, and detects human immunoglobulin (Ig) G against ADAMTS13. One significant limitation of this assay, however, is the potential to detect non-ADAMTS13 antibodies that may be present in patients with general autoimmune conditions, particularly if high levels of such antibodies are present. Dekimpe and colleagues assessed the influence of different rADAMTS13 presentation and autoAbs detection approaches in ELISA [45]. The authors concluded that although different methods of rADAMTS13 presentation for ADAMTS13 autoAb level determination correlate strongly, the detection of low ADAMTS13 autoAb levels can depend on the method of rADAMTS13 presentation.

ELISA-positive/Bethesda-negative results have been described in recovered iTTP patients who showed both ELISA- and Bethesda-positive autoAbs results at the time of acute iTTP diagnosis, confirming that inhibition is not necessarily the primary effect of some ADAMTS13 autoAbs. Thus, using only the Bethesda assay will lead to the underdetection of ADAMTS13 autoAbs [46] and generally cannot detect antibody titers below 0.5 BU. Bethesda and ELISA assays do not allow discrimination between free antibody and antibody bound to ADAMTS13 in circulating immune complexes in vivo. In conclusion, the literature data suggest that ELISA should be the preferred antibody assay at iTTP presentation, but that it requires supplementation with Bethesda assay to demonstrate the inhibitory function of the autoantibodies [46].

4. Anti-ADAMTS13 Autoantibodies and Prognostic Role

Together with ADAMTS13 activity and other potential prognostic markers, several authors have evaluated whether and what role ADAMTS13 autoAbs could have in a prognostic sense, considering both the impact on severity and mortality, and on the recurrence risk. Ferrari et al. observed that patients included in their study were less likely to survive their first iTTP event if they had IgG1 and very low or undetectable IgG4 levels plus higher titers of other classes of ADAMTS13 autoAbs (particularly IgA), suggesting that an immune response characterized by high levels of IgG4 could, at least partially, predict a more treatable form of iTTP [8]. The authors also investigated the possibility of an association between IgG subclasses and relapse and found that high levels of IgG4 with undetectable IgG1 was significantly associated with a trend towards iTTP recurrence. A different Italian group found that during acute-phase iTTP IgA represented the Ig class which most strongly associated with clinical severity (estimated in this study by the number of platelets at presentation) [47]. The authors suggested that IgA could contribute to the severity of the clinical manifestations by activating complement system through the mannose-binding lectin pathway, thus increasing complement-mediated inflammation [48]. In the same study, the IgG class and IgG subclass were also found to be predictive of the severity of the acute iTTP episode, as high IgG titers were associated with a higher number of PEXs and IgG1 and IgG3 were the classes most strongly associated with the clinical severity of acute-phase disease. Different authors have also suggested that high-titer inhibitors are associated with delayed response to PEX and refractory disease [49–51]. Alwan and colleagues demonstrated in a registry-based retrospective study that patients with ADAMTS13 autoAbs levels in the upper quartile had a mortality rate more than three times higher than that of patients with ADAMTS13 autoAbs in the lowest quartile. When comparing the upper and lower quartiles, those in the upper quartile were also more likely to have a raised troponin and a reduced Glasgow Coma Scale (GCS), and required a longer period of PEX to achieve platelet count normalization [52]. Another prospective multicenter study was conducted to assess the prognostic value of inhibitory ADAMTS13 autoAbs. It was found that patients with no detectable inhibitors usually displayed a more rapid and durable response to treatment, whereas patients with detectable inhibitors had a delayed improvement in ADAMTS13 activity and platelet count recovery, hence requiring significantly higher volumes of plasma to achieve durable complete remission [53]. In the same study, death was only observed in patients with an intermediate or high ADAMTS13 inhibitor titer at diagnosis, while all patients with a low inhibitor titer evolved favorably. This suggests that the strength of ADAMTS13 autoAbs may be associated with treatment responsiveness and outcome. A different group recently analyzed the role of ADAMTS13 autoAbs in the caplacizumab era. The authors first identified a delay in the normalization of ADAMTS13 activity (>30%) in a subgroup of caplacizumab-treated patients, which was not evident in the pre-caplacizumab era [54]. The authors then evaluated the potential role of ADAMTS13 autoAbs levels and ADAMTS13 antigen in predicting the delayed normalization of ADAMTS13 activity in patients with an ADAMTS13 activity < 10% at the time of stopping caplacizumab. Presenting anti-ADAMTS13 IgG levels were not predictive of ADAMTS13 activity delayed normalization, yet a rise in autoAbs levels from diagnosis to the time of stopping caplacizumab appeared relevant. Furthermore, concurrent ADAMTS13 antigen levels < 30% at the time of caplacizumab discontinuation were associated with a greater risk of recurrence (defined in this study as any exacerbation or relapse). However, raised anti-ADAMTS13 IgG levels were not predictive of TTP recurrence. Our group, on a retrospective analysis of 42 first iTTP episodes, identified ADAMTS13 autoAbs titer at diagnosis as a marker of iTTP burden of care, associated with higher total number of PEX sessions, PEXs needed to achieve clinical response, days of hospitalization and a higher probability of needing RTX rescue to achieve clinical response [55]. In other words, ADAMTS13 autoAbs titer could identify those iTTP cases in which caplacizumab, currently the standard of care, can bring the greatest benefits compared with standard of care in terms of cost-effective analysis, and the cases in which early intensification of immunosuppressive with RTX is indicated.

While the significance of reduced ADAMTS13 activity during remission is more consolidated, the predictive value of disease recurrence determined by the presence of ADAMTS13 autoAbs, their inhibitory activity and Ig classes and subclasses is still controversial. In different studies, ADAMTS13 autoAbs during remission emerged as one of the possible risk factors associated with an increased risk of iTTP relapse, together with young age, race, a previous relapse of iTTP and severely deficient ADAMTS13 activity in remission [56–58]. Peyvandi and colleagues reported that the prevalence of any ADAMTS13 autoAbs (whether or not they inhibited protease activity) was significantly different in patients with or without recurrence. In their study, 64% of patients with recurrent iTTP had ADAMTS13 autoAbs during remission, whereas only 36% of those without recurrence had ADAMTS13 autoAbs. The unadjusted odds ratios for recurrence indicated that the presence of ADAMTS13 autoAbs, regardless of neutralizing activity, increased the likelihood of TTP recurrence by approximately three-fold [59]. These data were also supported by another study in which the presence of ADAMTS13 autoAbs during remission appeared to predict the risk of recurrence [47]. The cited study added that anti-ADAMTS13 IgG had a strong predictive value for recurrence during both acute and remission phases; no association between IgG subclasses and recurrence risk or association between ADAMTS13 autoAbs levels and acute episode severity was detected, in disagreement with previous reports [53]. An Italian group proposed with their analysis that ADAMTS13 activity $\leq$ 20%, ADAMTS13 autoAbs titer $\geq$ 15 U/mL and inhibitory activity > 50% at the time of remission correlated with disease relapse. The multivariate analysis showed that in the group of patients achieving a complete remission with PEX and steroids the combination of ADAMTS13 activity $\leq$ 20% with ADAMTS13 autoAbs $\geq$ 15 U/mL at remission and a time to response to first-line treatment $\geq$ 13 days, were independent predictive factors of relapse. During the follow-up, ADAMTS13 activity $\leq$ 20% and autoAbs titer $\geq$ 15 U/mL at 3 and 6 months were also associated with disease relapse; the combination of ADAMTS13 activity $\leq$ 20% with ADAMTS13 autoAbs $\geq$ 15 U/mL measured at 3 and 6 months was again identified as an independent predictor of disease relapse. Cox regression analysis indicated that patients with ADAMTS13 activity $\leq$ 20% plus ADAMTS13 autoAbs $\geq$ 15 U/mL at remission have an increased risk of relapse compared to patients with ADAMTS13 activity > 20% plus ADAMTS13 autoAbs < 15 U/mL [60]. However, not all authors agree with the prognostic role of ADAMTS13 inhibitors. For example, Jin and colleagues did not find any predictive value for IgG anti-ADAMTS13 levels measured during remission and the risk of recurrence [61]. Mancini et al. focused on a different marker, namely ADAMTS13-specific circulating immune complexes (CICs) [62]. The presence of circulating ADAMTS13s specific CICs in patients with iTTP has been reported both in acute and remission phases [27,28]. In their analysis, ADAMTS13-specific CICs of IgG isotype were not found to be markers of disease severity, but they were found to have a possible prognostic role as predictors of recurrence. This was especially true in the first two years after iTTP onset, with a 4.2-fold increased risk. A prospective study and a case series [63,64] report on pre-emptive treatment with RTX in patients with iTTP and persistent ADAMTS13 autoAbs, confirming the efficacy of such therapy, but currently there are no published studies or clinical trials registered aiming to establish antibody titer or a precise timepoint at which to consider pre-emptive therapy.

Summing up, together with ADAMTS13 activity and other clinical and laboratory factors, the role of ADAMTS13 autoAbs has been and is currently an interesting object of research. Even if global agreement between authors has not been reached, ADAMTS13 autoAbs are emerging as possible markers of a more severe acute form of iTTP, associated with a longer time to platelet count recovery, a higher number of PEX sessions, mortality and burden of care. Such conclusions could also be used to optimize the selection of those patients needing early immunosuppressive treatment intensification with RTX or, on the other hand, those with good chance to achieve clinical response with only steroid therapy. Furthermore, ADAMTS13 autoAbs together with ADAMTS13 activity may also represent a useful tool in the remission phase, able to identify patients with higher recurrence risk and with possible indication for pre-emptive treatment.

5. Conclusions

ADAMTS13 autoAbs represent only one of the interesting and not fully understood aspects of iTTP. Much progress in understanding the pathophysiological mechanisms has been made. Interest in such mechanisms is growing given the important clinical implications they may have with the advent of new therapeutic molecules. Their prognostic value is another important aspect. Although a unanimous consensus cannot be drawn by published studies, ADAMTS13 autoAbs appear to play a role both in the identification of more severe forms of acute iTTP and as a marker of recurrence risk during the remission phase. Thus, the refinement of laboratory methods aimed at their detection and characterization as well as large data collections will represent a cornerstone in the world of iTTP for the coming years.

Author Contributions: C.D. contributed to conceptualization, writing, review and editing; F.V., B.B. and A.B. contributed to supervision. All authors have read and agreed to the published version of the manuscript.

Funding: This research received no external funding.

Institutional Review Board Statement: This review did not require ethical approval.

Informed Consent Statement: Not applicable.

Data Availability Statement: No new data were created or analyzed in this study. Data sharing is not applicable to this article.

Conflicts of Interest: The authors declare no conflict of interest.

References

1. Zheng, X.L. ADAMTS13 and von Willebrand factor in thrombotic thrombocytopenic purpura. *Annu. Rev. Med.* **2015**, *66*, 211–225. [PubMed]
2. Shin, J.S.; Subhan, M.O.; Cambridge, G.; Guo, Y. Alterations in B- and circulating T-follicular helper cell subsets in immune thrombotic thrombocytopenic purpura. *Blood Adv.* **2022**, *6*, 3792–3802. [CrossRef] [PubMed]
3. Sorvillo, N.; van Haren, S.D.; Kaijen, P.H.; ten Brinke, A. Preferential HLA-DRB1*11-dependent presentation of CUB2-derived peptides by ADAMTS13-pulsed dendritic cells. *Blood* **2013**, *121*, 3502–3510. [CrossRef] [PubMed]
4. Verbij, F.C.; Turksma, A.W.; de Heij, F.; Kaijen, P. CD4+ T cells from patients with acquired thrombotic thrombocytopenic purpura recognize CUB2 domain-derived peptides. *Blood* **2016**, *127*, 1606–1609. [PubMed]
5. Carsetti, R.; Rosado, M.M.; Wardmann, H. Peripheral development of B cells in mouse and man. *Immunol. Rev.* **2004**, *197*, 179–191. [CrossRef]
6. Sitaru, C.; Mihai, S.; Zillikens, D. The relevance of the IgG subclass of autoantibodies for blister induction in autoimmune bullous skin diseases. *Arch. Dermatol. Res.* **2007**, *299*, 1–8.
7. Maran, R.; Dueymes, M.; Le Corre, R.; Renaudineau, Y.; Shoenfeld, Y. IgG subclasses of human autoantibodies. *Ann. Med. Interne* **1997**, *148*, 29–38.
8. Ferrari, S.; Mudde, G.C.; Rieger, M.; Veyradier, A. IgG subclass distribution of anti-ADAMTS13 antibodies in patients with acquired thrombotic thrombocytopenic purpura. *J. Thromb. Haemost.* **2009**, *7*, 1703–1710. [CrossRef]
9. Zheng, X.; Chung, D.; Takayama, T.K.; Majerus, E.M. Structure of von Willebrand factor-cleaving protease (ADAMTS13), a metalloprotease involved in thrombotic thrombocytopenic purpura. *J. Biol. Chem.* **2001**, *276*, 41059–41063. [CrossRef]
10. South, K.; Luken, B.M.; Crawley, J.T.; Phillips, R. Conformational activation of ADAMTS13. *Proc. Natl. Acad. Sci. USA* **2014**, *111*, 18578–18583. [CrossRef]
11. Roose, E.; Schelpe, A.S.; Tellier, E.; Sinkovits, G. Open ADAMTS13, induced by antibodies, is a biomarker for subclinical immune-mediated thrombotic thrombocytopenic purpura. *Blood* **2020**, *136*, 353–361. [CrossRef] [PubMed]
12. Roose, E.; Vidarsson, G.; Kangro, K.; Verhagen, O.J.H.M. Anti-ADAMTS13 Autoantibodies against Cryptic Epitopes in Immune-Mediated Thrombotic Thrombocytopenic Purpura. *Thromb. Haemost.* **2018**, *118*, 1729–1742. [PubMed]
13. De Waele, L.; Curie, A.; Kangro, K.; Tellier, E. Anti-cysteine/spacer antibodies that open ADAMTS13 are a common feature in iTTP. *Blood Adv.* **2021**, *5*, 4480–4484. [CrossRef] [PubMed]
14. Luken, B.M.; Turenhout, E.A.; Hulstein, J.J.; Van Mourik, J.A. The spacer domain of ADAMTS13 contains a major binding site for antibodies in patients with thrombotic thrombocytopenic purpura. *Thromb. Haemost.* **2005**, *93*, 267–274. [CrossRef]
15. Luken, B.M.; Kaijen, P.H.; Turenhout, E.A.; Kremer Hovinga, J.A. Multiple B-cell clones producing antibodies directed to the spacer and disintegrin/thrombospondin type-1 repeat 1 (TSP1) of ADAMTS13 in a patient with acquired thrombotic thrombocytopenic purpura. *J. Thromb. Haemost.* **2006**, *4*, 2355–2364. [CrossRef]
16. Yamaguchi, Y.; Moriki, T.; Igari, A.; Nakagawa, T. Epitope analysis of autoantibodies to ADAMTS13 in patients with acquired thrombotic thrombocytopenic purpura. *Thromb. Res.* **2011**, *128*, 169–173. [CrossRef] [PubMed]
17. Velásquez Pereira, L.C.; Roose, E.; Graça, N.A.G.; Sinkovits, G. Immunogenic hotspots in the spacer domain of ADAMTS13 in immune-mediated thrombotic thrombocytopenic purpura. *J. Thromb. Haemost.* **2021**, *19*, 478–488. [CrossRef]
18. Klaus, C.; Plaimauer, B.; Studt, J.D.; Dorner, F. Epitope mapping of ADAMTS13 autoantibodies in acquired thrombotic thrombocytopenic purpura. *Blood* **2004**, *103*, 4514–4519. [CrossRef]
19. Ostertag, E.M.; Kacir, S.; Thiboutot, M.; Gulendran, G. ADAMTS13 autoantibodies cloned from patients with acquired thrombotic thrombocytopenic purpura: 1. Structural and functional characterization in vitro. *Transfusion* **2016**, *56*, 1763–1774. [CrossRef]
20. Thomas, M.R.; de Groot, R.; Scully, M.A.; Crawley, J.T. Pathogenicity of Anti-ADAMTS13 Autoantibodies in Acquired Thrombotic Thrombocytopenic Purpura. *EBioMedicine* **2015**, *2*, 942–952.
21. Kangro, K.; Roose, E.; Joly, B.S.; Sinkovits, G. Anti-ADAMTS13 autoantibody profiling in patients with immune-mediated thrombotic thrombocytopenic purpura. *Blood Adv.* **2021**, *5*, 3427–3435. [CrossRef] [PubMed]
22. Sakai, K.; Matsumoto, M.; De Waele, L.; Dekimpe, C. ADAMTS13 conformation and immunoprofiles in Japanese patients with immune-mediated thrombotic thrombocytopenic purpura. *Blood Adv.* **2023**, *7*, 131–140. [CrossRef] [PubMed]

23. Graça, N.A.G.; Ercig, B.; Carolina Velasquez Pereira, L.; Kangro, K. Modifying ADAMTS13 to modulate binding of pathogenic autoantibodies of patients with acquired thrombotic thrombocytopenic purpura. *Haematologica* **2020**, *105*, 2619–2630. [CrossRef]
24. Jian, C.; Xiao, J.; Gong, L.; Skipwith, C.G.; Jin, S.Y. Gain-of-function ADAMTS13 variants that are resistant to autoantibodies against ADAMTS13 in patients with acquired thrombotic thrombocytopenic purpura. *Blood* **2012**, *119*, 3836–3843. [CrossRef] [PubMed]
25. Soejima, K.; Matsumoto, M.; Kokame, K.; Yagi, H. ADAMTS-13 cysteine-rich/spacer domains are functionally essential for von Willebrand factor cleavage. *Blood* **2003**, *102*, 3232–3237. [CrossRef] [PubMed]
26. Ferrari, S.; Knöbl, P.; Kolovratova, V.; Plaimauer, B. Inverse correlation of free and immune complex-sequestered anti-ADAMTS13 antibodies in a patient with acquired thrombotic thrombocytopenic purpura. *J. Thromb. Haemost.* **2012**, *10*, 156–158. [CrossRef]
27. Ferrari, S.; Palavra, K.; Gruber, B.; Kremer Hovinga, J.A.; Knöbl, P.; Caron, C.; Cromwell, C.; Aledort, L.; Plaimauer, B.; Turecek, P.L.; et al. Persistence of circulating ADAMTS13-specific immune complexes in patients with acquired thrombotic thrombocytopenic purpura. *Haematologica* **2014**, *99*, 779–787. [CrossRef]
28. Lotta, L.A.; Valsecchi, C.; Pontiggia, S.; Mancini, I. Measurement and prevalence of circulating ADAMTS13-specific immune complexes in autoimmune thrombotic thrombocytopenic purpura. *J. Thromb. Haemost.* **2014**, *12*, 329–336. [CrossRef]
29. Vugmeyster, Y.; Xu, X.; Theil, F.P.; Khawli, L.A. Pharmacokinetics and toxicology of therapeutic proteins: Advances and challenges. *World J. Biol. Chem.* **2012**, *3*, 73–92. [CrossRef]
30. Schifferli, J.A.; Taylor, R.P. Physiological and pathological aspects of circulating immune complexes. *Kidney Int.* **1989**, *35*, 993–1003. [CrossRef]
31. Emlen, W.; Carl, V.; Burdick, G. Mechanism of transfer of immune complexes from red blood cell CR1 to monocytes. *Clin. Exp. Immunol.* **1992**, *89*, 8–17. [CrossRef] [PubMed]
32. Johansson, A.; Erlandsson, A.; Eriksson, D.; Ullén, A. Idiotypic-anti-idiotypic complexes and their in vivo metabolism. *Cancer* **2002**, *94* (Suppl. S4), 1306–1313. [CrossRef] [PubMed]
33. Kosugi, I.; Muro, H.; Shirasawa, H.; Ito, I. Endocytosis of soluble IgG immune complex and its transport to lysosomes in hepatic sinusoidal endothelial cells. *J. Hepatol.* **1992**, *16*, 106–114. [CrossRef]
34. Underwood, M.I.; Alwan, F.; Thomas, M.R.; Scully, M.A. Autoantibodies enhance ADAMTS-13 clearance in patients with immune thrombotic thrombocytopenic purpura. *J. Thromb. Haemost.* **2023**, *21*, 1544–1552. [CrossRef]
35. Smock, K.J. ADAMTS13 testing update: Focus on laboratory aspects of difficult thrombotic thrombocytopenic purpura diagnoses and effects of new therapies. *Int. J. Lab. Hematol.* **2021**, *43* (Suppl. S1), 103–108. [CrossRef]
36. Page, E.E.; Kremer Hovinga, J.A.; Terrell, D.R.; Vesely, S.K. Thrombotic thrombocytopenic purpura: Diagnostic criteria, clinical features, and long-term outcomes from 1995 through 2015. *Blood Adv.* **2017**, *1*, 590–600. [CrossRef]
37. Hubbard, A.R.; Heath, A.B.; Kremer Hovinga, J.A. Subcommittee on von Willebrand Factor. Establishment of the WHO 1st International Standard ADAMTS13, plasma (12/252): Communication from the SSC of the ISTH. *J. Thromb. Haemost.* **2015**, *13*, 1151–1153. [CrossRef]
38. George, J.N. The remarkable diversity of thrombotic thrombocytopenic purpura: A perspective. *Blood Adv.* **2018**, *2*, 1510–1516. [CrossRef]
39. Peyvandi, F.; Palla, R.; Lotta, L.A.; Mackie, I. ADAMTS-13 assays in thrombotic thrombocytopenic purpura. *J. Thromb. Haemost.* **2010**, *8*, 631–640. [CrossRef]
40. Moore, G.W.; Vetr, H.; Binder, N.B. ADAMTS13 Antibody and Inhibitor Assays. *Methods Mol. Biol.* **2023**, *2663*, 549–565.
41. Vendramin, C.; Thomas, M.; Westwood, J.P.; Scully, M. Bethesda Assay for Detecting Inhibitory Anti-ADAMTS13 Antibodies in Immune-Mediated Thrombotic Thrombocytopenic Purpura. *TH Open* **2018**, *2*, e329–e333. [CrossRef]
42. Kremer Hovinga, J.A.; Heeb, S.R.; Skowronska, M.; Schaller, M. Pathophysiology of thrombotic thrombocytopenic purpura and hemolytic uremic syndrome. *J. Thromb. Haemost.* **2018**, *16*, 618–629. [CrossRef]
43. Rieger, M.; Mannucci, P.M.; Kremer Hovinga, J.A.; Herzog, A. ADAMTS13 autoantibodies in patients with thrombotic microangiopathies and other immunomediated diseases. *Blood* **2005**, *106*, 1262–1267. [CrossRef] [PubMed]
44. Shelat, S.G.; Ai, J.; Zheng, X.L. Molecular biology of ADAMTS13 and diagnostic utility of ADAMTS13 proteolytic activity and inhibitor assays. *Semin. Thromb. Hemost.* **2005**, *31*, 659–672. [CrossRef] [PubMed]
45. Dekimpe, C.; Roose, E.; Kangro, K.; Bonnez, Q. Determination of anti-ADAMTS-13 autoantibody titers in ELISA: Influence of ADAMTS-13 presentation and autoantibody detection. *J. Thromb. Haemost.* **2021**, *19*, 2248–2255. [CrossRef] [PubMed]
46. Masias, C.; Cataland, S.R. The role of ADAMTS13 testing in the diagnosis and management of thrombotic microangiopathies and thrombosis. *Blood* **2018**, *132*, 903–910.
47. Bettoni, G.; Palla, R.; Valsecchi, C.; Consonni, D. ADAMTS-13 activity and autoantibodies classes and subclasses as prognostic predictors in acquired thrombotic thrombocytopenic purpura. *J. Thromb. Haemost.* **2012**, *10*, 1556–1565. [CrossRef]
48. Roos, A.; Bouwman, L.H.; van Gijlswijk-Janssen, D.J.; Faber-Krol, M.C. Human IgA activates the complement system via the mannan-binding lectin pathway. *J. Immunol.* **2001**, *167*, 2861–2868. [CrossRef]
49. Zheng, X.L.; Kaufman, R.M.; Goodnough, L.T.; Sadler, J.E. Effect of plasma exchange on plasma ADAMTS13 metalloprotease activity, inhibitor level, and clinical outcome in patients with idiopathic and nonidiopathic thrombotic thrombocytopenic purpura. *Blood* **2004**, *103*, 4043–4049. [CrossRef]

50. Vesely, S.K.; George, J.N.; Lämmle, B.; Studt, J.D. ADAMTS13 activity in thrombotic thrombocytopenic purpura-hemolytic uremic syndrome: Relation to presenting features and clinical outcomes in a prospective cohort of 142 patients. *Blood* **2003**, *102*, 60–68. [CrossRef]
51. Veyradier, A.; Obert, B.; Houllier, A.; Meyer, D. Specific von Willebrand factor-cleaving protease in thrombotic microangiopathies: A study of 111 cases. *Blood* **2001**, *98*, 1765–1772. [CrossRef] [PubMed]
52. Alwan, F.; Vendramin, C.; Vanhoorelbeke, K.; Langley, K. Presenting ADAMTS13 antibody and antigen levels predict prognosis in immune-mediated thrombotic thrombocytopenic purpura. *Blood* **2017**, *130*, 466–471. [CrossRef] [PubMed]
53. Coppo, P.; Wolf, M.; Veyradier, A.; Bussel, A. Réseau d'Etude des Microangiopathies Thrombotiques de l'Adulte. Prognostic value of inhibitory anti-ADAMTS13 antibodies in adult-acquired thrombotic thrombocytopenic purpura. *Br. J. Haematol.* **2006**, *132*, 66–74. [CrossRef]
54. Prasannan, N.; Thomas, M.; Stubbs, M.; Westwood, J.P. Delayed normalization of ADAMTS13 activity in acute thrombotic thrombocytopenic purpura in the caplacizumab era. *Blood* **2023**, *141*, 2206–2213. [PubMed]
55. Dainese, C.; Valeri, F.; Pizzo, E.; Valpreda, A. ADAMTS13 Autoantibodies and Burden of Care in Immune Thrombotic Thrombocytopenic purpura: New Evidence and Future Implications. *Clin. Appl. Thromb. Hemost.* **2022**, *28*, 10760296221125785. [CrossRef] [PubMed]
56. Jestin, M.; Benhamou, Y.; Schelpe, A.S.; Roose, E. French Thrombotic Microangiopathies Reference Center. Preemptive rituximab prevents long-term relapses in immune-mediated thrombotic thrombocytopenic purpura. *Blood* **2018**, *132*, 2143–2153.
57. Mai Falk, J.; Scharrer, I. Idiopathic thrombotic thrombocytopenic purpura: Strongest risk factor for relapse from remission is having had a relapse. *Transfusion* **2016**, *56*, 2819–2823.
58. Liu, A.; Mazepa, M.; Davis, E.; Johnson, A.; Antun, A.G.; Farland, A.M.; Woods, R.R.; Metjian, A.; Bagby, K.; Park, Y. African American race is associated with decreased relapse-free survival in immune thrombotic thrombocytopenic purpura. *Blood* **2019**, *134* (Suppl. S1), 1066.
59. Peyvandi, F.; Lavoretano, S.; Palla, R.; Feys, H.B. ADAMTS13 and anti-ADAMTS13 antibodies as markers for recurrence of acquired thrombotic thrombocytopenic purpura during remission. *Haematologica* **2008**, *93*, 232–239. [CrossRef]
60. Schieppati, F.; Russo, L.; Marchetti, M.; Barcella, L. Low levels of ADAMTS-13 with high anti-ADAMTS-13 antibodies during remission of immune-mediated thrombotic thrombocytopenic purpura highly predict for disease relapse: A multi-institutional study. *Am. J. Hematol.* **2020**, *95*, 953–959. [CrossRef]
61. Jin, M.; Casper, T.C.; Cataland, S.R.; Kennedy, M.S. Relationship between ADAMTS13 activity in clinical remission and the risk of TTP relapse. *Br. J. Haematol.* **2008**, *141*, 651–658. [CrossRef] [PubMed]
62. Mancini, I.; Ferrari, B.; Valsecchi, C.; Pontiggia, S. Italian Group of TTP Investigators. ADAMTS13-specific circulating immune complexes as potential predictors of relapse in patients with acquired thrombotic thrombocytopenic purpura. *Eur. J. Intern. Med.* **2017**, *39*, 79–83. [CrossRef] [PubMed]
63. Fakhouri, F.; Vernant, J.P.; Veyradier, A.; Wolf, M. Efficiency of curative and prophylactic treatment with rituximab in ADAMTS13-deficient thrombotic thrombocytopenic purpura: A study of 11 cases. *Blood* **2005**, *106*, 1932–1937. [CrossRef] [PubMed]
64. Bresin, E.; Gastoldi, S.; Daina, E.; Belotti, D. Rituximab as pre-emptive treatment in patients with thrombotic thrombocytopenic purpura and evidence of anti-ADAMTS13 autoantibodies. *Thromb. Haemost.* **2009**, *101*, 233–238.

Disclaimer/Publisher's Note: The statements, opinions and data contained in all publications are solely those of the individual author(s) and contributor(s) and not of MDPI and/or the editor(s). MDPI and/or the editor(s) disclaim responsibility for any injury to people or property resulting from any ideas, methods, instructions or products referred to in the content.

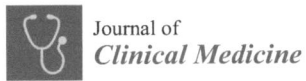

Review

Is Endothelial Activation a Critical Event in Thrombotic Thrombocytopenic Purpura?

Raphael Cauchois [1,2,*], Romain Muller [1], Marie Lagarde [2,3], Françoise Dignat-George [4], Edwige Tellier [2,3] and Gilles Kaplanski [1,2]

1. Aix Marseille University, Assistance Publique Hôpitaux de Marseille, INSERM, INRAE, C2VN, CHU Conception, Internal Medicine and Clinical Immunology, 13005 Marseille, France
2. French Reference Center for Thrombotic Microangiopathies, 75571 Paris, France
3. Aix Marseille University, INSERM, INRAE, C2VN, 13005 Marseille, France
4. Aix Marseille University, Assistance Publique Hôpitaux de Marseille, INSERM, INRAE, C2VN, CHU Conception, Hematology Laboratory, 13005 Marseille, France
* Correspondence: raphael.cauchois@ap-hm.fr

Abstract: Thrombotic thrombocytopenic purpura (TTP) is a severe thrombotic microangiopathy. The current pathophysiologic paradigm suggests that the ADAMTS13 deficiency leads to Ultra Large-Von Willebrand Factor multimers accumulation with generation of disseminated microthrombi. Nevertheless, the role of endothelial cells in this pathology remains an issue. In this review, we discuss the various clinical, in vitro and in vivo experimental data that support the important role of the endothelium in this pathology, suggesting that ADAMTS13 deficiency may be a necessary but not sufficient condition to induce TTP. The "second hit" model suggests that in TTP, in addition to ADAMTS13 deficiency, endogenous or exogenous factors induce endothelial activation affecting mainly microvascular cells. This leads to Weibel–Palade bodies degranulation, resulting in UL-VWF accumulation in microcirculation. This endothelial activation seems to be worsened by various amplification loops, such as the complement system, nucleosomes and free heme.

Keywords: thrombotic thrombocytopenic purpura; endothelial cells; Weibel–Palade bodies

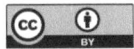

1. Introduction

Thrombotic thrombocytopenic purpura (TTP) is a rare and severe disease belonging to the thrombotic microangiopathies disorders and described for the first time in 1924 by Eli Moschcowitz. It is characterized by uncontrolled platelet aggregation and adhesion which will form microthrombi resulting in the clinical syndrome of TTP. Clinical presentation includes thrombocytopenia, mechanical hemolysis and organ damage. It can be fatal without prompt diagnosis and appropriate treatment [1]. Knowledge about TTP pathophysiology has considerably improved in recent decades: in 1982 Joel L Moake identified uncleaved von Willebrand Factor (VWF) multimers in patients with chronic relapsing TTP [2]. Nineteen years later, ADAMTS13 (A Disintegrin and Metalloproteinase with Thrombospondin-1 motifs, 13th member of the family) was related to the loss of function of the VWF multimers-cleaving metalloproteinase [3,4]. The severe ADAMTS-13 deficiency can be inherited as in congenital TTP (Upshaw–Schulmann syndrome [5]) or more commonly acquired due to inhibitory auto-antibodies against ADAMTS13 (i-TTP, for immune-mediated TTP) [6,7].

The current pathophysiological paradigm suggests that the ADAMTS13 deficiency leads to Ultra Large-VWF multimers (UL-VWF) accumulation on endothelial cells [8]. Flowing blood applies a tensile force that "unfolds" UL-VWF, which, therefore, form pro-thrombotic strings into micro vessels. They induce a massive platelet adhesion and aggregation with rapid generation of disseminated microthrombi, leading to the thrombotic microangiopathies characteristics triad: (i) organ ischemia, (ii) profound thrombocytopenia and (iii) hemolytic anemia. Organ ischemia affect mainly central nervous system but also heart, digestive tract and occasionally kidney. Thrombocytopenia (often < 30 G/L) is often associated with hemorrhagic risk because of platelet's consumption in thrombi. Furthermore, recent research has shown that thrombocytopenia is aggravated by insufficient bone marrow production of young platelets [9,10]. Anemia is accompanied with schistocytes on blood smear due to mechanical erythrocyte fragmentation on thrombi.

Due to its clinical severity, patients with i-TTP require urgent treatment in intensive care unit. Daily therapeutic plasma exchanges (TPE), commonly used since the 80's, represent the cornerstone of acute phase management and have significantly improved outcomes by drastically reducing mortality from 90% to 20% two weeks after diagnosis [11]. TPE are very effective by providing exogenous ADAMTS13 contained in donor's plasma and by removing anti-ADAMTS13 antibodies. Due to the autoimmune pathophysiology, corticosteroids are systematically associated with TPE during the acute phase. Rituximab, an anti-CD20 monoclonal antibody is another frontline therapy [12]. More recently, Caplacizumab, a nanobody inhibiting VWF-platelet interaction, provides an interesting protective effect during the acute phase [13–15]. Despite those recent therapeutic improvements, TTP remains a life-threatening disease with high morbidity [16] and relapse risk for patients who survive [17].

In addition to the central role of ADAMTS13 deficiency in TTP pathogenesis, the endothelial cells, which represent the main UL-VWF storage, have been long recognized as major actors in TMA and in TTP particularly [18,19]. Indeed, many TTP related studies have described endothelial damages, especially histopathological such as swelling/necrosis and subendothelial hyaline deposits, biomarkers association with endothelial activation and frequent environmental triggers. The existence of an endothelial activation during TTP acute phase is accepted by the scientific community. However, one question remains: is the endothelial activation a consequence of the micro-occlusive disease [20], i.e., an epiphenomenon, or is it a key initiating event that precipitates an individual susceptibility into an acute episode? Many clinical and experimental data support the hypothesis that endothelial activation is essential to the pathogenesis. This activation represents a "second hit" that induces a massive UL-VWF release into the microcirculation.

After a succinct presentation of the endothelium and the Weibel–Palade bodies, we will present elements that support or not this hypothesis. Then, we will discuss the nature of the suspected triggers and the existence of amplification loops increasing the severity degree of TTP.

2. The Endothelium
2.1. Endothelial Cells

The endothelium is a cellular monolayer that covers the luminal surface of the vascular tree [21]. Endothelial cells (ECs) are polarized through their actin cytoskeleton and constitute a dynamic interface between flowing blood (apical pole) and sub-endothelial tissues (basal pole). They play a central role in the regulation of major physiologic functions, such as hemostasis, vascular permeability, cellular and nutrient trafficking, inflammation, innate and adaptive immunity, vascular tone and angiogenesis.

Structure and function heterogeneity constitute key features of the endothelium. Depending on the vascular territory and vascular bed [22,23], endothelium presents a spatial phenotypic diversity. The morphology, secretory repertory and behavior of ECs differ between arteries and veins, and between microvascular (vessel size < 300 μm) and macrovascular (>300 μm) territories. Endothelial heterogeneity is also temporal: EC phenotype shows a high plasticity degree and phenotypical changes can occur in response to many physiological or pathological conditions, such as biomechanical signals, pH variations, hypoxemia, soluble mediators or cell–cell interactions.

2.2. Endothelial Activation

Quiescent ECs display a thromboresistant (anticoagulant and antiaggregant) and anti-inflammatory phenotype. They also protect flowing blood from the highly prothrombotic subendothelial matrix [24]. These features prevent spontaneous thrombi formation in blood vessels and result from antithrombotic molecules expression: TFPI (Tissue Factor Pathway Inhibitor), existing in transmembrane and soluble isoform, TM (Thrombomodulin), EPCR (Endothelial Protein C Receptor), t-PA (tissue-type Plasminogen Activator), NO (Nitric Oxide) and PGI2 (Prostacyclin). When exposed to various stress signals, such as cytokines, toxins, disturbed shear stress, etc., ECs acquire an "activated phenotype" which is prothrombotic (Figure 1). Consequences of this activation are multiple: VWF-multimers released from the Weibel–Palade bodies, reduced expression of the above-mentioned thromboresistant molecule and increased expression of Tissue Factor (TF), the main activator of the extrinsic coagulation pathway and Plasminogen-Activator Inhibitor-1 (PAI-1). Furthermore, activated ECs also acquire a pro-inflammatory phenotype characterized by leukocyte receptor expression, such as P-selectin, and an increase in intercellular permeability facilitating leukocyte trafficking.

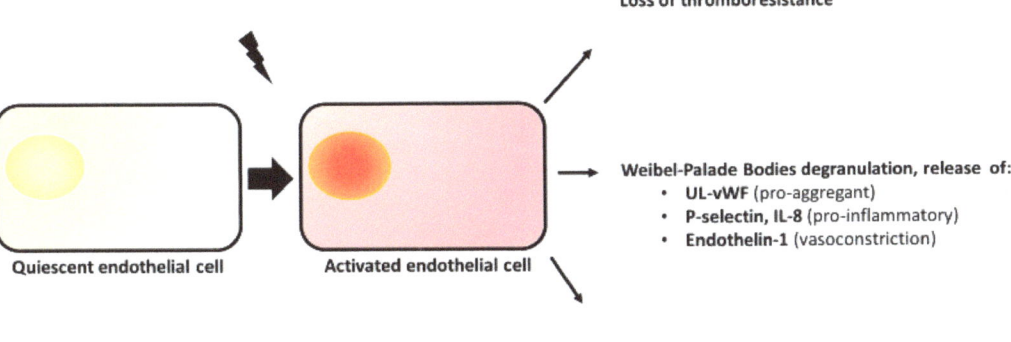

Figure 1. Consequences of endothelial cell activation. UL-VWF = Ultralarge von Willebrand factor; IL-8 = Interleukin-8.

Moreover, endothelial activation triggers cell vesiculation [25], leading to endothelial microvesicles (EMVs) generation and release in blood flow. These extracellular vesicles have a size ranging from 0.1 to 1 µm. EMV possess an essential role in intercellular communication. Their biogenesis occurs via the plasma membrane blebbing of ECs with whom they share common characteristic phenotypic features. EMVs have procoagulant properties because of the phosphatidylserine and TF, but they also seem to be involved in fibrinolysis with uPA or tPA [26]. They are generally pro-inflammatory and partly responsible for the dysregulation of vascular tone in endothelial dysfunction. Thus, EMVs, considered only as biomarkers for a long time, are likely to be also biologic effectors that actively participate to the endothelial activation consequences.

As pointed out by Roumenina et al. [27], ECs constitute all together a source, a barrier in well-regulated conditions and a target in pathologic conditions, for hemostasis and complement system actors. They form a "quiescent endothelium" different of the "activated endothelium" under regulated activation or in response to various stimuli. This activated endothelium can also lead to the "saturated endothelium" when ECs regulation capacity are exceeded. Then, two situations can occur: (1) the endothelial activation is too intense and it exceeds cells physiologic regulation potential (e.g., during septic shock) or (2) an acquired or innate susceptibility (e.g., ADAMTS13 deficiency) leads to disastrous repercussions: ECs are then the main target and actor of amplification loops.

A key point is that endothelial activation is a dynamic continuum between a quiescent and an activated phenotype. There is also a spatial heterogeneity of phenotypic features that would help us to distinguish between these two phenotypes [28] and a modulation of cytokines effects on ECs depending on the vascular site.

Finally, two types of endothelial activation have been usually described based on inflammatory context [29]. ECs type 1 activation typically occurs within few minutes. It does not involve gene expression modulation and is mediated by G-protein-coupled-receptors (GPCRs) leading to an intracellular calcium (Ca^{2+}) influx. ECs type 2 activation is mediated by a more sustained signal. It involves gene expression regulation. Tumor-Necrosis Factor (TNFα) and Interleukin-1 are the main mediators of this response. These signaling leads to the nuclear translocation of the transcription factor NFκB and AP-1, resulting in cytokine and chemokine production. Nevertheless, those two types of activation are mutually dependent and many crosstalk exist.

2.3. Weibel–Palade Bodies

Weibel–Palade Bodies (WPBs) are endothelial-specific storage organelles and their composition is closely linked to the physiological regulatory functions of the endothelium [30]. These cigar-shaped granules come from the Golgi apparatus. Their biogenesis is complex and is not fully understood but seems to depend on VWF multimerization process [31]. WPBs contain UL-VWF, which has a major role in hemostatic function. They also contain P-selectin, an important leukocyte adhesion molecule, Interleukin-8 (cytokine), eotaxin-3 (chemokine), Endothelin-1 (vasoconstrictor) and Angiopoietin-2 involved in angiogenesis. Other molecules have been identified in CWP, such as the Complement Factor H, Osteoprotegerin, t-PA, etc. However, this list is not exhaustive because of the spatial and temporal WPB heterogeneity similar to the ECs heterogeneity previously described [30–32].

The endothelial activation leads to WPBs fusion with the apical plasma membrane and the subsequent release of their content in the blood circulation. Two different pathways of WPB agonists-induced degranulation are described [32]:

- The Ca^{2+}-mediated pathway: agonists, such as thrombin and histamine activate G_qPCRs and G_iPCRs, leading to the activation of phospholipase Cβ and the formation of inositol triphosphate (IP3). The fixation of IP3 on the endoplasmic reticulum membrane IP-3 receptor generates a Ca^{2+} intracellular influx which triggers the degranulation of the cortical pool of WPBs. It also increases vascular permeability involving VE-Cadherin phosphorylation and myosin light-chain phosphorylation and participates in the vesiculation process [33].
- The cAMP-mediated pathway (cyclic adenosine monophosphate): other agonists, such as epinephrine and serotonin activate G_sPCRs, inducing an increase in cAMP intracellular level. This results in the activation of the PKA (protein kinase A) that triggers a lower degranulation of WPB microtubular pool. In contrast to the Ca^{2+}-mediated pathway, cAMP-mediated pathway is associated with a decrease in vascular permeability.

2.4. From Endothelial Activation to Endothelial Dysfunction

The endothelial activation is a well-regulated physiological stress-response. Nevertheless, it may have adverse impacts when it becomes chronic or uncontrolled. Indeed, the chronic EC activation leads to endothelial dysfunction affecting vascular tone, hemostasis, and inflammation. The term of endothelial dysfunction was initially used in the context of atherosclerosis [34,35], to describe the impaired NO-dependent vasodilatation to various biomechanical or chemical stimuli, such as an increase in blood flow or acetylcholine. However, a chronic EC activation also leads to an impaired regulation of other functions, resulting in a prothrombotic and pro-inflammatory phenotype. Chronic endothelial dysfunction involves a reduction in NO bioavailability and an oxidative stress which takes part in eNOS (endothelial NO-synthase) uncoupling. Disturbed flow can actively participate in endothelial dysfunction, inducing epigenetic modification in ECs [36,37]. Endothelial dysfunction is also associated with a greater endothelial senescence and apoptosis and it is a marker, and, most probably, also an actor of the global cardiovascular risk.

3. Evidence for Endothelial Activation in TTP

One of the key features of TTP pathogenesis is UL-VWF accumulation. The endothelial activation leads to UL-VWF massive release through CWPs degranulation. This phenomenon is supposed to be the trigger for TTP crisis when occurring in an ADAMTS13 deficiency context. In this part, we discuss clinical and experimental data that support or contradict this hypothesis.

3.1. Clinical Points

Patients with not treated hereditary TTP have a null or very low ADAMTS13 activity from birth. However, the first TTP crisis can occur at adulthood, especially during pregnancy [8,38,39]. Similarly, patients with i-TTP may have a very low ADAMTS13 activity (<5%) without displaying biological or clinical features of TMA [40,41]. These data suggest that ADAMTS13 deficiency is a necessary but not sufficient condition to induce TTP. Furthermore, an infectious episode is frequently reported few weeks before the crisis supporting the hypothesis of an environmental triggering factor.

3.2. Endothelial Exploration in Humans in TTP

Measurements of ECs activation degrees are possible by various in vitro studies, such as morphologic analysis, phenotypic markers analysis or functional tests. However, in clinical practice, evaluation of ECs activation degree is not easy. Nevertheless, some investigative methods exist soluble and cellular biomarkers analysis and histological studies.

Biomarkers analysis is a systemic approach of endothelial activation in clinical practice [42–44]. Classically plasmatic biomarkers analyzed are hemostatic biomarkers (soluble TM, soluble TF, VWF, t-PA and PAI-1), cytokines and soluble forms of adhesion proteins, such as VCAM, ICAM, E-selectin and P-selectin. High levels of soluble biomarkers of endothelial injury during the acute phase of TTP has been highlighted for a long time. Takahashi et al. reported in 1991 that plasmatic TM concentration was higher in TTP patients compared to healthy subjects, and decreased during remission [45]. Moreover, Mori et al. reported that plasmatic TM was associated with mortality in TTP patients, suggesting that TM plasmatic level could constitute a prognosis factor [46]. Soluble P-selectin [47,48], soluble t-PA [49], soluble PAI-1 and VWF:Ag (VWF antigen) have been proposed as EC activation markers in TTP patients plasma. Soluble P-selectin is also correlated to usual markers of TTP activity (platelet and LDH levels) [50]. Some authors support that endothelial activation leads to a procoagulant state [51] without high fibrinolysis level [52]. This idea is based on hemostatic parameters, such as sTFPI/sTF ratio, t-PA and PAI-1 analysis, although t-PA data differ between studies [49,52]. These parameters seem today obsolete in TTP context and their relevance questionable. Indeed, platelet-rich and fibrin-poor thrombi are the hallmark of the disease [53], suggesting a modest involvement of the coagulation system in TTP. Some data suggest that fibrinolytic system induced by ECs hypoxia may be a bypass pathway for VWF multimers cleavage [54]. Then, an alteration of ECs fibrinolytic potential has been proposed as a critical event for TTP crisis [55]. Van Mourik et al. proposed to analyze the VWF:Ag/VWF-propeptide ratio to distinguish between an acute or a chronic endothelial activation [56]. Indeed, the secretions of VWF:Ag and its propeptide are equimolar but their half-life are different: the propeptide is cleared from the circulation five times faster than the VWF:Ag. However, this ratio may be difficult to interpret in the TTP context: the ADAMTS13 deficiency modifies the half-life of VWF and the TPE provides de novo ADAMTS13. Furthermore, the dynamics for reconstitution of WPBs is not fully understood and a high level of circulating UL-VWF is not associated with TTP crisis [57]. The clinical relevance of these parameters is nowadays questionable [43].

Cellular biomarkers have been developed more recently. As mentioned, ECs activation and dysfunction are associated with EMVs production, but also with the detachment of ECs from the basal membrane. This results in generation of circulating endothelial cells (CEC). EMVs and CECs levels, which reflect endothelial injury, have been associated with an increase in global cardiovascular risk and may be poor prognosis factors for many diseases [25,44]. In addition to being biomarkers, they probably actively participate in vascular damage through vectorization of deleterious signals. Jimenez et al. were the first to document EMVs in TTP. They demonstrated that TTP plasmas induced a procoagulant EMVs generation from cultured brain and renal microvascular ECs (MVECs) [58]. They also shown elevated concentrations of EMVs in TTP patients during acute phase normalized during remission [59], shortly before LDH and platelet normalization. On the other hand, CEC were identified in 1993 in a TTP patient [60] and this was confirmed by Widemann et al. in a prospective multicentric study on 22 patients: CECs were elevated during acute phase of the TTP and normalized during remission and high CEC level at diagnosis was associated with clinical severity [50].

Biopsies with morphologic analysis and immuno-histological investigations of endothelium are rarely practiced. The procedure is invasive, and the subsequent analysis remains focal. However, histological features of endothelial lesions are frequently observed in other thrombotic microangiopathies, especially on renal biopsy. Above-mentioned data support that endothelial activation occurs in TTP and may be a prognosis factor. However, it remains to determine if ECs activation is a cause or a consequence of thrombi formation. Dang et al. provide responses elements [61]: they analyzed 8 spleens from TTP patients and highlighted thrombi and EC apoptosis overexpressed Fas as compared to control spleens. Interestingly, many apoptotic cells did not colocalize with thrombi, suggesting that ECs apoptosis precedes thrombi formation. However, as noticed by Jimenez [62], a percentage of ECs apoptosis should be interpreted with analysis of EC activation degree as Fas is also an ECs activation marker through NFκB pathway.

3.3. In Vitro Experimental Data

In 1982, Burns et al. reported that serum from TTP patients induced endothelial lesions in vitro as compared to serum from healthy volunteers [63]. They highlighted a pathogenic effect of the IgG fraction that fixed HUVECs (Human Umbilical Vein ECs) and induced ultrastructural lesions. Many other studies subsequently demonstrated a pathogenic effect of TTP plasmas on ECs. Laurence et al. reported the pro-apoptotic effect of 4 TTP plasmas on microvascular ECs, but not on macrovascular ECs. One of which was associated with HIV infection. This was not observed with plasmas from patients with disseminated intravascular coagulation or from asymptomatic HIV patients [64]. This pro-apoptotic effect seemed to be Fas-mediated and independent from TNFα or CD36 pathway. Mitra et al. then showed that this pro-apoptotic effect was induced with plasma from acute TTP patients, but not with plasma from patients in remission and only in restricted lineage of microvascular ECs [65]. Thus, Human Microvascular Endothelial Cells (HMVECs) from hepatic and pulmonary lineage were not affected, liver and lung being interestingly generally spared during TTP crisis. Jimenez et al. highlighted a mainly activator effect of TTP plasma on HMVECs, without a clear pro-apoptotic effect, based on phenotypic features of EMVs generated [59]. They also showed that EMVs generated in vitro carried VWF and induced platelet aggregation [66]. Discordances between these studies may be at least partly explained by the use of different experimental methods [62,67]. Finally, our team recently showed that plasmas from acute TTP patients induced a calcium and IgG WPB degranulation in vitro with a strong correlation with the pathology severity [68].

3.4. In Vivo Experimental Data

Motto et al. were the first to generate a TTP mice model, knocking-out ADAMTS13 gene on a mixed strain C57BL6/J–128X1/SvJ background [69]. Despite the loose of ADAMTS13 activity, mice did not present any clinical or biological TMA feature. These results were confirmed by Banno et al. [70]. Then, the mice were backcrossed on the CASA/Rk background which confers higher VWF levels. Consequently, a prothrombotic state was observed, with mild thrombocytopenia and a survey slightly decreased. TTP was finally induced through intravenous Shigatoxin administration. Shigatoxin is a bacterial toxin mainly produced by certain strains of Escherichia Coli and responsible for typical

Hemolytic and Uremic Syndrome (HUS), another TMA that principally affects the kidney. Shigatoxin exists on two isoforms and is composed of two subunits: the A-subunit induces a ribotoxic stress leading to EC death and the B-subunit induces the WPBs degranulation. This B-subunit is sufficient alone to induce TTP in this model [71]. Interestingly, double knock-out mice for ADAMTS13 and for VWF were protected from shigatoxin deleterious action [72], confirming that UL-VWF release is a key point of pathophysiology of TTP.

Feys et al. developed a TTP baboon model [73]. Authors generated murine blocking monoclonal antibodies (mAb) against human recombinant ADAMTS13. They injected this mAb to 6 healthy baboons. ADAMTS13 activity was lost and biological and histological features of TTP present, without clinical repercussion. Authors concluded that, contrary to observations in the mice model, an additional trigger was not necessary to induce TTP in baboons. The differences observed between the mice and the baboon models could be related to supplying protease in mice, such as plasmin, enough in case of isolated ADAMTS13 deficiency, but exceeded in case of massive endothelial activation. Nevertheless, ECs activation was not assessed in the baboon model and a direct effect of anti-ADAMTS13 antibodies on endothelial cells could not be excluded [74].

Le Besnerais et al. examined endothelial injury in another model of TTP, in which PTT was induced with administration of recombinant VWF, including UL-VWF, in ADAMTS13-deficient mice [74]. A systolic dysfunction was highlighted with a decrease in myocardial perfusion on magnetic resonance imaging, associated with an alteration of NO-mediated relaxation response in coronary and mesenteric arteries. These results reflected early endothelial dysfunction. Cardiac ECs presented a globally proadhesive state with overexpression of VCAM and E-Selectin and a pro-oxidative state.

Recently, Zheng et al. generated ADAMTS13 −/− zebrafish which exhibited spontaneously a mild thrombocytopenia with increased fragmentation of red blood cells and presented a prothrombotic state [75]. TTP was induced through a Lysine-rich histones injection, known to be WPBs calcium-dependent degranulation inducers [76]. Thrombocytopenia was more severe and microvascular VWF-rich microthrombi in the ADAMTS13 −/− zebrafish group more present compared to the wild type group. However, the Kaplan-Meyer survival analysis indicated a 2 week mortality rate after the histone challenge around 25% in the ADAMTS13 −/− group, which corresponds to a TTP model much less severe than in humans. The prothrombotic features (spontaneous or histones induced) of ADAMTS13 −/− zebrafish were—as expected—completely rescued in case of double knock out ADAMTS13 −/− and VWF −/−.

Other TTP rodent models have been developed, especially some auto-immune models [77–79]. In all of those, TTP induction needed recombinant VWF or Shigatoxin administration.

4. What Are the Suspected Triggers for the Second Hit Hypothesis?

Pregnancy is a common trigger of TTP crisis [80,81]. As mentioned above, patients with congenital ADAMTS13 deficiency may be asymptomatic and, thus, undiagnosed for decades until a first TTP crisis. Pregnancy is associated with an ad hoc prothrombotic state, linked to an increase in coagulation factors, circulating VWF levels and a concomitant low decrease in ADAMTS13 activity [82–84]. These additional variations may precipitate the TTP crisis.

Infections have often been suspected to be EC activation triggers in TMA disorders. Indeed, a flu-like episode is frequently reported during prodromes. In the literature, many cases reported TTP crisis occurring subsequently to infections, especially viral [85,86]. A prospective study conducted by the French Reference Center for Thrombotic Microangiopathies highlighted an infectious event within 2 weeks before the diagnosis in 41% of the 280 patients [87]. Different mechanisms may establish the link between the infectious process and TTP crisis:

- Some viruses, such as the Cytomegalovirus (CMV), have a tropism for ECs and can directly activate them [88].

- The cytokines secreted in response to the infectious process, especially γ-interferon, TNFα and Interleukin-8, may act as CWP degranulation inductors [89]. Type 1 interferons (α and β) may induce TMA, as shown in a murine model [90]. Furthermore, γ-interferon and TNFα are cytokines that downregulate *Adamts13* gene expression in the liver [91].
- TLR-9 (Toll-like receptor-9) is a molecule belonging to innate immunity expressed on neutrophils and ECs which recognizes DNA present in bacteria and viruses. TLR-9 polymorphisms have been suspected to be a genetic risk factor of TTP crisis [87].

In addition, HIV can lead to two distinct TMA [92]. HIV infection at the AIDS stage may induce a non-specific TMA with ADAMTS13 activity > 5%. This TMA has a very poor prognosis and may be mediated by angio-invasive infections in the context of major immunosuppression. However, HIV can also lead to i-TTP, with a better prognosis. Presence of p24 antigen in ECs from bone marrow has been reported in one patient [93], but this case seems isolated and pathogenesis of HIV-induced i-TTP is globally unknown.

Finally, many cases of TTP following COVID-19 have been reported [94]. SARS-CoV-2 is now well known as an endothelial activator [95] and may therefore precipitate TTP in susceptible individuals. ACE2, the main receptor of SARS-CoV-2, has been identified on endothelial cells, but other receptors also seem involved in viral entry (neuropilin 1, CD147) [96]. Viral entry in endothelial cells would even not be necessary, indeed Lei et al. described that proteins S and N would be sufficient to cause endothelial dysfunction [97]. Furthermore, endothelial damages in COVID-19 are also secondary to infection of neighboring cells and of hyper-inflammatory syndrome [98].

Many drugs have been incriminated for the development of TMA, such as calcineurin inhibitors, mitomycin, gemcitabine, anti-VEGF agents and quinine [8]. Generally, these drug-induced TMA are not associated with a profound ADAMTS13 activity deficiency. Many mechanisms are suspected and they overall involve ECs aggression, inducing an activated phenotype of ECs. For example, calcineurin inhibitors induce a prothrombotic and proinflammatory state with a decrease in NO and PGI2 production and an increase in endothelin-1 and thromboxane A2 synthesis [19]. Ticlopidine (a thienopyridine platelet-antagonist) seems to be an exception, as it induces TTP within 2 to 12 weeks after introduction of the drug [99]. Today, pathogenesis of this induced auto-immunity is very uncertain. Interestingly, Mauro et al. showed that pharmacological doses of ticlopidine induced in vitro EC apoptosis with the same restricted lineage affected as discussed above: macrovascular ECs and hepatic and pulmonary microvascular ECs were spared from this pro-apoptotic response. This study relied ticlopidine induced in vitro EC apoptosis to an alteration of ECs interaction with subendothelial matrix [100].

As previously mentioned, IgG fraction has been incriminated for long to explain endothelial aggression occurring in TTP. The mechanisms involved in auto-immunity in TTP remains unknown. The loss of tolerance to ADAMTS13 may be linked to a genetic predisposition involving the major histocompatibility complex class II (HLA DRB1*04 as protective and HLA DRB1*11 and DQB1*03 as predisposing) [101,102]. Interestingly, peptides from CUB2 domain of ADAMTS13 were presented on HLA DRB1*11 [103] and there is some evidence of involvement of CUB2 domain-reactive CD4+ T Cells in i-TTP [104]. Many studies highlighted the presence of antibodies against ECs (AECA) in plasmas of TTP patients. These antibodies have the property to induce CWP degranulation in vitro [105]. Even if the targeted epitope is not always known, two studies reported a significant proportion of TTP patients with anti-CD36 antibodies [106,107]. CD36 is an antigen present on microvascular ECs but not on macrovascular ECs. In 2000, Praprotnik et al. proposed a pathophysiology including two auto-immune hits: AECA would activate microvascular ECs, inducing a massive UL-VWF release, that, therefore, accumulate into microcirculation because of the immune-mediated ADAMTS13 deficiency [105]. Nevertheless, the proportion of patients with AECA is a controversial issue and a significant part of these antibodies are thought to target the major histocompatibility complex (MHC) [108]. Indeed, in allogeneic kidney transplantation, donor specific antibodies may induce ECs aggression, leading to acute or chronic humoral graft rejection with TMA histologic features [109]. Moreover, Ren et al. showed that administration of xenogeneic AECA to rats led to dose-dependent and complement-mediated TMA features [110]. We also demonstrated a potential role of ADAMTS13 antibodies: anti-ADAMTS13 monoclonal antibodies purified from iTTP patients B cells induced an ECs activation calcium dependent leading to a degranulation of WPBs [68].

Surgery or endovascular procedures have been described as trigger of TTP [111]. Endothelial activators (alpha-thrombin, nucleosomes, reactive oxygen species, etc.) generation during ischemia-reperfusion could lead to endothelial cell activation with vWF release [112].

Recently, TMA were observed after a snake bite in Sri Lanka, especially by *Hypnale hypnale*, as known as the hump-nosed viper [113]. Venom analysis highlights the presence of phospholipase A2, serine-proteases, metalloproteinases and of thrombin-like enzyme [114,115]. Effects of these venoms on ECs may be an interesting track to explore.

5. Amplification Loops of Endothelial Aggression

TTP is characterized by ADAMTS13 deficiency and the accumulation of UL-VWF following endothelial activation. This leads to the involvement of other actors that maintain and aggravate endothelial damage leading to a "saturated endothelium" stage. These amplification loops involve the alternative complement pathway, hemolysis and nucleosomes and are shown in Figure 2.

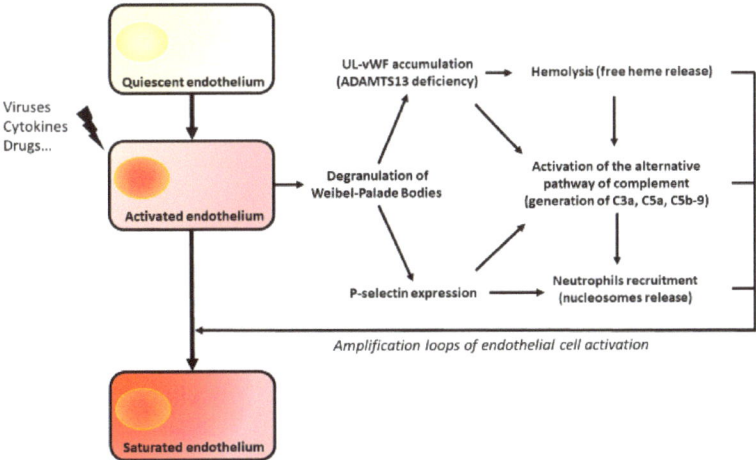

Figure 2. During PTT crisis, endothelium is the target of amplifications loops involving hemolysis, complement system and nucleosome UL-vWF = Ultralarge von Willebrand factor.

5.1. The Complement System

The complement system is an archaic defense system belonging to innate immunity. It is composed of a large number of proteins acting through a highly regulated cascade activation [116]. Complement activation leads to three main consequences: (i) pathogen agents' lysis through the action of C5b9, the membrane attack complex; (ii) apoptotic cells clearance through opsonization by C3b; and (iii) amplification of inflammatory response, through the action of C3a and C5a anaphylatoxins. The activation cascade can be initiated through a classical, lectin or alternative pathway. These pathways converge in a common terminal effector, the C5b9. The alternative pathway of the complement (APC) is characterized by a permanent low activation degree through spontaneous C3 hydrolysis. It needs to be regulated by soluble inhibitors, such as complement factor H and factor I, respectively, CFH and CFI and membranous inhibitors, such as Membranous Cofactor.

The complement system is involved in many thrombotic microangiopathies. Atypical HUS is a TMA affecting mainly kidneys and is a well-known "complementopathy" model [117]. Up to 60% of patients have an identified anomaly affecting APC: mutations leading to a loss of function affecting regulators (CFH, CFI, MCP and others) or an inhibitory antibody against CFH; mutations leading to a gain of function affecting activators C3 and Complement Factor B (CFB). This dysregulated activation of APC leads to ECs aggression, especially in the presence of an additional trigger, such as glycocalyx alteration or free heme release. This induces a strongly pro-thrombotic and pro-inflammatory endothelial phenotype with microthrombi formation, especially in glomerular endothelium. Eculizumab is a monoclonal antibody against the C5 fraction of complement targeting the common terminal pathway. It has dramatically improved outcomes of complement-mediated HUS. Other data support the complement involvement in pathogenesis of typical HUS [118,119], preeclampsia [120] and allogeneic hematopoietic stem-cell transplantation (HSCT) [121–123] related TMA. Thus, complement involvement in TTP pathogenesis has been supposed.

Many studies highlighted complement activation in TTP by indirect signs. C3a, C5a and soluble C5b9 are markedly elevated during acute phase and normalized during remission [124,125]. High levels of these markers are associated with poor outcome [126]. In accordance with these data, therapeutic plasma exchanges strongly decrease these markers even if their level are probably lower than in atypical HUS [127]. Only the APC seems to be involved in TTP. Indeed, Tati et al. have identified C3 and C5b9 in renal cortex of TTP patients and have highlighted that TTP plasma induced release of C3- and C9-coated EMVs in vitro [128]. Furthermore, Mikes et al. report a statistic correlation between the alternative pathway C3 convertase and endothelial degranulation, which was measured by carboxyterminal pro-endothelin-1 [129]. However, a causal link between APC activation and endothelial degranulation could not be establish because of the multitude of confounding factors, i.e., factors causally linked to APC and to ECs.

Moreover, UL-VWF is a platform for activation of the alternative pathway of complement. Tati et al. showed that administration of Shigatoxin to mice led to glomerular damage and C3 deposit only if mice were KO ADAMTS13 −/− [128]. Bettoni et al. showed that plasmas from hereditary TTP patients in acute phase induced C3 and C5b9 but not C4 deposits on HMVECs with comparable intensity of induced atypical HUS plasma deposits [125]. Remarkably, there were no more complement deposit with the adjunction of recombinant ADAMTS13. Yet, ADAMTS13 had no intrinsic inhibitory action on the alternative pathway C3 convertase formation. Turner et al. highlighted colocalization between APC components, especially C3, and UL-VWF. Thereafter, Bettoni et al. demonstrated a direct interaction between C3b and the A2 domain of VWF, leading to AP-C3/C5 convertase and C5b9 formation [125,130]. They also showed in vitro that the thrombus formation induced by TTP plasmas was corrected by restoring ADAMTS13 activity but also by complement inhibition. UL-VWF lose the ability of "normal" VWF multimers to act as cofactor of CFI, therefore losing the role of APC regulator [131]. Bettoni et al. proposed a mechanistic overview: during TTP crisis, UL-VWF pile up on the endothelial cell surface and act as platform for activation of the APC, leading to C5a and C5b9 formation that induce WPB degranulation resulting in an amplification loop. Furthermore, C5a induces shedding of TM, which downregulates coagulation cascade and indirectly inactivates C3b, as a cofactor of CFH and CFI, C3a and C5a, as a cofactor of the thrombin-activatable fibrinolysis inhibitor [27].

Recently, Zheng et al. demonstrated in a mice model that ADAMTS13 genetic deficiency had synergistic effect with APC over-activation resulting from heterozygous mutation of CFH, leading to severe TMA. Each of these genetic defects were asymptomatic when isolated [132].

P-selectin is another compound of WPBs and is expressed on activated ECs. It is a platelet and leukocyte adhesion molecule and may also serve as a platform for APC activation [133]. Thus, P-selectin may act as an amplification loop through different ways.

P-selectin interacts with C3b [27,134], leading to the formation of C3a, C5a and C5b9 and the endothelial activation [135,136]. Furthermore, P-selectin participates to neutrophils recruitment, which are more cytotoxic during TTP crisis and seem to induce a complement-dependent loss of thromboresistance in vitro [137]. Finally, P-selectin is also expressed on activated platelets, which may also act as a platform for APC activation [138].

Nevertheless, Eculizumab has exceptionally been used in TTP. One case reported a very rare overlap syndrome: the patient had auto-antibodies against ADAMTS13 and against CFH [139,140]; one case was a hereditary TTP [141]; two recent cases were i-TTP with heterozygous variants of CFH, CFI and C3 [142]. These few observations do not allow us to conclude on the interest of Eculizumab in TTP.

5.2. Hemolysis

Intravascular hemolysis has been for long suspected to act as an amplification loop of ECs activation in TMA. Hemoglobin released induces NO consumption and produces reactive oxygen species [143], leading to endothelial dysfunction and CWP degranulation [144,145]. Hemoglobin also participates to decrease ADAMTS13 activity [146]. Furthermore, free heme has been suspected to be a critical event leading to atypical HUS when occurring on a deleterious underlying condition. Free heme induces (i) WPB degranulation in a TLR4-dependant manner [147], (ii) APC activation on ECs and (iii) APC activation in the fluid phase through facilitation of C3-C3 homophilic interaction [148,149]. We have recently shown high levels of plasmatic free heme in TTP patients. Furthermore, ECs treatment with hemopexin mildly decreased calcium influx and WPB degranulation in vitro, which supports a modest amplification role of free heme [68].

5.3. Nucleosomes

In response to inflammatory or infectious stimuli, neutrophils can release Neutrophils Extracellular Traps (NETs), composed of nucleosomes (DNA and histone) and of proteins, such as myeloperoxidase (MPO), neutrophil-elastase and cathepsin G. NETs have anti-infectious properties as they are "trapping" bacteria [150]. However, they also seem to have prothrombotic properties [151]. Furthermore, histones can induce consumptive thrombocytopenia in mice [152]. In 2012, Fuchs et al. showed that in patient with TMA disorders, high levels of circulating DNA and MPO were associated with low platelet counts and a low ADAMTS13 activity. These markers normalized during remission [153]. Moreover, nucleosomes are incriminated for endothelial activation in typical HUS and in allogeneic HSCT related TMA [154,155]. In this context, interleukin-8 released from endothelium may induce NETs production, which act as platform for APC [156]. As discussed above, Lysine-rich histones are used to trigger TTP in a zebrafish model. This suggests a potent mechanistic link between inflammation and TTP crisis. Moreover, Michels et al. have shown that Lysine-rich histones may act as WPB degranulation inducers by a Ca^{2+}-, caspase- and charge-dependent mechanism [76]. Furthermore, ischemic damages can also lead to DNA and histones release [157], therefore acting as another prothrombotic amplification loop. Our team recently confirmed high levels of nucleosomes in plasma from acute TTP patients and a participation of these nucleosomes in iTTP patient's plasma ECs activation [68].

6. Conclusions

Currently, we admit that chronic endothelial activation leads to major endothelium dysfunctions implying deregulation of hemostasis, inflammation and vascular tone. Similarly, in some circumstances, such as TMA, an acute endothelial activation can also have deleterious consequences. However, in some circumstances, such as TMA, an acute endothelial activation can also lead to deleterious consequences. We suggest that in TTP, endogenous factors, such as antibodies, cytokines, heme, histones or exogenous factors, such as virus, drug or toxin, induce an endothelial activation affecting mainly microvascular cells. This leads to a Ca^{2+}-dependent WPB degranulation, resulting in UL-VWF accumulation in the microcirculation. These events may be cumulative and may be associated with amplification loops, to reach an activation level such as balance is disrupted and TMA occurs. P-selectin expression is a consequence of ECs activation, and may be a key point of pathogenesis because UL-VWF are thought to be anchored on ECs through it [158]. EMVs may also participate of amplification and systematization of the TMA process.

Despite recent therapeutic advances, mortality and morbidity during TTP remain major concerns. We have exposed clinical and experimental data supporting the "second hit hypothesis". Furthermore, endothelium is strategically located between blood and tissues and, therefore, preferentially accessible to drugs. Its plasticity may be an interesting feature for pharmacological modulation, making endothelial cells an attractive therapeutic target [159]. Thus, we think that there is a rational basis to pharmacologically inhibit endothelial cell activation. This would be a new therapeutic axis.

Funding: This research received no external funding.

Institutional Review Board Statement: Not applicable.

Informed Consent Statement: Not applicable.

Data Availability Statement: Not applicable.

Conflicts of Interest: The authors declare no conflict of interest.

References

1. George, J.N.; Nester, C.M. Syndromes of Thrombotic Microangiopathy. *N. Engl. J. Med.* **2014**, *371*, 654–666. [CrossRef] [PubMed]
2. Moake, J.L.; Rudy, C.K.; Troll, J.H.; Weinstein, M.J.; Colannino, N.M.; Azocar, J.; Seder, R.H.; Hong, S.L.; Deykin, D. Unusually Large Plasma Factor VIII: Von Willebrand Factor Multimers in Chronic Relapsing Thrombotic Thrombocytopenic Purpura. *N. Engl. J. Med.* **1982**, *307*, 1432–1435. [CrossRef] [PubMed]
3. Fujikawa, K.; Suzuki, H.; McMullen, B.; Chung, D. Purification of human von Willebrand factor–cleaving protease and its identification as a new member of the metalloproteinase family. *Blood* **2001**, *98*, 1662–1666. [CrossRef] [PubMed]
4. Zheng, X.; Chung, D.; Takayama, T.K.; Majerus, E.M.; Sadler, J.E.; Fujikawa, K. Structure of von Willebrand Factor-cleaving Protease (ADAMTS13), a Metalloprotease Involved in Thrombotic Thrombocytopenic Purpura. *J. Biol. Chem.* **2001**, *276*, 41059–41063. [CrossRef] [PubMed]
5. Lotta, L.A.; Garagiola, I.; Palla, R.; Cairo, A.; Peyvandi, F. ADAMTS13 mutations and polymorphisms in congenital thrombotic thrombocytopenic purpura. *Hum. Mutat.* **2010**, *31*, 11–19. [CrossRef] [PubMed]
6. Tsai, H.-M.; Lian, E.C.-Y. Antibodies to von Willebrand Factor–Cleaving Protease in Acute Thrombotic Thrombocytopenic Purpura. *N. Engl. J. Med.* **1998**, *339*, 1585–1594. [CrossRef] [PubMed]
7. Scully, M.; Yarranton, H.; Liesner, R.; Cavenagh, J.; Hunt, B.; Benjamin, S.; Bevan, D.; Mackie, I.; Machin, S. Regional UK TTP Registry: Correlation with laboratory ADAMTS 13 analysis and clinical features. *Br. J. Haematol.* **2008**, *142*, 819–826. [CrossRef]
8. Kremer Hovinga, J.A.; Coppo, P.; Lämmle, B.; Moake, J.L.; Miyata, T.; Vanhoorelbeke, K. Thrombotic thrombocytopenic purpura. *Nat. Rev. Dis. Prim.* **2017**, *3*, 17020. [CrossRef]
9. Reeves, H.M.; Maitta, R.W. Comparison of absolute immature platelet count to the PLASMIC score at presentation in predicting ADAMTS13 deficiency in suspected thrombotic thrombocytopenic purpura. *Thromb. Res.* **2022**, *215*, 30–36. [CrossRef]
10. Zhu, M.-L.; Reeves, H.M.; Maitta, R.W. Immature platelet dynamics correlate with ADAMTS13 deficiency and predict therapy response in immune-mediated thrombotic thrombocytopenic purpura. *Thromb. Res.* **2021**, *198*, 72–78. [CrossRef]
11. George, J.N. How I treat patients with thrombotic thrombocytopenic purpura: 2010. *Blood* **2010**, *116*, 4060–4069. [CrossRef] [PubMed]
12. Coppo, P. Treatment of autoimmune thrombotic thrombocytopenic purpura in the more severe forms. *Transfus. Apher. Sci.* **2017**, *56*, 52–56. [CrossRef] [PubMed]
13. Peyvandi, F.; Scully, M.; Kremer Hovinga, J.A.; Cataland, S.; Knöbl, P.; Wu, H.; Artoni, A.; Westwood, J.-P.; Mansouri Taleghani, M.; Jilma, B.; et al. Caplacizumab for Acquired Thrombotic Thrombocytopenic Purpura. *N. Engl. J. Med.* **2016**, *374*, 511–522. [CrossRef] [PubMed]
14. Scully, M.; Cataland, S.R.; Peyvandi, F.; Coppo, P.; Knöbl, P.; Kremer Hovinga, J.A.; Zeldin, R.K. Caplacizumab Treatment for Acquired Thrombotic Thrombocytopenic Purpura. *N. Engl. J. Med.* **2019**, *380*, 335–346. [CrossRef] [PubMed]
15. Poullin, P.; Bornet, C.; Veyradier, A.; Coppo, P. Caplacizumab to treat immune-mediated thrombotic thrombocytopenic purpura. *Drugs Today* **2019**, *55*, 367–376. [CrossRef] [PubMed]
16. Deford, C.C.; Reese, J.A.; Schwartz, L.H.; Perdue, J.J.; Kremer Hovinga, J.A.; Lämmle, B.; George, J.N. Multiple major morbidities and increased mortality during long-term follow-up after recovery from thrombotic thrombocytopenic purpura. *Blood* **2013**, *122*, 2023–2029. [CrossRef]

17. Kremer Hovinga, J.A.; Vesely, S.K.; Terrell, D.R.; Lämmle, B.; George, J.N. Survival and relapse in patients with thrombotic thrombocytopenic purpura. *Blood* **2010**, *115*, 1500–1511. [CrossRef] [PubMed]
18. Ruggenenti, P.; Noris, M.; Remuzzi, G. Thrombotic microangiopathy, hemolytic uremic syndrome, and thrombotic thrombocytopenic purpura. *Kidney Int.* **2001**, *60*, 831–846. [CrossRef] [PubMed]
19. Goldberg, R.J.; Nakagawa, T.; Johnson, R.J.; Thurman, J.M. The Role of Endothelial Cell Injury in Thrombotic Microangiopathy. *Am. J. Kidney Dis.* **2010**, *56*, 1168–1174. [CrossRef]
20. Tsai, H.M. Thrombotic Thrombocytopenic Purpura and the Hemolytic-Uremic Syndrome. In *Platelets*; Elsevier: Amsterdam, The Netherlands, 2013; pp. 883–907. Available online: https://linkinghub.elsevier.com/retrieve/pii/B9780123878373000432 (accessed on 2 August 2019).
21. Jaffe, E.A. Cell biology of endothelial cells. *Hum. Pathol.* **1987**, *18*, 234–239. [CrossRef] [PubMed]
22. Aird, W.C. Phenotypic heterogeneity of the endothelium: I. Structure, function, and mechanisms. *Circ. Res.* **2007**, *100*, 158–173. [CrossRef] [PubMed]
23. Aird, W.C. Phenotypic heterogeneity of the endothelium: II. Representative vascular beds. *Circ. Res.* **2007**, *100*, 174–190. [CrossRef] [PubMed]
24. Sturtzel, C. Endothelial Cells. *Adv. Exp. Med. Biol.* **2017**, *1003*, 71–91. [PubMed]
25. Sabatier, F.; Camoin-Jau, L.; Anfosso, F.; Sampol, J.; Dignat-George, F. Circulating endothelial cells, microparticles and progenitors: Key players towards the definition of vascular competence. *J. Cell Mol. Med.* **2009**, *13*, 454–471. [CrossRef] [PubMed]
26. Vallier, L.; Cointe, S.; Lacroix, R.; Bonifay, A.; Judicone, C.; Dignat-George, F.; Kwaan, H.C. Microparticles and Fibrinolysis. *Semin. Thromb. Hemost.* **2017**, *43*, 129–134. [CrossRef] [PubMed]
27. Roumenina, L.T.; Rayes, J.; Frimat, M.; Fremeaux-Bacchi, V. Endothelial cells: Source, barrier, and target of defensive mediators. *Immunol. Rev.* **2016**, *274*, 307–329. [CrossRef] [PubMed]
28. Pober, J.S.; Sessa, W.C. Evolving functions of endothelial cells in inflammation. *Nat. Rev. Immunol.* **2007**, *7*, 803–815. [CrossRef]
29. Pober, J.S.; Cotran, R.S. The role of endothelial cells in inflammation. *Transplantation* **1990**, *50*, 537–544. [CrossRef]
30. Lowenstein, C.J.; Morrell, C.N.; Yamakuchi, M. Regulation of Weibel–Palade Body Exocytosis. *Trends Cardiovasc. Med.* **2005**, *15*, 302–308. [CrossRef]
31. Mourik, M.; Eikenboom, J. Lifecycle of Weibel-Palade bodies. *Hamostaseologie* **2017**, *37*, 13–24. [CrossRef]
32. Rondaij, M.G.; Bierings, R.; Kragt, A.; Van Mourik, J.A.; Voorberg, J. Dynamics and Plasticity of Weibel-Palade Bodies in Endothelial Cells. *Arter. Thromb. Vasc. Biol.* **2006**, *26*, 1002–1007. [CrossRef] [PubMed]
33. Tiruppathi, C.; Minshall, R.D.; Paria, B.C.; Vogel, S.M.; Malik, A.B. Role of Ca^{2+} signaling in the regulation of endothelial permeability. *Vasc. Pharmacol.* **2002**, *39*, 173–185. [CrossRef] [PubMed]
34. Ludmer, P.L.; Selwyn, A.P.; Shook, T.L.; Wayne, R.R.; Mudge, G.H.; Alexander, R.W.; Ganz, P. Paradoxical Vasoconstriction Induced by Acetylcholine in Atherosclerotic Coronary Arteries. *N. Engl. J. Med.* **1986**, *315*, 1046–1051. [CrossRef] [PubMed]
35. Poredos, P. Endothelial dysfunction in the pathogenesis of atherosclerosis. *Int. Angiol.* **2002**, *21*, 109–116. [PubMed]
36. Endemann, D.H.; Schiffrin, E.L. Endothelial dysfunction. *J. Am. Soc. Nephrol.* **2004**, *15*, 1983–1992. [CrossRef]
37. Huynh, D.T.N.; Heo, K.-S. Therapeutic targets for endothelial dysfunction in vascular diseases. *Arch. Pharmacal Res.* **2019**, *42*, 848–861. [CrossRef]
38. Moatti-Cohen, M.; Garrec, C.; Wolf, M.; Boisseau, P.; Galicier, L.; Azoulay, E.; Stepanian, A.; Delmas, Y.; Rondeau, E.; Bezieau, S.; et al. Unexpected frequency of Upshaw-Schulman syndrome in pregnancy-onset thrombotic thrombocytopenic purpura. *Blood* **2012**, *119*, 5888–5897. [CrossRef]
39. Mariotte, E.; Azoulay, E.; Galicier, L.; Rondeau, E.; Zouiti, F.; Boisseau, P.; Poullin, P.; de Maistre, E.; Provôt, F.; Delmas, Y.; et al. Epidemiology and pathophysiology of adulthood-onset thrombotic microangiopathy with severe ADAMTS13 deficiency (thrombotic thrombocytopenic purpura): A cross-sectional analysis of the French national registry for thrombotic microangiopathy. *Lancet Haematol.* **2016**, *3*, e237–e245. [CrossRef]
40. Page, E.E.; Hovinga, J.A.K.; Terrell, D.R.; Vesely, S.K.; George, J.N. Clinical importance of ADAMTS13 activity during remission in patients with acquired thrombotic thrombocytopenic purpura. *Blood* **2016**, *128*, 2175–2178. [CrossRef]
41. George, J.N. Measuring ADAMTS13 activity in patients with suspected thrombotic thrombocytopenic purpura: When, how, and why? *Transfusion* **2015**, *55*, 11–13. [CrossRef]
42. Jourde-Chiche, N.; Fakhouri, F.; Dou, L.; Bellien, J.; Burtey, S.; Frimat, M.; Jarrot, P.-A.; Kaplanski, G.; Le Quintrec, M.; Pernin, V.; et al. Endothelium structure and function in kidney health and disease. *Nat. Rev. Nephrol.* **2019**, *15*, 87–108. [CrossRef] [PubMed]
43. Lekakis, J.; Abraham, P.; Balbarini, A.; Blann, A.; Boulanger, C.M.; Cockcroft, J.; Cosentino, F.; Deanfield, J.; Gallino, A.; Ikonomidis, I.; et al. Methods for evaluating endothelial function: A position statement from the European Society of Cardiology Working Group on Peripheral Circulation. *Eur. J. Cardiovasc. Prev. Rehabil.* **2011**, *18*, 775–789. [CrossRef] [PubMed]
44. Horstman, L.L.; Jy, W.; Jimenez, J.J.; Ahn, Y.S. Endothelial microparticles as markers of endothelial dysfunction. *Front. Biosci.* **2004**, *9*, 1118–1135. [CrossRef] [PubMed]
45. Takahashi, H.; Hanano, M.; Wada, K.; Tatewaki, W.; Niwano, H.; Shibata, A.; Tsubouchi, J.; Nakano, M.; Nakamura, T. Circulating thrombomodulin in thrombotic thrombocytopenic purpura. *Am. J. Hematol.* **1991**, *38*, 174–177. [CrossRef]

46. Mori, Y.; Wada, H.; Okugawa, Y.; Tamaki, S.; Nakasaki, T.; Watanabe, R.; Gabazza, E.C.; Nishikawa, M.; Minami, N.; Shiku, H. Increased Plasma Thrombomodulin as a Vascular Endothelial Cell Marker in Patients with Thrombotic Thrombocytopenic Purpura and Hemolytic Uremic Syndrome. *Clin. Appl. Thromb.* **2001**, *7*, 5–9. [CrossRef]
47. Chong, B.H.; Murray, B.; Berndt, M.C.; Dunlop, L.C.; Brighton, T.; Chesterman, C.N. Plasma P-selectin is increased in thrombotic consumptive platelet disorders. *Blood* **1994**, *83*, 1535–1541. [CrossRef]
48. Katayama, M.; Handa, M.; Araki, Y.; Ambo, H.; Kawai, Y.; Watanabe, K.; Ikeda, Y. Soluble P-selectin is present in normal circulation and its plasma level is elevated in patients with thrombotic thrombocytopenic purpura and haemolytic uraemic syndrome. *Br. J. Haematol.* **1993**, *84*, 702–710. [CrossRef]
49. Wada, H.; Kaneko, T.; Ohiwa, M.; Tanigawa, M.; Hayashi, T.; Tamaki, S.; Minami, N.; Deguchi, K.; Suzuki, K.; Nakano, T.; et al. Increased levels of vascular endothelial cell markers in thrombotic thrombocytopenic purpura. *Am. J. Hematol.* **1993**, *44*, 101–105. [CrossRef]
50. Widemann, A.; Pasero, C.; Arnaud, L.; Poullin, P.; Loundou, A.D.; Choukroun, G.; Sanderson, F.; Lacroix, R.; Sabatier, F.; Coppo, P.; et al. Circulating endothelial cells and progenitors as prognostic factors during autoimmune thrombotic thrombocytopenic purpura: Results of a prospective multicenter French study. *J. Thromb. Haemost.* **2014**, *12*, 1601–1609. [CrossRef]
51. Kobayashi, M.; Wada, H.; Wakita, Y.; Shimura, M.; Nakase, T.; Hiyoyama, K.; Nagaya, S.; Minami, N.; Nakano, T.; Shiku, H. Decreased plasma tissue factor pathway inhibitor levels in patients with thrombotic thrombocytopenic purpura. *Thromb. Haemost.* **1995**, *73*, 10–14.
52. Glas-Greenwalt, P.; Hall, J.M.; Panke, T.W.; Kant, K.S.; Allen, C.M.; Pollak, V.E. Fibrinolysis in health and disease: Abnormal levels of plasminogen activator, plasminogen activator inhibitor, and protein C in thrombotic thrombocytopenic purpura. *J. Lab. Clin. Med.* **1986**, *108*, 415–422. [PubMed]
53. Asada, Y.; Sumiyoshi, A.; Hayashi, T.; Suzumiya, J.; Kaketani, K. Immunohistochemistry of vascular lesion in thrombotic thrombocytopenic purpura, with special reference to factor VIII related antigen. *Thromb. Res.* **1985**, *38*, 469–479. [CrossRef] [PubMed]
54. Tersteeg, C.; de Maat, S.; De Meyer, S.F.; Smeets, M.W.; Barendrecht, A.D.; Roest, M.; Pasterkamp, G.; Fijnheer, R.; Vanhoorelbeke, K.; de Groot, P.G.; et al. Plasmin Cleavage of von Willebrand Factor as an Emergency Bypass for ADAMTS13 Deficiency in Thrombotic Microangiopathy. *Circulation* **2014**, *129*, 1320–1331. [CrossRef] [PubMed]
55. Lian, E.C.-Y. Pathogenesis of Thrombotic Thrombocytopenic Purpura: ADAMTS13 Deficiency and Beyond. *Semin. Thromb. Hemost.* **2005**, *31*, 625–632. [CrossRef] [PubMed]
56. van Mourik, J.A.; Boertjes, R.; Huisveld, I.A.; Fijnvandraat, K.; Pajkrt, D.; van Genderen, P.J.; Fijnheer, R. von Willebrand factor propeptide in vascular disorders: A tool to distinguish between acute and chronic endothelial cell perturbation. *Blood* **1999**, *94*, 179–185. [CrossRef] [PubMed]
57. Béranger, N.; Benghezal, S.; Savigny, S.; Capdenat, S.; Joly, B.S.; Coppo, P.; Stepanian, A.; Veyradier, A. Loss of von Willebrand factor high-molecular-weight multimers at acute phase is associated with detectable anti-ADAMTS13 IgG and neurological symptoms in acquired thrombotic thrombocytopenic purpura. *Thromb. Res.* **2019**, *181*, 29–35. [CrossRef]
58. Jimenez, J.J.; Jy, W.; Mauro, L.M.; Horstman, L.L.; Ahn, Y.S. Elevated endothelial microparticles in thrombotic thrombocytopenic purpura: Findings from brain and renal microvascular cell culture and patients with active disease. *Br. J. Haematol.* **2001**, *112*, 81–90. [CrossRef]
59. Jimenez, J.J.; Jy, W.; Mauro, L.M.; Horstman, L.L.; Soderland, C.; Ahn, Y.S. Endothelial microparticles released in thrombotic thrombocytopenic purpura express von Willebrand factor and markers of endothelial activation. *Br. J. Haematol.* **2003**, *123*, 896–902. [CrossRef]
60. Lefevre, P.; George, F.; Durand, J.M.; Sampol, J. Detection of Circulating Endothelial Cells in Thrombotic Thrombocytopenic Purpura. *Thromb. Haemost.* **1993**, *69*, 522. [CrossRef]
61. Dang, C.T.; Magid, M.S.; Weksler, B.; Chadburn, A.; Laurence, J. Enhanced endothelial cell apoptosis in splenic tissues of patients with thrombotic thrombocytopenic purpura. *Blood* **1999**, *93*, 1264–1270. [CrossRef]
62. Jimenez, J.J.; Jy, W.; Mauro, L.M.; Horstman, L.L.; Soderland, C.; Ahn, Y.S. Response to Laurence. *Br. J. Haematol.* **2004**, *125*, 416–417. [CrossRef]
63. Burns, E.R.; Zucker-Franklin, D. Pathologic effects of plasma from patients with thrombotic thrombocytopenic purpura on platelets and cultured vascular endothelial cells. *Blood* **1982**, *60*, 1030–1037. [CrossRef] [PubMed]
64. Laurence, J.; Mitra, D.; Steiner, M.; Staiano-Coico, L.; Jaffe, E. Plasma from patients with idiopathic and human immunodeficiency Virus-Associated thrombotic thrombocytopenic purpura induces apoptosis in microvascular endothelial cells. *Transfus. Med. Rev.* **1996**, *10*, 315. [CrossRef]
65. Mitra, D.; Jaffe, E.A.; Weksler, B.; Hajjar, K.A.; Soderland, C.; Laurence, J. Thrombotic thrombocytopenic purpura and sporadic hemolytic-uremic syndrome plasmas induce apoptosis in restricted lineages of human microvascular endothelial cells. *Blood* **1997**, *89*, 1224–1234. [CrossRef]
66. Jy, W.; Jimenez, J.J.; Mauro, L.M.; Horstman, L.L.; Cheng, P.; Ahn, E.R.; Bidot, C.J.; Ahn, Y.S. Endothelial microparticles induce formation of platelet aggregates via a von Willebrand factor/ristocetin dependent pathway, rendering them resistant to dissociation. *J. Thromb. Haemost.* **2005**, *3*, 1301–1308. [CrossRef]
67. Laurence, J. Endothelial cell activation and apoptosis in the thrombotic microangiopathies. *Br. J. Haematol.* **2004**, *125*, 415–416. [CrossRef]

68. Tellier, E.; Widemann, A.; Cauchois, R.; Faccini, J.; Lagarde, M.; Brun, M.; Kaplanski, G. Immune thrombotic thrombocytopenic purpura plasmas induce calcium- and IgG-dependent endothelial activation: Correlations with disease severity. *Haematologica* **2022**. [CrossRef]
69. Motto, D.G.; Chauhan, A.K.; Zhu, G.; Homeister, J.; Lamb, C.B.; Desch, K.C.; Zhang, W.; Tsai, H.-M.; Wagner, D.D.; Ginsburg, D. Shigatoxin triggers thrombotic thrombocytopenic purpura in genetically susceptible ADAMTS13-deficient mice. *J. Clin. Investig.* **2005**, *115*, 2752–2761. [CrossRef]
70. Banno, F.; Kokame, K.; Okuda, T.; Honda, S.; Miyata, S.; Kato, H.; Tomiyama, Y.; Miyata, T. Complete deficiency in ADAMTS13 is prothrombotic, but it alone is not sufficient to cause thrombotic thrombocytopenic purpura. *Blood* **2006**, *107*, 3161–3166. [CrossRef]
71. Huang, J.; Motto, D.G.; Bundle, D.R.; Sadler, J.E. Shiga toxin B subunits induce VWF secretion by human endothelial cells and thrombotic microangiopathy in ADAMTS13-deficient mice. *Blood* **2010**, *116*, 3653–3659. [CrossRef]
72. Chauhan, A.K.; Walsh, M.T.; Zhu, G.; Ginsburg, D.; Wagner, D.D.; Motto, D.G. The combined roles of ADAMTS13 and VWF in murine models of TTP, endotoxemia, and thrombosis. *Blood* **2008**, *111*, 3452–3457. [CrossRef] [PubMed]
73. Feys, H.B.; Liu, F.; Dong, N.; Pareyn, I.; Vauterin, S.; Vandeputte, N.; Noppe, W.; Ruan, C.; Deckmyn, H.; Vanhoorelbeke, K. ADAMTS-13 plasma level determination uncovers antigen absence in acquired thrombotic thrombocytopenic purpura and ethnic differences. *J. Thromb. Haemost.* **2006**, *4*, 955–962. [CrossRef]
74. Le Besnerais, M.; Favre, J.; Denis, C.V.; Mulder, P.; Martinet, J.; Nicol, L.; Benhamou, Y. Assessment of endothelial damage and cardiac injury in a mouse model mimicking thrombotic thrombocytopenic purpura. *J. Thromb. Haemost.* **2016**, *14*, 1917–1930. [CrossRef] [PubMed]
75. Zheng, L.; Abdelgawwad, M.S.; Di Zhang, L.X.; Wei, S.; Cao, W.; Zheng, X.L. Histone-induced thrombotic thrombocytopenic purpura in adamts13-/- zebrafish depends on von Willebrand factor. *Haematologica* **2019**, *105*, 1107. [CrossRef] [PubMed]
76. Michels, A.; Albánez, S.; Mewburn, J.; Nesbitt, K.; Gould, T.J.; Liaw, P.C.; James, P.D.; Swystun, L.L.; Lillicrap, D. Histones link inflammation and thrombosis through the induction of Weibel-Palade body exocytosis. *J. Thromb. Haemost.* **2016**, *14*, 2274–2286. [CrossRef] [PubMed]
77. Tersteeg, C.; Schiviz, A.; De Meyer, S.F.; Plaimauer, B.; Scheiflinger, F.; Rottensteiner, H.; Vanhoorelbeke, K. Potential for Recombinant ADAMTS13 as an Effective Therapy for Acquired Thrombotic Thrombocytopenic Purpura. *Arter. Thromb. Vasc. Biol.* **2015**, *35*, 2336–2342. [CrossRef]
78. Deforche, L.; Tersteeg, C.; Roose, E.; Vandenbulcke, A.; Vandeputte, N.; Pareyn, I.; De Cock, E.; Rottensteiner, H.; Deckmyn, H.; De Meyer, S.F.; et al. Generation of Anti-Murine ADAMTS13 Antibodies and Their Application in a Mouse Model for Acquired Thrombotic Thrombocytopenic Purpura. *PLoS ONE* **2016**, *11*, e0160388. [CrossRef]
79. Pickens, B.; Mao, Y.; Li, D.; Siegel, N.L.; Ponczm, M.; Cines, U.B.; Zheng, X.L. Platelet-delivered ADAMTS13 inhibits arterial thrombosis and prevents thrombotic thrombocytopenic purpura in murine models. *Blood* **2015**, *125*, 3326–3334. [CrossRef]
80. Fujimura, Y.; Matsumoto, M.; Kokame, K.; Isonishi, A.; Soejima, K.; Akiyama, N.; Tomiyama, J.; Natori, K.; Kuranishi, Y.; Imamura, Y.; et al. Pregnancy-induced thrombocytopenia and TTP, and the risk of fetal death, in Upshaw-Schulman syndrome: A series of 15 pregnancies in 9 genotyped patients. *Br. J. Haematol.* **2009**, *144*, 742–754. [CrossRef]
81. Falter, T.; Hovinga, J.A.K.; Lackner, K.; Füllemann, H.-G.; Lämmle, B.; Scharrer, I. Late onset and pregnancy-induced congenital thrombotic thrombocytopenic purpura. *Hamostaseologie* **2014**, *34*, 244–248. [CrossRef]
82. Stirling, Y.; Woolf, L.; North, W.R.; Seghatchian, M.J.; Meade, T.W. Haemostasis in normal pregnancy. *Thromb. Haemost.* **1984**, *52*, 176–182. [CrossRef] [PubMed]
83. Furlan, M.; Robles, R.; Galbusera, M.; Remuzzi, G.; Kyrle, P.A.; Brenner, B.; Krause, M.; Scharrer, I.; Aumann, V.; Mittler, U.; et al. von Willebrand Factor–Cleaving Protease in Thrombotic Thrombocytopenic Purpura and the Hemolytic–Uremic Syndrome. *N. Engl. J. Med.* **1998**, *339*, 1578–1584. [CrossRef] [PubMed]
84. George, J.N. The association of pregnancy with thrombotic thrombocytopenic purpura–hemolytic uremic syndrome. *Curr. Opin. Hematol.* **2003**, *10*, 339–344. [CrossRef] [PubMed]
85. Morioka, M.; Matsumoto, M.; Saito, M.; Kokame, K.; Miyata, T.; Fujimura, Y. A first bout of thrombotic thrombocytopenic purpura triggered by herpes simplex infection in a 45-year-old nulliparous female with Upshaw-Schulman syndrome. *Blood Transfus.* **2014**, *12* (Suppl. 1), s153–s155. [PubMed]
86. Bitzan, M.; Zieg, J. Influenza-associated thrombotic microangiopathies. *Pediatr. Nephrol.* **2018**, *33*, 2009–2025. [CrossRef] [PubMed]
87. Morgand, M.; Buffet, M.; Busson, M.; Loiseau, P.; Malot, S.; Amokrane, K.; Fortier, C.; London, J.; Bonmarchand, G.; Wynckel, A.; et al. High prevalence of infectious events in thrombotic thrombocytopenic purpura and genetic relationship with toll-like receptor 9 polymorphisms: Experience of the French Thrombotic Microangiopathies Reference Center. *Transfusion* **2014**, *54*, 389–397. [CrossRef]
88. Popović, M.; Smiljanić, K.; Dobutović, B.; Syrovets, T.; Simmet, T.; Isenović, E.R. Human cytomegalovirus infection and atherothrombosis. *J. Thromb. Thrombolysis* **2012**, *33*, 160–172. [CrossRef]
89. Bernardo, A.; Ball, C.; Nolasco, L.; Moake, J.F.; Dong, J.-F. Effects of inflammatory cytokines on the release and cleavage of the endothelial cell–derived ultralarge von Willebrand factor multimers under flow. *Blood* **2004**, *104*, 100–106. [CrossRef]
90. Kavanagh, D.; McGlasson, S.; Jury, A.; Williams, J.; Scolding, N.; Bellamy, C.; Gunther, C.; Ritchie, D.; Gale, D.; Kanwar, Y.S.; et al. Type I interferon causes thrombotic microangiopathy by a dose-dependent toxic effect on the microvasculature. *Blood* **2016**, *128*, 2824–2833. [CrossRef]

91. Cao, W.J.; Niiya, M.; Zheng, X.W.; Shang, D.Z. Inflammatory cytokines inhibit ADAMTS13 synthesis in hepatic stellate cells and endothelial cells. *J. Thromb. Haemost.* **2008**, *6*, 1233–1235. [CrossRef]
92. Malak, S.; Wolf, M.; Millot, G.A.; Mariotte, E.; Veyradier, A.; Meynard, J.-L.; Korach, J.-M.; Malot, S.; Bussel, A.; Azoulay, E.; et al. Human Immunodeficiency Virus-Associated Thrombotic Microangiopathies: Clinical Characteristics and Outcome According to ADAMTS13 Activity. *Scand. J. Immunol.* **2008**, *68*, 337–344. [CrossRef] [PubMed]
93. del Arco, A.; Martinez, M.A.; Peña, J.M.; Gamallo, C.; González, J.J.; Barbado, F.J.; Vazquez, J.J. Thrombotic thrombocytopenic purpura associated with human immunodeficiency virus infection: Demonstration of p24 antigen in endothelial cells. *Clin. Infect. Dis.* **1993**, *17*, 360–363. [CrossRef] [PubMed]
94. Tehrani, H.A.; Darnahal, M.; Vaezi, M.; Haghighi, S. COVID-19 associated thrombotic thrombocytopenic purpura (TTP); A case series and mini-review. *Int. Immunopharmacol.* **2021**, *93*, 107397. [CrossRef]
95. Ward, S.E.; Curley, G.F.; Lavin, M.; Fogarty, H.; Karampini, E.; McEvoy, N.L.; Clarke, J.; Boylan, M.; Alalqam, R.; Worrall, A.P.; et al. Von Willebrand factor propeptide in severe coronavirus disease 2019 (COVID-19): Evidence of acute and sustained endothelial cell activation. *Br. J. Haematol.* **2021**, *192*, 714–719. [CrossRef] [PubMed]
96. Flaumenhaft, R.; Enjyoji, K.; Schmaier, A.A. Vasculopathy in COVID-19. *Blood* **2022**, *140*, 222–235. [CrossRef] [PubMed]
97. Lei, Y.; Zhang, J.; Schiavon, C.R.; He, M.; Chen, L.; Shen, H.; Shyy, J.Y. SARS-CoV-2 Spike Protein Impairs Endothelial Function via Downregulation of ACE 2. *Circ. Res.* **2021**, *128*, 1323–1326. [CrossRef] [PubMed]
98. McCracken, I.R.; Saginc, G.; He, L.; Huseynov, A.; Daniels, A.; Fletcher, S.; Randi, A.M. Lack of Evidence of Angiotensin-Converting Enzyme 2 Expression and Replicative Infection by SARS-CoV-2 in Human Endothelial Cells. *Circulation* **2021**, *143*, 865–868. [CrossRef]
99. Zakarija, A.; Kwaan, H.C.; Moake, J.L.; Bandarenko, N.; Pandey, D.K.; McKoy, J.M.; Yarnold, P.R.; Raisch, D.W.; Winters, J.L.; Raife, T.J.; et al. Ticlopidine- and clopidogrel-associated thrombotic thrombocytopenic purpura (TTP): Review of clinical, laboratory, epidemiological, and pharmacovigilance findings (1989–2008). *Kidney Int.* **2009**, *75*, S20–S24. [CrossRef]
100. Mauro, M.; Zlatopolskiy, A.; Raife, T.J.; Laurence, J. Thienopyridine-linked thrombotic microangiopathy: Association with endothelial cell apoptosis and activation of MAP kinase signalling cascades. *Br. J. Haematol.* **2004**, *124*, 200–210. [CrossRef]
101. Coppo, P.; Busson, M.; Veyradier, A.; Wynckel, A.; Poullin, P.; Azoulay, E.; Galicier, L.; Loiseau, P. HLA-DRB1*11: A strong risk factor for acquired severe ADAMTS13 deficiency-related idiopathic thrombotic thrombocytopenic purpura in Caucasians. *J. Thromb. Haemost.* **2010**, *8*, 856–859. [CrossRef]
102. Scully, M.; Brown, J.; Patel, R.; Mcdonald, V.; Brown, C.J.; Machin, S. Human leukocyte antigen association in idiopathic thrombotic thrombocytopenic purpura: Evidence for an immunogenetic link. *J. Thromb. Haemost.* **2010**, *8*, 257–262. [CrossRef] [PubMed]
103. Sorvillo, N.; van Haren, S.; Kaijen, P.H.; Brinke, A.T.; Fijnheer, R.; Meijer, A.B.; Voorberg, J. Preferential HLA-DRB1*11–dependent presentation of CUB2-derived peptides by ADAMTS13-pulsed dendritic cells. *Blood* **2013**, *121*, 3502–3510. [CrossRef] [PubMed]
104. Verbij, F.C.; Turksma, A.W.; de Heij, F.; Kaijen, P.; Lardy, N.; Fijnheer, R.; Sorvillo, N.; Brinke, A.T.; Voorberg, J. CD4+ T cells from patients with acquired thrombotic thrombocytopenic purpura recognize CUB2 domain-derived peptides. *Blood* **2016**, *127*, 1606–1609. [CrossRef] [PubMed]
105. Praprotnik, S.; Blank, M.; Levy, Y.; Tavor, S.; Boffa, M.-C.; Weksler, B.; Eldor, A.; Shoenfeld, Y. Anti-endothelial cell antibodies from patients with thrombotic thrombocytopenic purpura specifically activate small vessel endothelial cells. *Int. Immunol.* **2001**, *13*, 203–210. [CrossRef] [PubMed]
106. Wright, J.F.; Wang, H.; Hornstein, A.; Hogarth, M.; Mody, M.; Garvey, M.B.; Blanchette, V.; Rock, G.; Freedman, J. Characterization of platelet glycoproteins and platelet/endothelial cell antibodies in patients with thrombotic thrombocytopenic purpura. *Br. J. Haematol.* **1999**, *107*, 546–555. [CrossRef] [PubMed]
107. Tandon, N.N.; Rock, G.; Jamieson, G.A. Anti-CD36 antibodies in thrombotic thrombocytopenic purpura. *Br. J. Haematol.* **1994**, *88*, 816–825. [CrossRef]
108. Raife, T.J.; Atkinson, B.; Aster, R.H.; McFarland, J.G.; Gottschall, J.L. Minimal evidence of platelet and endothelial cell reactive antibodies in thrombotic thrombocytopenic purpura. *Am. J. Hematol.* **1999**, *62*, 82–87. [CrossRef]
109. Drachenberg, C.B.; Papadimitriou, J.C. Endothelial injury in renal antibody-mediated allograft rejection: A schematic view based on pathogenesis. *Transplantation* **2013**, *95*, 1073–1083. [CrossRef]
110. Rena, G.; Hack, B.K.; Minto, A.W.; Cunningham, P.N.; Alexander, J.J.; Haasb, M.; Quigg, R.J. A Complement-Dependent Model of Thrombotic Thrombocytopenic Purpura Induced by Antibodies Reactive with Endothelial Cells. *Clin. Immunol.* **2002**, *103*, 43–53. [CrossRef]
111. Chang, J.C.; Shipstone, A.; Llenado-Lee, M.A. Postoperative thrombotic thrombocytopenic purpura following cardiovascular surgeries. *Am. J. Hematol.* **1996**, *53*, 11–17. [CrossRef]
112. Jackson, S.P.; Darbousset, R.; Schoenwaelder, S.M. Thromboinflammation: Challenges of therapeutically targeting coagulation and other host defense mechanisms. *Blood* **2019**, *133*, 906–918. [CrossRef] [PubMed]
113. Namal Rathnayaka, R.; Ranathunga, P.A.N.; Kularatne, S.A. Thrombotic Microangiopathy, Hemolytic Uremic Syndrome, and Thrombotic Thrombocytopenic Purpura Following Hump-nosed Pit Viper (Genus: Hypnale) Envenoming in Sri Lanka. *Wilderness Environ. Med.* **2019**, *30*, 66–78. [CrossRef] [PubMed]
114. Tan, C.H.; Tan, N.H.; Sim, S.M.; Fung, S.Y.; Gnanathasan, C.A. Proteomic investigation of Sri Lankan hump-nosed pit viper (Hypnale hypnale) venom. *Toxicon* **2015**, *93*, 164–170. [CrossRef]

115. Vanuopadath, M.; Sajeev, N.; Murali, A.R.; Sudish, N.; Kangosseri, N.; Sebastian, I.R.; Jain, N.D.; Pal, A.; Raveendran, D.; Nair, B.G.; et al. Mass spectrometry-assisted venom profiling of Hypnale hypnale found in the Western Ghats of India incorporating de novo sequencing approaches. *Int. J. Biol. Macromol.* **2018**, *118*, 1736–1746. [CrossRef] [PubMed]
116. Noris, M.; Remuzzi, G. Overview of Complement Activation and Regulation. *Semin. Nephrol.* **2013**, *33*, 479–492. [CrossRef] [PubMed]
117. Fakhouri, F.; Zuber, J.; Frémeaux-Bacchi, V.; Loirat, C. Haemolytic uraemic syndrome. *Lancet* **2017**, *390*, 681–696. [CrossRef] [PubMed]
118. Orth, D.; Khan, A.B.; Naim, A.; Grif, K.; Brockmeyer, J.; Karch, H.; Joannidis, M.; Clark, S.J.; Day, A.J.; Fidanzi, S.; et al. Shiga Toxin Activates Complement and Binds Factor H: Evidence for an Active Role of Complement in Hemolytic Uremic Syndrome. *J. Immunol.* **2009**, *182*, 6394–6400. [CrossRef] [PubMed]
119. Brady, T.M.; Pruette, C.; Loeffler, L.F.; Weidemann, D.; Strouse, J.J.; Gavriilaki, E.; Brodsky, R.A. Typical Hus: Evidence of Acute Phase Complement Activation from a Daycare Outbreak. *J. Clin. Exp. Nephrol.* **2016**, *1*, 11. [CrossRef]
120. Burwick, R.M.; Fichorova, R.N.; Dawood, H.Y.; Yamamoto, H.S.; Feinberg, B.B. Urinary excretion of C5b-9 in severe preeclampsia: Tipping the balance of complement activation in pregnancy. *Hypertension* **2013**, *62*, 1040–1045. [CrossRef]
121. Jodele, S.; Licht, C.; Goebel, J.; Dixon, B.; Zhang, K.; Sivakumaran, T.A.; Davies, S.M.; Pluthero, F.; Lu, L.; Laskin, B.L. Abnormalities in the alternative pathway of complement in children with hematopoietic stem cell transplant-associated thrombotic microangiopathy. *Blood* **2013**, *122*, 2003–2007. [CrossRef]
122. Jodele, S.; Zhang, K.; Zou, F.; Laskin, B.; Dandoy, C.; Myers, K.C.; Lane, A.; Meller, J.; Medvedovic, M.; Chen, J.; et al. The genetic fingerprint of susceptibility for transplant-associated thrombotic microangiopathy. *Blood* **2016**, *127*, 989–996. [CrossRef] [PubMed]
123. de Fontbrune, F.S.; Galambrun, C.; Sirvent, A.; Huynh, A.; Faguer, S.; Nguyen, S.; de Latour, R.P. Use of Eculizumab in Patients with Allogeneic Stem Cell Transplant-Associated Thrombotic Microangiopathy: A Study From the SFGM-TC. *Transplantation* **2015**, *99*, 1953–1959. [CrossRef] [PubMed]
124. Westwood, J.-P.; Langley, K.; Heelas, E.; Machin, S.J.; Scully, M. Complement and cytokine response in acute Thrombotic Thrombocytopenic Purpura. *Br. J. Haematol.* **2014**, *164*, 858–866. [CrossRef] [PubMed]
125. Bettoni, S.; Galbusera, M.; Gastoldi, S.; Donadelli, R.; Tentori, C.; Spartà, G.; Bresin, E.; Mele, C.; Alberti, M.; Tortajada, A.; et al. Interaction between Multimeric von Willebrand Factor and Complement: A Fresh Look to the Pathophysiology of Microvascular Thrombosis. *J. Immunol.* **2017**, *199*, 1021–1040. [CrossRef] [PubMed]
126. Wu, T.C.; Yang, S.; Haven, S.; Holers, V.M.; Lundberg, A.S.; Wu, H.; Cataland, S.R. Complement activation and mortality during an acute episode of thrombotic thrombocytopenic purpura. *J. Thromb. Haemost.* **2013**, *11*, 1925–1927. [CrossRef] [PubMed]
127. Cataland, S.R.; Holers, V.M.; Geyer, S.; Yang, S.; Wu, H.M. Biomarkers of terminal complement activation confirm the diagnosis of aHUS and differentiate aHUS from TTP. *Blood* **2014**, *123*, 3733–3738. [CrossRef]
128. Tati, R.; Kristoffersson, A.-C.; Ståhl, A.-L.; Rebetz, J.; Wang, L.; Licht, C.; Motto, D.; Karpman, D. Complement Activation Associated with ADAMTS13 Deficiency in Human and Murine Thrombotic Microangiopathy. *J. Immunol.* **2013**, *191*, 2184–2193. [CrossRef]
129. Sinkovits, G.; Farkas, P.; Csuka, D.; Rázsó, K.; Réti, M.; Radványi, G.; Demeter, J.; Prohászka, Z.; Mikes, B. Carboxiterminal pro-endothelin-1 as an endothelial cell biomarker in thrombotic thrombocytopenic purpura. *Thromb. Haemost.* **2016**, *115*, 1034–1043. [CrossRef]
130. Turner, N.; Sartain, S.; Moake, J. Ultralarge Von Willebrand Factor–Induced Platelet Clumping and Activation of the Alternative Complement Pathway in Thrombotic Thrombocytopenic Purpura and the Hemolytic-Uremic Syndromes. *Hematol. Clin. North Am.* **2015**, *29*, 509–524. [CrossRef]
131. Feng, S.; Liang, X.; Kroll, M.H.; Chung, D.W.; Afshar-Kharghan, V. von Willebrand factor is a cofactor in complement regulation. *Blood* **2015**, *125*, 1034–1037. [CrossRef]
132. Zheng, L.; Zhang, D.; Cao, W.; Song, W.-C.; Zheng, X.L. Synergistic effects of ADAMTS13 deficiency and complement activation in pathogenesis of thrombotic microangiopathy. *Blood* **2019**, *134*, 1095–1105. [CrossRef] [PubMed]
133. Lorant, D.E.; Topham, M.K.; Whatley, R.E.; McEver, R.P.; McIntyre, T.M.; Prescott, S.M.; Zimmerman, G.A. Inflammatory roles of P-selectin. *J. Clin. Investig.* **1993**, *92*, 559–570. [CrossRef] [PubMed]
134. Morigi, M.; Galbusera, M.; Gastoldi, S.; Locatelli, M.; Buelli, S.; Pezzotta, A.; Pagani, C.; Noris, M.; Gobbi, M.; Stravalaci, M.; et al. Alternative Pathway Activation of Complement by Shiga Toxin Promotes Exuberant C3a Formation That Triggers Microvascular Thrombosis. *J. Immunol.* **2011**, *187*, 172–180. [CrossRef] [PubMed]
135. Foreman, K.E.; Vaporciyan, A.A.; Bonish, B.K.; Jones, M.L.; Johnson, K.J.; Glovsky, M.M.; Eddy, S.M.; A Ward, P. C5a-induced expression of P-selectin in endothelial cells. *J. Clin. Investig.* **1994**, *94*, 1147–1155. [CrossRef] [PubMed]
136. Tedesco, F.; Pausa, M.; Nardon, E.; Introna, M.; Mantovani, A.; Dobrina, A. The Cytolytically Inactive Terminal Complement Complex Activates Endothelial Cells to Express Adhesion Molecules and Tissue Factor Procoagulant Activity. *J. Exp. Med.* **1997**, *185*, 1619–1628. [CrossRef]
137. Ruiz-Torres, M.P.; Casiraghi, F.; Galbusera, M.; Macconi, D.; Gastoldi, S.; Todeschini, M.; Porrati, F.; Belotti, D.; Pogliani, E.M.; Remuzzi, G.; et al. Complement activation: The missing link between ADAMTS-13 deficiency and microvascular thrombosis of thrombotic microangiopathies. *Thromb. Haemost.* **2005**, *93*, 443–452. [CrossRef]
138. del Conde, I.; Crúz, M.A.; Zhang, H.; López, J.A.; Afshar-Kharghan, V. Platelet activation leads to activation and propagation of the complement system. *J. Exp. Med.* **2005**, *201*, 871–879. [CrossRef]

139. Chapin, J.; Weksler, B.; Magro, C.; Laurence, J. Eculizumab in the treatment of refractory idiopathic thrombotic thrombocytopenic purpura. *Br. J. Haematol.* **2012**, *157*, 772–774. [CrossRef]
140. Tsai, E.; Chapin, J.; Laurence, J.C.; Tsai, H.-M. Use of eculizumab in the treatment of a case of refractory, ADAMTS13-deficient thrombotic thrombocytopenic purpura: Additional data and clinical follow-up. *Br. J. Haematol.* **2013**, *162*, 558–559. [CrossRef]
141. Pecoraro, C.; Ferretti, A.V.S.; Rurali, E.; Galbusera, M.; Noris, M.; Remuzzi, G. Treatment of Congenital Thrombotic Thrombocytopenic Purpura with Eculizumab. *Am. J. Kidney Dis.* **2015**, *66*, 1067–1070. [CrossRef]
142. Vigna, E.; Petrungaro, A.; Perri, A.; Terzi, D.; Recchia, A.G.; Mendicino, F.; La Russa, A.; Bossio, S.; De Stefano, L.; Zinno, F.; et al. Efficacy of eculizumab in severe ADAMTS13-deficient thrombotic thrombocytopenic purpura (TTP) refractory to standard therapies. *Transfus. Apher. Sci.* **2018**, *57*, 247–249. [CrossRef] [PubMed]
143. Rother, R.P.; Bell, L.; Hillmen, P.; Gladwin, M.T. The clinical sequelae of intravascular hemolysis and extracellular plasma hemoglobin: A novel mechanism of human disease. *JAMA* **2005**, *293*, 1653–1662. [CrossRef] [PubMed]
144. Vinchi, F.; De Franceschi, L.; Ghigo, A.; Townes, T.; Cimino, J.; Silengo, L.; Hirsch, E.; Altruda, F.; Tolosano, E. Hemopexin Therapy Improves Cardiovascular Function by Preventing Heme-Induced Endothelial Toxicity in Mouse Models of Hemolytic Diseases. *Circulation* **2013**, *127*, 1317–1329. [CrossRef] [PubMed]
145. Matsushita, K.; Morrell, C.N.; Cambien, B.; Yang, S.-X.; Yamakuchi, M.; Bao, C.; Hara, M.R.; Quick, R.A.; Cao, W.; O'Rourke, B.; et al. Nitric Oxide Regulates Exocytosis by S-Nitrosylation of N-ethylmaleimide-Sensitive Factor. *Cell* **2003**, *115*, 139–150. [CrossRef] [PubMed]
146. Studt, J.-D.; Hovinga, J.A.K.; Antoine, G.; Hermann, M.; Rieger, M.; Scheiflinger, F.; Lämmle, B. Fatal congenital thrombotic thrombocytopenic purpura with apparent ADAMTS13 inhibitor: In vitro inhibition of ADAMTS13 activity by hemoglobin. *Blood* **2005**, *105*, 542–544. [CrossRef]
147. Merle, N.S.; Paule, R.; Leon, J.; Daugan, M.; Robe-Rybkine, T.; Poillerat, V.; Roumenina, L.T. P-selectin drives complement attack on endothelium during intravascular hemolysis in TLR-4/heme-dependent manner. *Proc. Natl. Acad. Sci. USA* **2019**, *116*, 6280–6285. [CrossRef]
148. May, O.; Merle, N.S.; Grunenwald, A.; Gnemmi, V.; Leon, J.; Payet, C.; Robe-Rybkine, T.; Paule, R.; Delguste, F.; Satchell, S.C.; et al. Heme Drives Susceptibility of Glomerular Endothelium to Complement Overactivation Due to Inefficient Upregulation of Heme Oxygenase-1. *Front. Immunol.* **2018**, *9*, 3008. [CrossRef]
149. Frimat, M.; Tabarin, F.; Dimitrov, J.; Poitou, C.; Halbwachs-Mecarelli, L.; Fremeaux-Bacchi, V.; Roumenina, L. Complement activation by heme as a secondary hit for atypical hemolytic uremic syndrome. *Blood* **2013**, *122*, 282–292. [CrossRef]
150. Brinkmann, V.; Reichard, U.; Goosmann, C.; Fauler, B.; Uhlemann, Y.; Weiss, D.S.; Weinrauch, Y.; Zychlinsky, A. Neutrophil extracellular traps kill bacteria. *Science* **2004**, *303*, 1532–1535. [CrossRef]
151. Fuchs, T.A.; Brill, A.; Duerschmied, D.; Schatzberg, D.; Monestier, M.; Myers, D.D., Jr.; Wrobleski, S.K.; Wakefield, T.W.; Hartwig, J.H.; Wagner, D.D. Extracellular DNA traps promote thrombosis. *Proc. Natl. Acad. Sci. USA* **2010**, *107*, 15880–15885. [CrossRef]
152. Fuchs, T.A.; Bhandari, A.A.; Wagner, D.D. Histones induce rapid and profound thrombocytopenia in mice. *Blood* **2011**, *118*, 3708–3714. [CrossRef] [PubMed]
153. Fuchs, T.A.; Hovinga, J.A.K.; Schatzberg, D.; Wagner, D.D.; Lämmle, B. Circulating DNA and myeloperoxidase indicate disease activity in patients with thrombotic microangiopathies. *Blood* **2012**, *120*, 1157–1164. [CrossRef] [PubMed]
154. Ramos, M.V.; Mejias, M.P.; Sabbione, F.; Fernandez-Brando, R.J.; Santiago, A.P.; Amaral, M.M.; Exeni, R.; Trevani, A.S.; Palermo, M.S. Induction of Neutrophil Extracellular Traps in Shiga Toxin-Associated Hemolytic Uremic Syndrome. *J. Innate Immun.* **2016**, *8*, 400–411. [CrossRef] [PubMed]
155. Gloude, N.J.; Khandelwal, P.; Luebbering, N.; Lounder, D.T.; Jodele, S.; Alder, M.N.; Lane, A.; Wilkey, A.; Lake, K.E.; Litts, B.; et al. Circulating dsDNA, endothelial injury, and complement activation in thrombotic microangiopathy and GVHD. *Blood* **2017**, *130*, 1259–1266. [CrossRef]
156. Yuen, J.; Pluthero, F.G.; Douda, D.N.; Riedl, M.; Cherry, A.; Ulanova, M.; Kahr, W.H.A.; Palaniyar, N.; Licht, C. NETosing Neutrophils Activate Complement Both on Their Own NETs and Bacteria via Alternative and Non-alternative Pathways. *Front. Immunol.* **2016**, *7*, 137. [CrossRef] [PubMed]
157. Miyata, T.; Fan, X. A second hit for TMA. *Blood* **2012**, *120*, 1152–1154. [CrossRef]
158. Padilla, A.; Moake, J.L.; Bernardo, A.; Ball, C.; Wang, Y.; Arya, M.; Nolasco, L.; Turner, N.; Berndt, M.C.; Anvari, B.; et al. P-selectin anchors newly released ultralarge von Willebrand factor multimers to the endothelial cell surface. *Blood* **2004**, *103*, 2150–2156. [CrossRef]
159. El-Mansi, S.; Nightingale, T.D. Emerging mechanisms to modulate VWF release from endothelial cells. *Int. J. Biochem. Cell Biol.* **2021**, *131*, 105900. [CrossRef]

Disclaimer/Publisher's Note: The statements, opinions and data contained in all publications are solely those of the individual author(s) and contributor(s) and not of MDPI and/or the editor(s). MDPI and/or the editor(s) disclaim responsibility for any injury to people or property resulting from any ideas, methods, instructions or products referred to in the content.

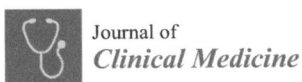

Review

The Specificities of Thrombotic Thrombocytopenic Purpura at Extreme Ages: A Narrative Review

Adrien Joseph [1,2,†], Bérangère S. Joly [2,3,4,†], Adrien Picod [1,2], Agnès Veyradier [2,3,4] and Paul Coppo [2,5,*]

1. Medical Intensive Care Unit, Saint-Louis Hospital, Public Assistance Hospitals of Paris, 75010 Paris, France; adrien.joseph@aphp.fr (A.J.); adrien.picod@aphp.fr (A.P.)
2. French Reference Center for Thrombotic Microangiopathies, 75012 Paris, France; berangere.joly@aphp.fr (B.S.J.); agnes.veyradier@aphp.fr (A.V.)
3. Hematology Biology Department, Lariboisière Hospital, Public Assistance Hospitals of Paris, 75006 Paris, France
4. EA-3518, Clinical Research in Hematology, Immunology and Transplantation, Institut de Recherche Saint-Louis, Université de Paris, 75571 Paris, France
5. Hematology Department, Saint-Antoine hospital, Public Assistance Hospitals of Paris, 75571 Paris, France
* Correspondence: paul.coppo@aphp.fr; Tel.: +33-1-49-28-34-39
† These authors contributed equally to this work.

Abstract: Thrombotic thrombocytopenic purpura (TTP) is a rare and life-threatening thrombotic microangiopathy (TMA) related to a severe ADAMTS13 deficiency, the specific von Willebrand factor (VWF)-cleaving protease. This deficiency is often immune-mediated (iTTP) and related to the presence of anti-ADAMTS13 autoantibodies that enhance its clearance or inhibit its VWF processing activity. iTTP management may be challenging at extreme ages of life. International cohorts of people with TTP report delayed diagnoses and misdiagnoses in children and elderly people. Child-onset iTTP shares many features with adult-onset iTTP: a female predominance, an idiopathic presentation, and the presence of neurological disorders and therapeutic strategies. Long-term follow-ups and a transition from childhood to adulthood are crucial to preventing iTTP relapses, in order to identify the occurrence of other autoimmune disorders and psychosocial sequelae. In contrast, older iTTP patients have an atypical clinical presentation, with delirium, an atypical neurological presentation, and severe renal and cardiac damages. They also have a poorer response to treatment and prognosis. Long-term sequelae are highly prevalent in older patients. Prediction scores for iTTP diagnoses are not used for children and have a lower sensitivity and specificity in patients over 60 years old. ADAMTS13 remains the unique biological marker that is able to definitely confirm or rule out the diagnosis of iTTP and predict relapses during follow-ups.

Keywords: thrombotic microangiopathy; thrombotic thrombocytopenic purpura; ADAMTS13 protein; diagnosis; prognosis; child; aging; plasma exchange; caplacizumab; von Willebrand factor

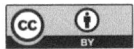

1. Introduction

Thrombotic thrombocytopenic purpura (TTP) is a thrombotic microangiopathy caused by a severe functional deficiency in a disintegrin and metalloprotease with thrombospondin type I repeats-13 (ADAMTS13), the specific von Willebrand factor (VWF)-cleaving protease [1]. TTP is associated with microangiopathic hemolytic anemia, severe thrombocytopenia, and end-organ ischemia, which is linked to the spontaneous formation of microvascular VWFs and platelet-rich thrombi, particularly in the central nervous system [2].

In its most frequent form, immune-mediated TTP (iTTP) is caused by autoantibodies, mainly IgG, which are directed against ADAMTS13, where they inhibit its function or enhance its clearance. The anti-ADAMTS13 autoimmune response is polyclonal. Similar to other autoimmune diseases [3], iTTP predominantly affects women of reproductive age (30–40 years). In its presentation, iTTP is idiopathic in 60% of cases and is associated with another preexisting or concomitant clinical condition in 40% of cases [4]. In its non-idiopathic forms, infections, systemic autoimmune diseases, cancer, transplantation, antiplatelet drugs, immunosuppressive agents, HIV, and pregnancy are the most commonly listed triggers for iTTP [4].

French and PLASMIC scores, both of which are based on platelet counts and serum creatinine levels at diagnosis, have been developed for the early identification of adult patients with severe ADAMTS13 activity, in order to guide the clinical and therapeutic decisions when ADAMTS13 testing is not available in an emergency [5,6]. The measurement of ADAMTS13 activity is crucial to confirming an iTTP diagnosis (activity <10 IU/dL) [1,7]. Additional investigations into the presence of anti-ADAMTS13 autoantibodies (mainly ELISAs to detect anti-ADAMTS13 IgG) are required to document the auto-immune mechanism of ADAMTS13 deficiency [2,7,8].

Due to its rarity (a prevalence of around 5–13 cases/1,000,000) [4,9,10], the initial description of iTTP was focused on prototypical patients [11]. As larger cohorts were reported, it appeared clear that younger and older patients represented an appreciable share of iTTP patients. In the French National Registry for TTP, 4% of cases occurred in individuals below 18 years, and 17% to 23% of cases in individuals above 60 years (Figure 1). Moreover, differences in the phenotypes and outcomes of such patients were described.

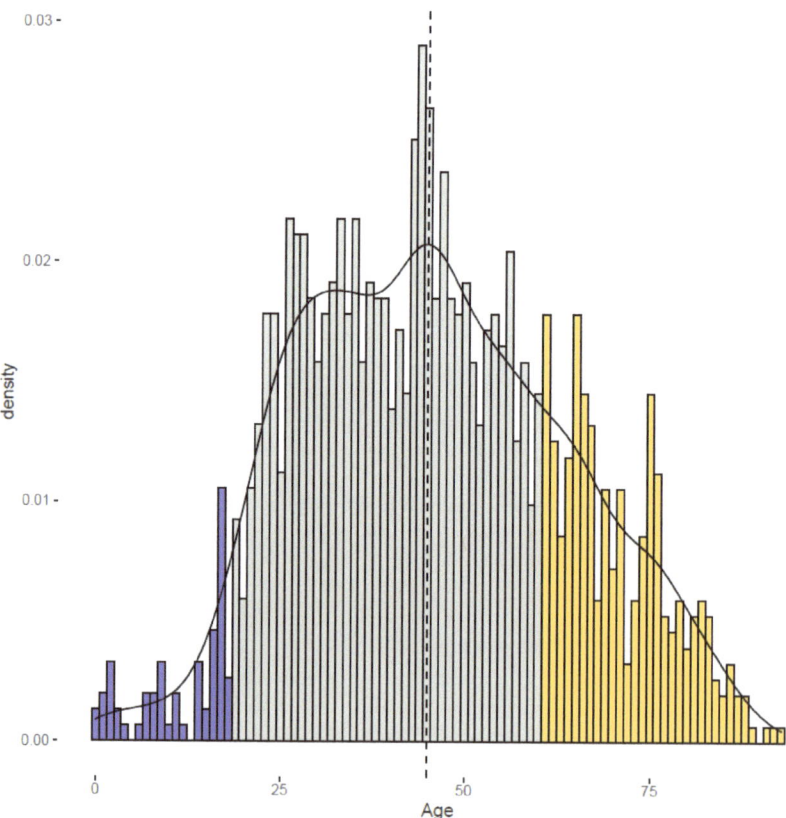

Figure 1. Distribution of immune-mediated thrombotic thrombocytopenic purpura cases according to age of onset.

The proportions of adulthood- (73%, grey), old-age- (23%, orange), and childhood (4%, blue)-onset iTTP that are presented in this figure have been extracted from the data of the

French Registry for TTP (inclusion period 2000–2020, 1514 patients). The median age is represented as a dashed line.

In this review, we will describe the particular characteristics of iTTP occurring at extreme ages, i.e., below 18 years and above 60 years of age. We will also describe the implications in terms of their outcomes and the recommendations for providing optimal care to these patients and preventing delayed management.

2. Immune-Mediated Thrombotic Thrombocytopenic Purpura in Children

In 1924, Eli Moschcowitz described the first case of iTTP in a 16-year-old girl who had suddenly developed weakness, pain, pallor, fever, and petechiae (no platelet count available). A few days later, she developed neurological disorders and died. The autopsy revealed the presence of disseminated hyaline thrombi in the microcirculation of her heart, kidney, spleen, and liver [12]. Based on the scope of the scientific literature and the national registries for TTP since 2001, ~150 different cases of child-onset iTTP with a documented severe functional deficiency of ADAMTS13 (activity < 10 IU/dL per definition) and the presence of anti-ADAMTS13 autoantibodies have been reported [13–25]. The prevalence of child-onset iTTP is ~1 case per million children and its diagnosis remains challenging [13,25].

2.1. Clinical Presentation and Diagnosis

Child-onset iTTP is rare and life-threatening. Besides an early onset in the neonatal period of the congenital form of TTP (~1/3 of child-onset TTP cases), iTTP may occur in ~2/3 of child-onset TTP cases, with a frequency that is two times greater for older compared to younger children [2,13,21,25] (Figure 2). Physicians have to rule out the possibility of congenital TTP before starting treatment for iTTP with immunosuppressive drugs or anti-VWF agents.

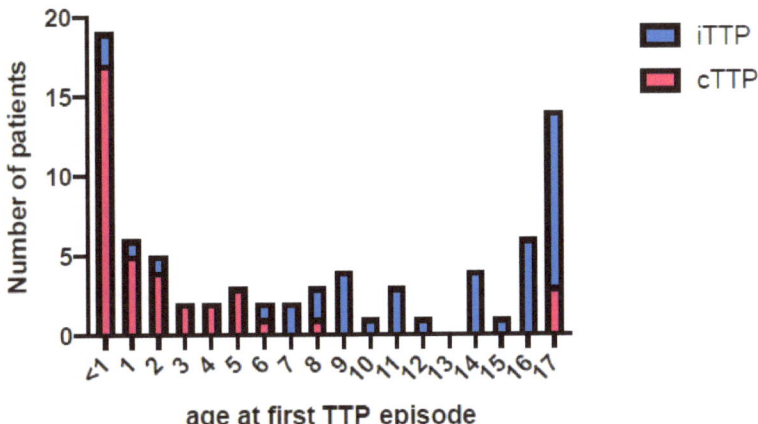

Figure 2. Proportion of child-onset congenital (cTTP) and immune thrombotic thrombocytopenic purpura (iTTP) according to age at first TTP episode.

The proportions presented in this figure have been extracted from the data of the French Registry for TTP (inclusion period 2000–2020).

In children, the median age of the first iTTP episode is ~12 years and the sex ratio is ~2–2.5 F/1 M [13–25]. The clinical presentation of iTTP is mainly idiopathic (~56% with a median age of 15 years), but other clinical contexts such as infection, systemic autoimmune disease (mainly systemic lupus erythematosus), neoplasia, or organ transplantation are sometimes associated with its inaugural episode (~44% with a median age of 8 years) [13,21]. iTTP remains rare before 6 years.

In child-onset iTTP, fever and neurological symptoms (such as headache, confusion, coma, seizures, strokes, or transient focal defects) are frequent (~40% and 40–55%, respectively), while renal or cardiac injury are less common (~40% and ~6–7%, respectively) [13–25].

The most important laboratory features are severe consumption thrombocytopenia (a platelet count typically of $<30 \times 10^9/L$) and microangiopathic hemolytic anemia (hemoglobin levels usually of 6–7 g/dL), with the presence of schistocytes on the peripheral blood smear. The first episode of iTTP may be sudden and severe. By definition [7], all iTTP patients have an ADAMTS13 activity of less than 10 IU/dL and positive anti-ADAMTS13 autoantibodies at diagnosis [13–25].

In 20–25% of children, iTTP can be misdiagnosed as autoimmune cytopenia (idiopathic thrombocytopenic purpura, Evans syndrome) or another thrombotic microangiopathy (TMA) syndrome, such as shigatoxin-mediated hemolytic uremic syndrome (HUS) or atypical HUS, due to the dysregulation of the complement alternative pathway or a malignant hemopathy [13]. An iTTP diagnosis should be suspected when microangiopathic hemolytic anemia and consumption thrombocytopenia are associated with organ failure or a previous diagnosis of autoimmune cytopenia is not responding to specific treatments.

An ADAMTS13 activity measurement is the unique biological marker that is able to differentiate iTTP from other TMA syndromes or immune cytopenias [2,7]. In adult patients, both French and PLASMIC scores facilitate the rapid recognition of a severe ADAMTS13 deficiency and guide the clinical decisions when ADAMTS13 testing is not available [5,6]. The performances of these scores with age-related variables should be evaluated in children to improve iTTP diagnoses.

2.2. Treatment

The treatment of the acute phase of iTTP is an emergency because major stroke and organ failure can subsequently occur. The therapeutic targets used in child-onset iTTP are ADAMTS13, anti-ADAMTS13 IgG, and VWF [26].

A therapeutic plasma exchange (TPE) or plasma infusion, allowing for an exogenous supply of ADAMTS13 deficiency and the saturation of anti-ADAMTS13 autoantibodies, is the first-line treatment for acute iTTP in children, as soon as an iTTP diagnosis is made or even suspected [27].

Corticosteroids are usually used as an adjunctive treatment to curative first-line plasmatherapy. When iTTP is confirmed, an immunomodulation with rituximab (a chimeric anti-CD20 monoclonal antibody) may be considered together with TPE and corticosteroids to decrease the autoimmune response and normalize the ADAMTS13 levels [27]. Rituximab is typically effective after 2 weeks following the first infusion; therefore, it does not prevent early death [2].

Caplacizumab, a nanobody directed against the A1 domain of VWF, immediately inhibits the interactions between platelet GPIb and VWF and prevents the formation of microvascular thrombosis in the microcirculation. Caplacizumab has shown safety and efficacy in adult-onset iTTP [20,28]. Immunosuppressive therapies are still required to control the underlying disease process [27]. In total, thirteen cases of iTTP being successfully treated by caplacizumab have been recently reported in children, with a faster normalization of their platelet counts and favorable outcomes [15,17,18,20,22–24]. The pediatric dosing recommendations were developed using model-based simulations and the results of this modeling and simulation analysis constituted the basis for the European extension of indication for caplacizumab (10 mg) to children over 12 years with a body weight of $\geq$40 kg [29].

Platelet transfusions are relatively contraindicated in children with iTTP and should be limited to the treatment of life-threatening bleeding [13,20].

Thus, several child-onset iTTP cases have reported similar therapeutic experiences when compared to adults over the past 20 years.

2.3. Prognosis

Before the caplacizumab era, the mortality rate of the first iTTP episode was ~4% in children [13,21,25]. These epidemiological data need to be updated in the coming years.

Disease relapse is recognized as a risk in iTTP. Child-onset iTTP requires a long-term follow-up to avoid a clinical relapse that is preventable by preemptive rituximab injections when the ADAMTS13 activity drops below 10 IU/dL [7,13,27].

Physical examinations and biological (hemoglobin levels, platelet counts, ADAMTS13 activity monitoring, and autoimmunity) and psychological follow-ups are recommended to evaluate the emergence of autoimmune diseases and the physical and/or psychological sequelae of the disease. Some children have neurologic or renal sequelae. Some of them need psychomotor support and others have familial, social, schooling, or working difficulties. Similar to other autoimmune diseases, iTTP is a life-long disorder with potential psychological, cognitive, and social consequences [13,21].

The pathogenesis of an autoimmune disorder is considered to be multifactorial and a strong association between the HLA region, the generation of autoantibodies against self-antigens, and autoimmune diseases has been described [30]. In children, HLA-DRB1*11 may be a susceptibility factor for iTTP, while HLA-DRB1*04, when not associated with HLA-DQB1*03, may be protective [31]. Pediatricians should also be aware of the occurrence of another systemic autoimmune disease many years following remission [13,32]. Systemic lupus erythematosus is the most common additional autoimmune disorder that has been reported in older girls, in line with the increased frequency of autoimmune disorders at the beginning of puberty.

The transition period from childhood to adulthood is usually difficult and presents many challenges for many young adults with a past history of iTTP. Transition programs are necessary and should include specific actions that patients consider to be priorities, including awareness about relapse prevention, the occurrence of comorbidities (ischemic strokes or other cardiovascular events, hypertension, becoming overweight, etc.), and pregnancy planning.

3. Immune Mediated Thrombotic Thrombocytopenic Purpura in Older Patients

The prevalence of older patients with iTTP is increasing due to the aging of the general population and the possibly of improvements in disease recognition. Recent, dedicated studies [33–35] have underlined that older iTTP patients have an atypical clinical presentation and a poorer response to treatment and prognosis, which are detailed hereafter.

3.1. Clinical Presentation and Diagnosis

As expected, older patients more often present with comorbidities, especially cardiovascular diseases, diabetes, and osteoporosis. The conditions associated with iTTP more frequently involve cancer than autoimmune diseases, while infectious triggers do not seem to be more prevalent [33,34].

Delirium and behavioral abnormalities are often at the forefront of iTTP's clinical presentation in older patients, as opposed to headache and abdominal pain, which are more frequent in younger patients. Renal and cardiac involvement are more frequent and severe in older patients, whereas hematologic features such as thrombocytopenia and anemia are less pronounced [33], despite a seemingly increased gastro-enteral bleeding rate [35].

These differences translate into poorer performances of both the French and PLASMIC scores [33,36] and a longer time from admission to diagnosis for older patients (3 versus 1 day) [33,35], even though the proportion of iTTP amongst TMA does not seem to decrease with advanced age [35]. Recently, proteinuria and blood pressure were reported as potential leads for improving the performances of these scores [37–40], but these results warrant confirmation and their added value for older patients more frequently affected by hypertension, diabetes mellitus, and/or chronic kidney disease remains to be evaluated.

3.2. Treatment

The current standard of care for iTTP patients relies on TPE, immunosuppressive therapies with corticosteroids and rituximab, and the anti-von Willebrand factor caplacizumab [41]. In the French National Registry, treatment decisions do not differ between older and younger patients, although older patients receive fewer rituximab doses [33] and corticosteroids are less prescribed for patients ≥65 years in the Milan TTP Registry [42].

The combination of TPE and immunosuppressive therapies has resulted in a dramatic improvement in the outcome of iTTP acute episodes [20,41]. Nevertheless, several cohorts with diverse populations have shown that short-term mortality remains significant in older compared to younger iTTP patients (37% versus 9% in one month), due to the higher risks of renal, cardiac, and neurological events [33,43,44], as well as unresponsiveness [45,46]. These studies were published before the caplacizumab era and it would be interesting to evaluate the impact of this new therapeutic approach on the age-related short-term mortality of iTTP patients. In a cluster analysis of 666 patients from the Optum-Humedica database, older patients formed two clusters, with a higher mortality and episodes of a longer duration [47].

A decreased efficacy or increased side effects of caplacizumab have never been described [20,28,41], even though the risk of gastrointestinal or intracranial bleeding calls for caution in frail patients. In a retrospective series of four patients with intracranial hemorrhages after caplacizumab therapy, only one was over 60 years of age [48].

Polypharmacy [34] represents a risk factor for drug interactions and warrants medication optimization upon discharge from the hospital. Particular attention should be paid to antiplatelet agents and anticoagulants, which are more often prescribed to older patients [33], as such treatments could increase the risk of bleeding in association with caplacizumab.

Catheter self-removal as a result of delirium is also an important issue in older iTTP patients; thus, attention should be paid to limit the duration of central venous access to the strict minimum, i.e., it is usually limited to the period of the therapeutic plasma exchange [33].

Current guidelines recommend starting TPE and steroids for patients with TMA after an evaluation of the pretest probability of iTTP, based on a clinical judgement or a risk assessment model [7]. In the elderly, however, poorer diagnostic score performances may render an iTTP diagnosis challenging for clinicians. In older patients with an intermediate probability (French score = 1 or PLASMIC score 5) and/or an atypical clinical presentation, we consider that treatment decisions should rely on knowledge of the older patients' clinical specificities, a thorough evaluation of alternate diagnoses, and expert opinions. As the proportion of intermediate diagnostic probabilities is increased in elderly patients, clinicians should initiate TPE in these patients even in the presence of an atypical presentation, given the increased risk of short-term mortality and in spite of the increased risk of treatment-related complications.

3.3. Prognosis

After an acute episode, relapse rates do not seem to differ between older and younger iTTP patients [33]. However, a growing body of evidence has demonstrated that, in general, iTTP patients require a long-term follow-up due to late-occurring complications. Life expectancy is decreased in iTTP survivors and cardiovascular and neurological complications can occur independently of relapses [49–53]. The pathophysiology of these late complications is thought to rely on both the sequelae of microvascular thrombosis during the acute phase and also a subnormal, non-severe, chronic ADAMTS13 deficiency, with an accumulation of hyper-adhesive, ultra-large VWF multimers released from the endothelium, leading to subclinical vasculopathy and cumulative vascular injury [51]. This last finding appears to be of particular importance in the elderly population and suggests that the risk of cardiac and cerebrovascular events could be mitigated by the careful control of the cardiovascular risk factors and a strict monitoring of the ADAMTS13 activity in remission with the use of preemptive rituximab.

In addition, the psychological, cognitive, and social consequences of iTTP are being increasingly recognized [54–56]. Even though there are currently no data comparing older and younger iTTP patients' cognitive prognoses, older patients are likely to experience a more severe cognitive decline. Delirium, which is more frequent as a presenting feature in older iTTP patients, has been consistently associated with long-term cognitive decline in other contexts [57]. Subclinical vasculopathy related to large, circulating von Willebrand factor multimers may also accelerate this cognitive decline, as evidenced in population cohorts [58]. It is important to note that 26% of patients > 60 years are institutionalized 1 year after their initial episode of iTTP [33].

Infectious complications after the resolution of an iTTP flare-up are scarce, but one worry is that the immunosuppressive effects of corticosteroids and rituximab may lead to a clinically significant infectious risk for older individuals and for those with comorbidities, as shown with other systemic autoimmune diseases [59].

Consistently, long-term survival rates are poorer for older iTTP survivors compared to the general older population (a multivariable HR for death of 3.44, 95% CI [2.02; 5.87]) [33], and these patients experience more frequent long-term cardiovascular and cerebrovascular diseases [34]. Moreover, alike to younger patients, autoimmune diseases can occur months or years after an iTTP diagnosis and warrant a specific follow-up [34,60]. Lastly, older patients have a poorer understanding of the disease, potentially impacting their adherence to the follow-up and their identification of high-risk situations [61]. These data argue for a comprehensive geriatric assessment of older iTTP survivors in order to identify and manage the modifiable risk factors of poor long-term outcomes accordingly (Table 1).

Table 1. Recommendations and research agenda (italic) for optimal care of iTTP in older patients.

	Recommendations
Diagnosis	Physician awareness of atypical neurological presentations Adaptation of clinical scores for older patients specificities
Treatment	Rapid identification and intensification in unresponsive patients Medication optimization to avoid drug interactions Reassessment of prognostic factors in the caplacizumab era
Long-term follow-up	Comprehensive geriatric assessment and management of associated (cardiovascular) risk factors Careful ADAMTS13 monitoring ± preemptive rituximab Characterization of cognitive impairment in older patients following iTTP episode

4. Conclusions

An iTTP diagnosis can be challenging at extreme ages, resulting in frequently delayed diagnoses. The prediction scores of iTTP are not used for children and have a lower sensitivity and specificity in patients over 60 years old. ADAMTS13 therefore remains the unique biological marker that is able to definitely confirm the diagnosis of iTTP in these patients. The treatment of iTTP in children and elderly patients should not differ from that in other age groups. In both populations, an assessment of caplacizumab's efficacy and tolerance is urgently needed. While the efficacy and safety of caplacizumab in children are likely to be similar to those of the drug in adults, additional safety data are required for the elderly, where patients are typically polymedicated and more exposed to bleeding complications. In all cases, long-term follow-up is crucial to preventing relapses of the disease, to identifying the occurrence of systemic autoimmune disorders, and to evaluating its consequences for social life. In children, helping patients during their transition period to adulthood is key (Figure 3).

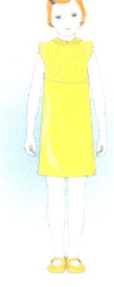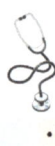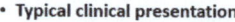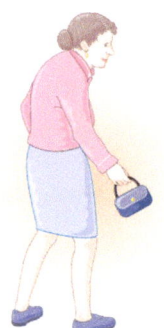

Figure 3. Difference in clinical presentation, biological features, treatment, and outcomes between immune-mediated thrombotic thrombocytopenic purpura at extreme ages.

Funding: This research received no external funding.

Institutional Review Board Statement: Not applicable.

Informed Consent Statement: Not applicable.

Data Availability Statement: Not applicable.

Conflicts of Interest: P.C. is member of the advisory board for SANOFI, ALEXION and TAKEDA. A.V. is a member of the French advisory board for caplacizumab (SANOFI) and for recombinant vwf and Adamts13 (TAKEDA). B.S.J. received speaker fees from SANOFI and TAKEDA. The other authors declare no conflict of interest.

References

1. Furlan, M.; Robles, R.; Galbusera, M.; Remuzzi, G.; Kyrle, P.A.; Brenner, B.; Krause, M.; Scharrer, I.; Aumann, V.; Mittler, U.; et al. Von Willebrand factor-cleaving protease in thrombotic thrombocytopenic purpura and the hemolytic-uremic syndrome. *N. Engl. J. Med.* **1998**, *339*, 1578–1584. [CrossRef] [PubMed]
2. Joly, B.S.; Coppo, P.; Veyradier, A. Thrombotic thrombocytopenic purpura. *Blood* **2017**, *129*, 2836–2846. [CrossRef] [PubMed]
3. Quintero, O.L.; Amador-Patarroyo, M.J.; Montoya-Ortiz, G.; Rojas-Villarraga, A.; Anaya, J.M. Autoimmune disease and gender: Plausible mechanisms for the female predominance of autoimmunity. *J. Autoimmun.* **2012**, *38*, J109–J119. [CrossRef]
4. Mariotte, E.; Azoulay, E.; Galicier, L.; Rondeau, E.; Zouiti, F.; Boisseau, P.; Poullin, P.; de Maistre, E.; Provôt, F.; Delmas, Y.; et al. Epidemiology and pathophysiology of adulthood-onset thrombotic microangiopathy with severe ADAMTS13 deficiency (thrombotic thrombocytopenic purpura): A cross-sectional analysis of the French national registry for thrombotic microangiopathy. *Lancet Haematol.* **2016**, *3*, e237–e245. [CrossRef] [PubMed]
5. Coppo, P.; Schwarzinger, M.; Buffet, M.; Wynckel, A.; Clabault, K.; Presne, C.; Poullin, P.; Malot, S.; Vanhille, P.; Azoulay, E.; et al. Predictive features of severe acquired ADAMTS13 deficiency in idiopathic thrombotic microangiopathies: The French TMA reference center experience. *PLoS ONE* **2010**, *5*, e10208. [CrossRef]
6. Bendapudi, P.K.; Hurwitz, S.; Fry, A.; Marques, M.B.; Waldo, S.W.; Li, A.; Sun, L.; Upadhyay, V.; Hamdan, A.; Brunner, A.M.; et al. Derivation and external validation of the PLASMIC score for rapid assessment of adults with thrombotic microangiopathies: A cohort study. *Lancet Haematol.* **2017**, *4*, e157–e164. [CrossRef]

7. Zheng, X.L.; Vesely, S.K.; Cataland, S.R.; Coppo, P.; Geldziler, B.; Iorio, A.; Matsumoto, M.; Mustafa, R.A.; Pai, M.; Rock, G.; et al. ISTH guidelines for the diagnosis of thrombotic thrombocytopenic purpura. *J. Thromb. Haemost.* **2020**, *18*, 2486–2495. [CrossRef]
8. Tsai, H.M.; Lian, E.C. Antibodies to von Willebrand factor-cleaving protease in acute thrombotic thrombocytopenic purpura. *N. Engl. J. Med.* **1998**, *339*, 1585–1594. [CrossRef] [PubMed]
9. Miller, D.P.; Kaye, J.A.; Shea, K.; Ziyadeh, N.; Cali, C.; Black, C.; Walker, A.M. Incidence of thrombotic thrombocytopenic purpura/hemolytic uremic syndrome. *Epidemiology* **2004**, *15*, 208–215. [CrossRef]
10. Terrell, D.R.; Williams, L.A.; Vesely, S.K.; Lämmle, B.; Hovinga, J.A.K.; George, J.N. The incidence of thrombotic thrombocytopenic purpura-hemolytic uremic syndrome: All patients, idiopathic patients, and patients with severe ADAMTS-13 deficiency. *J. Thromb. Haemost.* **2005**, *3*, 1432–1436. [CrossRef]
11. Amorosi, E.L.; Ultmann, J.E. Thrombotic thrombocytopenic purpura: Report of 16 cases and review of the literature. *Medicine* **1966**, *45*, 139–160. [CrossRef]
12. Moschcowitz, E.L.I. Hyaline thrombosis of the terminal arterioles and capillaries: A hitherto undescribed disease. *Proc. N. Y. Pathol. Soc.* **1924**, *24*, 21–24.
13. Joly, B.S.; Stepanian, A.; Leblanc, T.; Hajage, D.; Chambost, H.; Harambat, J.; Fouyssac, F.; Guigonis, V.; Leverger, G.; Ulinski, T.; et al. Child-onset and adolescent-onset acquired thrombotic thrombocytopenic purpura with severe ADAMTS13 deficiency: A cohort study of the French national registry for thrombotic microangiopathy. *Lancet Haematol.* **2016**, *3*, e537–e546. [CrossRef] [PubMed]
14. Saleem, R.; Rogers, Z.R.; Neunert, C.; George, J.N. Maintenance rituximab for relapsing thrombotic thrombocytopenic purpura: A case report. *Transfusion* **2019**, *59*, 921–926. [CrossRef]
15. Bhoopalan, S.V.; Hankins, J.; George, J.; Ryder, A.; Onder, A.M.; Puri, L. Use of caplacizumab in a child with refractory thrombotic thrombocytopenic purpura. *Pediatr. Blood Cancer* **2019**, *66*, e27737. [CrossRef] [PubMed]
16. Sakai, K.; Kuwana, M.; Tanaka, H.; Hosomichi, K.; Hasegawa, A.; Uyama, H.; Nishio, K.; Omae, T.; Hishizawa, M.; Matsui, M.; et al. HLA loci predisposing to immune TTP in Japanese: Potential role of the shared ADAMTS13 peptide bound to different HLA-DR. *Blood* **2020**, *135*, 2413–2419. [CrossRef]
17. Nagel, M.B.; Ryder, A.; Lobbins, M.; Bhatt, N. Refractory acquired thrombotic thrombocytopenic purpura treated with caplacizumab in a pediatric patient with systemic lupus erythematosus. *Pediatr. Blood Cancer* **2021**, *68*, e28534. [CrossRef]
18. Tripiciano, C.; Zangari, P.; Montanari, M.; Leone, G.; Massella, L.; Garaboldi, L.; Massoud, M.; Lancellotti, S.; Strocchio, L.; Manno, E.C.; et al. Case Report: Two Cases of Pediatric Thrombotic Thrombocytopenic Purpura Treated with Combined Therapy. *Front. Pediatr.* **2021**, *9*, 743206. [CrossRef]
19. Azapağası, E.; Yazici, M.U.; Eroğlu, N.; Albayrak, M.; Kucur, Ö.; Fettah, A. Successful Treatment with Bortezomib for Refractory and Complicated Acquired Thrombotic Thrombocytopenic Purpura in an Adolescent Girl. *J. Pediatr. Hematol. Oncol.* **2021**, *43*, e587–e591. [CrossRef]
20. Dutt, T.; Shaw, R.J.; Stubbs, M.; Yong, J.; Bailiff, B.; Cranfield, T.; Crowley, M.P.; Desborough, M.; Eyre, T.A.; Gooding, R.; et al. Real-world experience with caplacizumab in the management of acute TTP. *Blood* **2021**, *137*, 1731–1740. [CrossRef]
21. Siddiqui, A.; Journeycake, J.M.; Borogovac, A.; George, J.N. Recognizing and managing hereditary and acquired thrombotic thrombocytopenic purpura in infants and children. *Pediatr. Blood Cancer* **2021**, *68*, e28949. [CrossRef] [PubMed]
22. Boudali, J.; Hallak, B.; Haeck, M.; Sellier-Leclerc, A.L.; Ulrich, M.; Coppo, P.; Tellier, S.; Provôt, F. Immune-mediated thrombotic thrombocytopenic purpura in childhood treated by caplacizumab, about 3 cases. *J. Nephrol.* **2022**, *35*, 653–656. [CrossRef] [PubMed]
23. Kirpalani, A.; Garabon, J.; Amos, K.; Patel, S.; Sharma, A.P.; Ganesan, S.L.; Barton, M.; Cacciotti, C.; Leppington, S.; Bakovic, L.; et al. Thrombotic thrombocytopenic purpura temporally associated with BNT162b2 vaccination in an adolescent successfully treated with caplacizumab. *Br. J. Haematol.* **2022**, *196*, e11–e14. [CrossRef]
24. Veltroni, M.; Pegoraro, F.; Scappini, B.; Brugnolo, F.; Allegro, E.; Ermini, S.; Tondo, A.; Fotzi, I.; Bambi, F.; Favre, C. Off-label caplacizumab as add-on therapy in a 9-year-old boy with refractory aTTP. *Ann. Hematol.* **2022**, *101*, 1369–1371. [CrossRef]
25. Reese, J.A.; Muthurajah, D.S.; Hovinga, J.A.K.; Vesely, S.K.; Terrell, D.R.; George, J.N. Children and adults with thrombotic thrombocytopenic purpura associated with severe, acquired Adamts13 deficiency: Comparison of incidence, demographic and clinical features. *Pediatr. Blood Cancer* **2013**, *60*, 1676–1682. [CrossRef] [PubMed]
26. Joly, B.S.; Vanhoorelbeke, K.; Veyradier, A. Understanding therapeutic targets in thrombotic thrombocytopenic purpura. *Intensive Care Med.* **2017**, *43*, 1398–1400. [CrossRef]
27. Zheng, X.L.; Vesely, S.K.; Cataland, S.R.; Coppo, P.; Geldziler, B.; Iorio, A.; Matsumoto, M.; Mustafa, R.A.; Pai, M.; Rock, G.; et al. ISTH guidelines for treatment of thrombotic thrombocytopenic purpura. *J. Thromb. Haemost.* **2020**, *18*, 2496–2502. [CrossRef]
28. Scully, M.; Cataland, S.R.; Peyvandi, F.; Coppo, P.; Knöbl, P.; Hovinga, J.A.K.; Metjian, A.; de la Rubia, G.; Pavenski, K.; Callewaert, F.; et al. Caplacizumab Treatment for Acquired Thrombotic Thrombocytopenic Purpura. *N. Engl. J. Med.* **2019**, *380*, 335–346. [CrossRef]
29. Bergstrand, M.; Hansson, E.; Delaey, B.; Callewaert, F.; De Passos Sousa, R.; Sargentini-Maier, M.L. Caplacizumab Model-Based Dosing Recommendations in Pediatric Patients with Acquired Thrombotic Thrombocytopenic Purpura. *J. Clin. Pharmacol.* **2022**, *62*, 409–421. [CrossRef]
30. Amin Asnafi, A.; Jalali, M.T.; Pezeshki, S.M.S.; Jaseb, K.; Saki, N. The Association Between Human Leukocyte Antigens and ITP, TTP, and HIT. *J. Pediatr. Hematol. Oncol.* **2019**, *41*, 81–86. [CrossRef]

31. Joly, B.S.; Loiseau, P.; Darmon, M.; Leblanc, T.; Chambost, H.; Fouyssac, F.; Guigonis, V.; Harambat, G.; Stepanian, A.; Coppo, P.; et al. HLA-DRB1*11 is a strong risk factor for acquired thrombotic thrombocytopenic purpura in children. *Haematologica* **2020**, *105*, e531. [CrossRef]
32. Hassan, A.; Iqbal, M.; George, J.N. Additional autoimmune disorders in patients with acquired autoimmune thrombotic thrombocytopenic purpura. *Am. J. Hematol.* **2019**, *94*, E172–E174. [CrossRef] [PubMed]
33. Prevel, R.; Roubaud-Baudron, C.; Gourlain, S.; Jamme, M.; Peres, K.; Benhamou, Y.; Galicier, L.; Azoulay, E.; Poullin, P.; Provôt, F.; et al. Immune thrombotic thrombocytopenic purpura in older patients: Prognosis and long-term survival. *Blood* **2019**, *134*, 2209–2217. [CrossRef]
34. Agosti, P.; Mancini, I.; Gianniello, F.; Bucciarelli, P.; Artoni, A.; Ferrari, B.; Pontiggia, S.; Trisolini, S.M.; Facchini, L.; Carbone, C.; et al. Prevalence of the age-related diseases in older patients with acquired thrombotic thrombocytopenic purpura. *Eur. J. Intern. Med.* **2020**, *75*, 79–83. [CrossRef] [PubMed]
35. Schmidt, J.; Zafrani, L.; Lemiale, V.; Stepanian, A.; Joly, B.; Azoulay, E.; Mariotte, E. The clinical picture of thrombotic microangiopathy in patients older than 60 years of age. *Br. J. Haematol.* **2021**, *192*, e25–e28. [CrossRef]
36. Liu, A.; Dhaliwal, N.; Upreti, H.; Kasmani, J.; Dane, K.; Moliterno, A.; Braunstein, E.; Brodsky, R.; Chaturvedi, S. Reduced sensitivity of PLASMIC and French scores for the diagnosis of thrombotic thrombocytopenic purpura in older individuals. *Transfusion* **2021**, *61*, 266–273. [CrossRef]
37. Joseph, A.; Eloit, M.; Azoulay, E.; Kaplanski, G.; Provot, F.; Presne, C.; Wynckel, A.; Grangé, S.; Rondeau; Pène, F.; et al. Immune-mediated thrombotic thrombocytopenic purpura prognosis is affected by blood pressure. *Res. Pract. Thromb. Haemost.* **2022**, *6*, e12702. [CrossRef]
38. Fage, N.; Orvain, C.; Henry, N.; Mellaza, C.; Beloncle, F.; Tuffigo, M.; Geneviève, F.; Coppo, P.; Augusto, J.F.; Brilland, B.; et al. Proteinuria Increases the PLASMIC and French Scores Performance to Predict Thrombotic Thrombocytopenic Purpura in Patients with Thrombotic Microangiopathy Syndrome. *Kidney Int. Rep.* **2022**, *7*, 221–231. [CrossRef]
39. Burguet, L.; Taton, B.; Prezelin-Reydit, M.; Rubin, S.; Picard, W.; Gruson, D.; Ryman, A.; Contin-Bordes, C.; Coppo, P.; Combe, C.; et al. Urine Protein/Creatinine Ratio in Thrombotic Microangiopathies: A Simple Test to Facilitate Thrombotic Thrombocytopenic Purpura and Hemolytic and Uremic Syndrome Diagnosis. *J. Clin. Med.* **2022**, *11*, 648. [CrossRef]
40. Joseph, A.; Brilland, B.; Burguet, L.; Eloit, M.; Fage, N.; Augusto, J.F.; Delmas, Y.; Veyradier, A.; Halimi, J.-M.; Coppo, P. Predictive Scores for Early Identification of Immune-Mediated Thrombotic Thrombocytopenic Purpura: Room for Improvement? *Kidney Int. Rep.* **2022**, *7*, 2541–2542. [CrossRef]
41. Coppo, P.; Bubenheim, M.; Azoulay, E.; Galicier, L.; Malot, S.; Bigé, N.; Poullin, P.; Provôt, F.; Martis, N.; Presne, C.; et al. A regimen with caplacizumab, immunosuppression, and plasma exchange prevents unfavorable outcomes in immune-mediated TTP. *Blood* **2021**, *137*, 733–742. [CrossRef] [PubMed]
42. Agosti, P.; Mancini, I.; Artoni, A.; Ferrari, B.; Pontiggia, S.; Trisolini, S.M.; Facchini, L.; Peyvandi, F.; Italian Group of TTP Investigators. The features of acquired thrombotic thrombocytopenic purpura occurring at advanced age. *Thromb. Res.* **2020**, *187*, 197–201. [CrossRef]
43. De Louw, A.V.; Mariotte, E.; Darmon, M.; Cohrs, A.; Leslie, D.; Azoulay, E. Outcomes in 1096 patients with severe thrombotic thrombocytopenic purpura before the Caplacizumab era. *PLoS ONE* **2021**, *16*, e0256024. [CrossRef]
44. Matsumoto, M.; Bennett, C.L.; Isonishi, A.; Qureshi, Z.; Hori, Y.; Hayakawa, M.; Yoshida, Y.; Yagi, H.; Fujimura, Y. Acquired idiopathic ADAMTS13 activity deficient thrombotic thrombocytopenic purpura in a population from Japan. *PLoS ONE* **2012**, *7*, e33029. [CrossRef] [PubMed]
45. Mariotte, E.; Blet, A.; Galicier, L.; Darmon, M.; Parquet, N.; Lengline, E.; Boutboul, D.; Canet, E.; Traineau, R.; Schlemmer, B.; et al. Unresponsive thrombotic thrombocytopenic purpura in critically ill adults. *Intensive Care Med.* **2013**, *39*, 1272–1281. [CrossRef]
46. Gui, R.; Huang, Q.; Cai, X.; Wu, J.; Liu, H.; Liu, Y.; Yang, L.; Zhang, J.; Cheng, Y.; Jiang, M.; et al. Development and validation of a prediction model (AHC) for early identification of refractory thrombotic thrombocytopenic purpura using nationally representative data. *Br. J. Haematol.* **2020**, *191*, 269–281. [CrossRef] [PubMed]
47. Adeyemi, A.; Razakariasa, F.; Chiorean, A.; de Passos Sousa, R. Epidemiology, treatment patterns, clinical outcomes, and disease burden among patients with immune-mediated thrombotic thrombocytopenic purpura in the United States. *Res. Pract. Thromb. Haemost.* **2022**, *6*, e12802. [CrossRef] [PubMed]
48. Schofield, J.; Shaw, R.J.; Lester, W.; Thomas, W.; Toh, C.H.; Dutt, T. Intracranial hemorrhage in immune thrombotic thrombocytopenic purpura treated with caplacizumab. *J. Thromb. Haemost.* **2021**, *19*, 1922–1925. [CrossRef] [PubMed]
49. Deford, C.C.; Reese, J.A.; Schwartz, L.H.; Perdue, J.J.; Hovinga, J.A.K.; Lämmle, B.; Terrell, D.; Vesely, S.; George, J.N. Multiple major morbidities and increased mortality during long-term follow-up after recovery from thrombotic thrombocytopenic purpura. *Blood* **2013**, *122*, 2023–2029. [CrossRef] [PubMed]
50. Sukumar, S.; Brodsky, M.A.; Hussain, S.; Yanek, L.R.; Moliterno, A.R.; Brodsky, R.A.; Cataland, S.R.; Chaturvedi, S. Cardiovascular disease is a leading cause of mortality among TTP survivors in clinical remission. *Blood Adv.* **2022**, *6*, 1264–1270. [CrossRef]
51. Upreti, H.; Kasmani, J.; Dane, K.; Braunstein, E.M.; Streiff, M.B.; Shanbhag, S.; Moliterno, A.R.; Sperati, C.J.; Gottesman, R.F.; Brodsky, R.A.; et al. Reduced ADAMTS13 activity during TTP remission is associated with stroke in TTP survivors. *Blood* **2019**, *134*, 1037–1045. [CrossRef]
52. Chaturvedi, S.; Abbas, H.; McCrae, K.R. Increased morbidity during long-term follow-up of survivors of thrombotic thrombocytopenic purpura. *Am. J. Hematol.* **2015**, *90*, E208. [CrossRef]

53. Brodsky, M.A.; Sukumar, S.; Selvakumar, S.; Yanek, L.; Hussain, S.; Mazepa, M.A.; Braunstein, E.M.; Moliterno, A.R.; Kickler, T.S.; Brodsky, R.A.; et al. Major adverse cardiovascular events in survivors of immune-mediated thrombotic thrombocytopenic purpura. *Am. J. Hematol.* **2021**, *96*, 1587–1594. [CrossRef]
54. Chaturvedi, S.; Oluwole, O.; Cataland, S.; McCrae, K.R. Post-traumatic stress disorder and depression in survivors of thrombotic thrombocytopenic purpura. *Thromb. Res.* **2017**, *151*, 51–56.
55. Falter, T.; Schmitt, V.; Herold, S.; Weyer, V.; von Auer, C.; Wagner, S.; Hefner, G.; Beutel, M.; Lackner, K.; Lämmle, B.; et al. Depression and cognitive deficits as long-term consequences of thrombotic thrombocytopenic purpura. *Transfusion* **2017**, *57*, 1152–1162. [CrossRef]
56. Han, B.; Page, E.E.; Stewart, L.M.; Deford, C.C.; Scott, J.G.; Schwartz, L.H.; Perdue, J.J.; Terrell, D.R.; Vesely, S.K.; George, J.N. Depression and cognitive impairment following recovery from thrombotic thrombocytopenic purpura. *Am. J. Hematol.* **2015**, *90*, 709–714. [CrossRef]
57. Goldberg, T.E.; Chen, C.; Wang, Y.; Jung, E.; Swanson, A.; Ing, C.; Garcia, P.S.; Whittington, R.A.; Moitra, V. Association of Delirium with Long-term Cognitive Decline: A Meta-analysis. *JAMA Neurol.* **2020**, *77*, 1373–1381. [CrossRef] [PubMed]
58. Wolters, F.J.; Boender, J.; de Vries, P.S.; Sonneveld, M.A.; Koudstaal, P.J.; de Maat, M.P.; Franco, O.H.; Ikram, M.K.; Leebeek, F.W. Von Willebrand factor and ADAMTS13 activity in relation to risk of dementia: A population-based study. *Sci. Rep.* **2018**, *8*, 5474. [CrossRef] [PubMed]
59. Stabler, S.; Giovannelli, J.; Launay, D.; Cotteau-Leroy, A.; Heusele, M.; Lefèvre, G.; Terriou, L.; Lambert, M.; Dubucquoi, S.; Hachulla, E.; et al. Serious Infectious Events and Immunoglobulin Replacement Therapy in Patients with Autoimmune Disease Receiving Rituximab: A Retrospective Cohort Study. *Clin. Infect. Dis.* **2021**, *72*, 727–737. [PubMed]
60. Roriz, M.; Landais, M.; Desprez, J.; Barbet, C.; Azoulay, E.; Galicier, L.; Wynckel, A.; Baudel, J.-L.; Provôt, F.; Pène, F.; et al. Risk Factors for Autoimmune Diseases Development After Thrombotic Thrombocytopenic Purpura. *Medicine* **2015**, *94*, e1598. [CrossRef]
61. Pereira, L.C.V.; Ercig, B.; Kangro, K.; Jamme, M.; Malot, S.; Galicier, L.; Poullin, P.; Provôt, F.; Presne, C.; Kanouni, T.; et al. Understanding the Health Literacy in Patients with Thrombotic Thrombocytopenic Purpura. *Hemasphere* **2020**, *4*, e462. [CrossRef] [PubMed]

Disclaimer/Publisher's Note: The statements, opinions and data contained in all publications are solely those of the individual author(s) and contributor(s) and not of MDPI and/or the editor(s). MDPI and/or the editor(s) disclaim responsibility for any injury to people or property resulting from any ideas, methods, instructions or products referred to in the content.

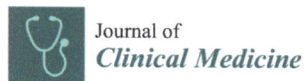

Review

Cardiovascular Disease and Stroke in Immune TTP–Challenges and Opportunities

Senthil Sukumar [1], Marshall A. Mazepa [2] and Shruti Chaturvedi [3,*]

[1] Division of Hematology/Oncology, Department of Medicine, Baylor College of Medicine, Houston, TX 77098, USA; senthil.sukumar@bcm.edu
[2] Division of Hematology, Oncology, and Transplantation, Department of Medicine, University of Minnesota, Minneapolis, MN 55455, USA; mmazepa@umn.edu
[3] Division of Hematology, Department of Medicine, Johns Hopkins University School of Medicine, Baltimore, MD 21287, USA
* Correspondence: schatur3@jhmi.edu; Tel.: +410-502-6686; Fax: +410-955-0185

Abstract: Advances in the management of immune thrombotic thrombocytopenic purpura (iTTP) have dramatically improved outcomes of acute TTP episodes, and TTP is now treated as a chronic, relapsing disorder. It is now recognized that iTTP survivors are at high risk for vascular disease, with stroke and myocardial infarction occurring at younger ages than in the general population, and cardiovascular disease is the leading cause of premature death in this population. iTTP appears to have a phenotype of accelerated vascular aging with a particular predilection for cerebral circulation, and stroke is much more common than myocardial infarction. In addition to traditional cardiovascular risk factors, low ADAMTS13 activity during clinical remission may be a risk factor for some of these outcomes, such as stroke. Recent studies also suggest that Black patients, who are disproportionately affected by iTTP in the United States, are at higher risk of adverse cardiovascular outcomes, likely due to multifactorial reasons. Additional research is required to establish the risk factors and mechanisms underlying these complications in order to institute optimal screening strategies and identify interventions to improve outcomes.

Keywords: TTP; TMA; cardiovascular disease; stroke

Citation: Sukumar, S.; Mazepa, M.A.; Chaturvedi, S. Cardiovascular Disease and Stroke in Immune TTP–Challenges and Opportunities. *J. Clin. Med.* **2023**, *12*, 5961. https://doi.org/10.3390/jcm12185961

Academic Editors: Ilaria Mancini and Andrea Artoni

Received: 29 June 2023
Revised: 29 August 2023
Accepted: 9 September 2023
Published: 14 September 2023

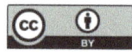

Copyright: © 2023 by the authors. Licensee MDPI, Basel, Switzerland. This article is an open access article distributed under the terms and conditions of the Creative Commons Attribution (CC BY) license (https://creativecommons.org/licenses/by/4.0/).

1. Introduction

Nearly a century ago, Eli Moschowitz described the case of a 16-year-old girl with fever and hemolytic anemia accompanied by progressive neurologic dysfunction resulting in coma and ultimately death, which is now recognized as the first description of thrombotic thrombocytopenic purpura (TTP) [1]. Over the last century, our understanding of this devastating condition has evolved immensely. Severe deficiency of the von Willebrand factor-cleaving protease, ADAMTS13, which leads to the formation of VWF–platelet microthrombi, has been elucidated as the underlying mechanism of TTP [2]. TTP may be congenital due to biallelic pathogenic mutations in ADAMTS13 or due to an antibody against ADAMTS13. This review focuses on immune-mediated TTP (iTTP), which is more common and represents 95% of TTP. Mortality of acute TTP episodes has reduced from >90% to <10% with rapid diagnosis and prompt treatment with plasma exchange and immunosuppression [3,4]. With a growing population of TTP survivors, immune-mediated TTP (iTTP) is recognized as a chronic disorder that requires long-term care [5–8]. Importantly, iTTP is a thrombotic vascular disorder, and thromboembolic events such as stroke are a leading cause of mortality and morbidity in acute iTTP [9,10]. Even after surviving acute iTTP, survivors have shortened overall survival, with a nearly two-fold increased rate of mortality when compared to an age-, sex-, and race-matched control population [11,12]. Cardiovascular disease is a leading driver of this increase in mortality [11,12]. Recent epidemiological investigations in both congenital and immune TTP reveal a pattern of accelerated vascular disease and early ischemic events, such as stroke and myocardial infarction, that contribute to mortality and morbidity [13–17]. In this review, we discuss the epidemiology of cardiovascular disease in iTTP, potential risk factors and underlying mechanisms, and review opportunities to improve cardiovascular outcomes in this vulnerable population.

2. Cardiovascular Involvement in Acute iTTP

Cardiac involvement in acute episodes of iTTP is heterogeneous and underrecognized [10,18]. Cardiac arrest and myocardial infarction are the most common immediate causes of death in iTTP, and autopsy studies commonly show cardiac involvement [9]. Microthrombosis is the most common finding in autopsy studies, which is the most likely mechanism of ischemic cardiac injury in iTTP [19]. In a systematic review of 111 patients with iTTP, Hawkins et al. reported that the most common cardiac symptoms in iTTP were chest pain (11.7%), CHF (9.0%), and syncope (0.9%), and the most frequent clinical cardiac events were myocardial infarction (23.4%), congestive heart failure (15.3%), arrhythmias (9.0%), cardiogenic shock (5.4%), and sudden cardiac death (7.2%). Overall acute MI rates of approximately 5–15% have been reported in acute iTTP, and non-ST segment elevation MI is more common than ST segment elevation MI [20,21]. While a smaller study did not find an association of traditional risk factors with MI in iTTP, a larger analysis from the United States Nationwide Inpatient Sample suggests that older age, smoking, known coronary artery disease, and congestive heart failure are associated with increased risk of MI with acute iTTP, and overt cardiovascular complications are associated with substantially higher in-hospital mortality [21,22]. Even patients without overt symptoms may have cardiac involvement of iTTP evidenced by troponin elevation and electrocardiogram changes [23]. Troponinemia is associated with acute mortality and refractoriness in iTTP [23,24]. Given the association of symptomatic and asymptomatic cardiac involvement with adverse outcomes in acute iTTP [25], and the contribution of cardiac events as a proximate cause of death [10], we suggest that all patients should undergo at least baseline evaluation with cardiac troponin measurement and an electrocardiogram. Patients with confirmed cardiac involvement may benefit from added telemetry and echocardiography during the acute episode [26].

The management of acute MI in iTTP is made more challenging by coexisting thrombocytopenia and drugs such as caplacizumab, which increase bleeding risk and may preclude aggressive antithrombotic measures. Most patients with non-ST elevation MI can be managed with iTTP-directed therapy, along with medical management of MI with beta-blockers and vasodilators, with the consideration of adding antiplatelet therapy once the platelet count increases to over $30–50^9$/L. Antiplatelet therapy appears to be safe in iTTP. In the seminal trial that established plasma exchange as the standard treatment for iTTP [4], all the patients received either aspirin or dipyridamole; however, the safety of aspirin in patients who are also receiving caplacizumab, a novel anti-VWF nanobody approved for acute iTTP, needs to be established [27]. Caplacizumab binds to the A1 domain of VWF, thus preventing VWF platelet interactions and consequently inhibiting the formation of microthrombi; however, as a result of this mechanism of action, caplacizumab also increases bleeding risk. Targeted coronary interventions have not been widely studied in the context of acute iTTP, which is not surprising since iTTP is an extremely rare, high-risk disorder. However, successful percutaneous coronary intervention has been reported in iTTP with acute STEMI [28].

While neurologic symptoms such as headache and altered mental status attributed to microvascular injury are most commonly recognized in acute iTTP, stroke is reported in 5–10% of acute iTTP episodes [7,29]. The pattern of stroke is heterogeneous, affecting different parts of the cerebral circulation, and is multifocal in 30–40% [30]. When a stroke occurs in the context of acute iTTP, the mainstay of treatment is treatment of the iTTP with plasma exchange and immunosuppression. Similar to acute MI, stroke-specific interventions have not been studied widely in the setting of iTTP. Measures such as thrombolysis carry increased bleeding risk in patients with thrombocytopenia, but rare cases of stroke in iTTP treated with thrombolysis have been reported.

3. Cardiovascular Disease Burden in Chronic iTTP

3.1. Cardiovascular Disease Contributes to Shortened Survival in iTTP Survivors

Recent reports from multiple iTTP registries show that iTTP survivors are at a higher risk of premature death and, rather than acute iTTP relapse, cardiovascular disease is the leading cause of mortality and morbidity (Table 1) [6,11,12]. For example, of 57 patients followed after iTTP diagnosis in the Oklahoma iTTP registry, 19% died over a median follow-up of 7.8 years, which is higher than expected based on age- and sex-matched U.S. or Oklahoma reference populations [6,11]. The majority (64%) of deaths were attributed to cardiovascular and/or cerebrovascular complications, while only 18% of deaths were attributed to iTTP relapse [6]. Subsequently, we compiled a 222-patient cohort from the Johns Hopkins University and Ohio State University, which also had higher all-cause mortality in iTTP survivors compared to age- and sex-matched reference populations [12]. Similar to the Oklahoma registry, cardiovascular disease (27.6%, 8 of 29) and iTTP relapse (27.6%, 8 of 29) were the leading causes of death [12]. Finally, Prevel et al. reported that older (>60 years) iTTP patients in the French iTTP registry had increased short- and long-term mortality [31]. In addition to the iTTP diagnosis itself, traditional cardiovascular risk factors such as male sex, diabetes, tobacco use, malignancy, hypertension, cerebrovascular events, dementia, and COPD were risk factors for one-year mortality among older iTTP survivors [31].

3.2. Epidemiology of Stroke and Myocardial Infarction in iTTP Survivors

In a cohort of 137 iTTP survivors followed for a median observation period of 3.08 years, the risk of stroke during clinical remission was increased nearly five-fold (13.1% vs. 2.6%) compared with an age- and sex-matched control population, and this risk was strongly associated with suboptimal ADAMTS13 recovery during clinical remission [15]. Subsequently, we showed that major adverse cardiovascular events (stroke, non-fatal and fatal MI, and cardiac revascularization) occurred in 24% of iTTP survivors followed for a median of 7.6 years [14]. This rate is more than double previously reported high-risk cohorts including populations with known underlying vascular disease or genetic predispositions [32,33]. Notably, stroke was much more common than myocardial infarction (18.2% vs. 6.8%), a pattern that has also been reported in patients with congenital iTTP, who have a much higher burden of stroke compared to cardiac ischemic disease [13–17]. Additionally, neurologic involvement is also more common in acute iTTP. These observations suggest that the brain is particularly vulnerable to TTP-associated (or ADAMTS13 deficiency-associated) vascular injury. Finally, the age at the first MACE event was 1–2 decades younger than the age at the first MACE event in populations without iTTP [34]. These differences are more striking in young female iTTP survivors, who would not typically be considered at high risk for MACE events compared with usual at-risk populations such as older males. For example, age at first stroke event was younger for individuals with iTTP than individuals in the general population without iTTP for both males (56.5 years versus 68.6 years, $p = 0.031$) and females (49.7 years versus 72.9 years, $p < 0.001$). Similarly, the mean age at first myocardial infarction was lower for males (56.5 years versus 65.6 years, $p < 0.001$) and females (53.1 years versus 72.0 years, $p < 0.001$) with iTTP compared with individuals in the general population without iTTP [14]. This pattern of early cerebrovascular disease has also been reported in cTTP, suggesting that TTP or ADAMTS13 deficiency is characterized by a phenotype of accelerated vascular aging.

3.3. Silent Cerebral Infarction in iTTP Survivors and Impact on Functional Outcomes

Most recently, a study reported that in a prospectively enrolled cohort of iTTP survivors, 50% demonstrated silent cerebral infarction, which is defined as magnetic resonance imaging (MRI) evidence of brain ischemic infarction without a corresponding neuro-deficit [35]. Silent cerebral infarction was strongly associated with cognitive impairment, including both major and mild cognitive impairment [35]. Given that silent cerebral infarctions are a risk factor for both cognitive impairment [36] and stroke [37] in the general population, it is likely that silent cerebral infarction also contributes to neurocognitive deficits that are a common complaint in TTP survivors (60–80%) [38–42]. Similar to stroke, the rate of silent cerebral infarction in this relatively young iTTP cohort with a median age of 48 years was much higher than in older cohorts of individuals without iTTP, where the prevalence of silent cerebral infarction ranges from approximately 10% to 20% at a mean age of 60–70 years and increases with age [43–49]. While this was a small study that did not measure serial ADAMTS13 activity for the entire period since iTTP diagnosis, the patients with SCI had lower mean ADAMTS13 activity than those without SCI in the year preceding evaluation, suggesting again that lower remission ADAMTS13 activity contributes to the risk of cerebrovascular disease in iTTP survivors. The findings of this study are also supported by a previous study from Ohio State University and University College London that reported ischemic findings on brain MRI in 9 of 23 patients with iTTP in clinical remission [41]. Silent cerebral infarction is a risk factor for stroke in the general population [37,50] and individuals with sickle cell disease [51]. This observation as well as shared risk factors with stroke, such as increasing age and hypertension, suggest that silent cerebral infarction is on the spectrum of cerebrovascular disease that culminates in stroke. Moreover, the strong association of silent cerebral infarction with cognitive impairment makes it an attractive target for interventions aimed at reducing neurocognitive morbidity in iTTP survivors.

3.4. Factors Contributing to Risk of CV Disease in iTTP

Multiple heterogeneous factors, both related to iTTP as well as other patient characteristics and comorbidities, contribute to the increased risk of cardiovascular disease in iTTP (Figure 1) In a retrospective cohort study from the United States, increasing age and diabetes mellitus were associated with increased rates of MACE in iTTP survivors [14]. This study did not find an association between other traditional risk factors for MACE such as hypertension, obesity, and CKD; however, this may be due to the relatively small sample size. In contrast, a report from the French iTTP registry found that older iTTP patients had 3.4 times higher long-term mortality compared with an age-matched reference population from the same geographic area (a population-based cohort on aging and dementia, the Three City Study) and attributed shortened survival to coexisting disorders, such as hypertension, depression, and cognitive decline [31]. Coupled with the finding that cardiovascular disease is a leading cause of death, these findings suggest that these comorbidities may contribute to lower survival in iTTP survivors. Indeed, compared to a reference population, iTTP survivors have higher rates of comorbidities such as autoimmune disorders [6], obesity [6], hypertension [6], and depression, which are recognized as predictors of all-cause and cardiovascular mortality [52]. The factors driving the higher prevalence of these comorbidities in iTTP are complex and incompletely understood. iTTP is associated with depression and other mood disorders, which are independent risk factors for obesity [53], which may in turn increase cardiovascular morbidity [54]. Obesity is also a risk factor for hypertension, cardiovascular disease, and mortality [55,56]. iTTP more commonly affects women and Black people, the same patient demographic susceptible to autoimmune conditions like SLE [57,58]. In the single study that examined risk factors for major adverse cardiovascular events in iTTP in the United States, Black patients had a 2.3 times higher hazard of adverse cardiovascular events than White patients with iTTP [14]. However, race is not simply a biological construct and is often a surrogate for socioeconomic status, education level, access to resources, and other social determinants of health that have marked impacts on the risk of chronic disease development, as well as overall survival [59,60]. These factors likely also contribute to the increased risk of relapse in Black TTP survivors, which may in turn increase their risk for cardiovascular events.

Recent research links racism and discrimination to chronic stress [61], which can have an independent effect on promoting autoimmunity and inflammation [62,63].

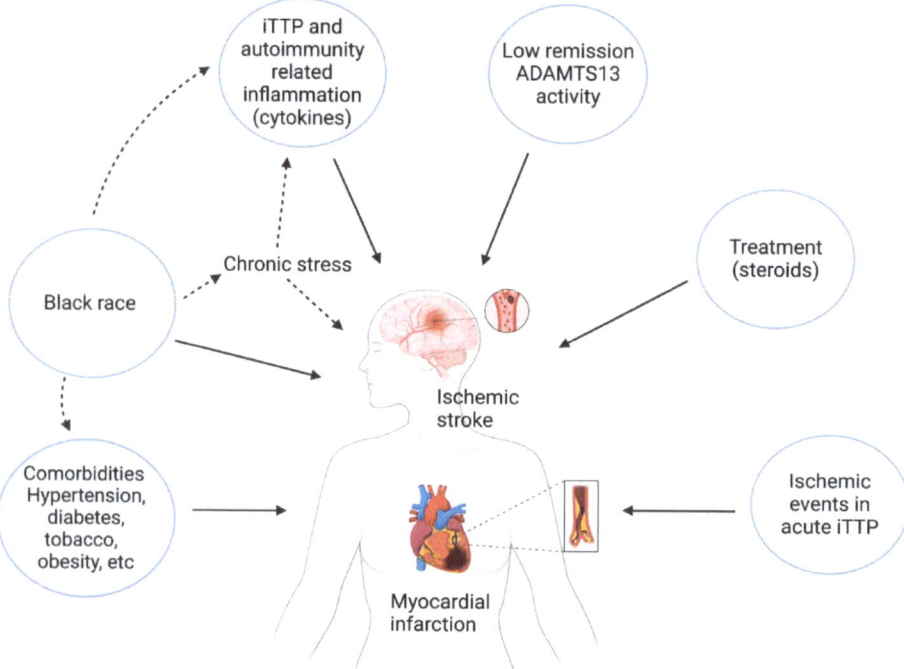

Figure 1. Potential risk factors for cardiovascular disease (stroke and myocardial infarction) in individuals with immune thrombotic thrombocytopenic purpura.

One of the more provocative findings from observational studies is the association of lower remission ADAMTS13 activity in iTTP survivors with a number of adverse health outcomes, including stroke [15], silent cerebral infarction [35], and a trend towards higher all-cause mortality [12]. Thus, patients with both immune and congenital TTP, who share a phenotype of partial or complete ADAMTS13 deficiency, develop accelerated vascular aging and atherosclerosis that predominantly affects the cerebral circulation. The rate of vascular events, particularly stroke, is higher than expected based on traditional risk factors. In this setting, remission ADAMTS13 activity is an attractive biomarker to explain the additional risk. This premise is also supported by large population-based cohort studies from the Netherlands, where lower ADAMTS13 activity has been identified as a risk factor for coronary heart disease, stroke, and all-cause and cardiovascular mortality [64–66]. The potential mechanism for these findings is that lower ADAMTS13 levels lead to an accumulation of larger, more physiologically active von Willebrand factor multimers that promote platelet activation [67], complement activation [68,69], and accelerate atherosclerosis [65,66,70,71]. This may be pronounced among iTTP survivors, who often do not fully recover ADAMTS13 activity during clinical remission (dubbed partial or incomplete ADAMTS13 remission) [64,72].

3.5. Future Directions—Opportunities to Improve Cardiovascular and Neurologic Outcomes

The pathobiology and risk factors for cerebrovascular disease and cardiac ischemia are diverse, and thus potential therapeutic avenues are also diverse and will depend on the phase of the disease (acute iTTP versus remission) and an individual patient's risk factors. During acute iTTP, microthrombi due to iTTP itself are the main cause of ischemic injury to the brain, heart, and other organs. Cardiovascular assessment and the management of acute MI or stroke during acute iTTP have been discussed above. Novel agents such as caplacizumab that target VWF and theoretically reduce microthrombi formation have been developed and are approved for use in acute iTTP [73]. While clinical trials of caplacizumab did not specifically examine ischemic events as a primary outcome, the Phase 3 HERCULES trial did show that normalization of markers associated with organ damage (including cardiac troponin I) occurred sooner among patients who received caplacizumab than among those who received a placebo [73]. Whether caplacizumab reduces clinically significant cardiac or cerebral ischemia has not been evaluated. It is plausible that the ischemic insults of acute iTTP may be reduced by the prompt use of therapies targeting microthrombi, such as the anti-VWF nanobody, caplacizumab (and novel agents under development such as Microlyse, a VWF-targeting thrombolytic fusion protein) [74]. Analogous to the use of thrombolytics in acute stroke and myocardial infarction, these VWF/microthrombi-targeting drugs may not prevent all ischemic injury but are likely to reduce it, which still needs to be shown in clinical studies.

Remission ADAMTS13 activity is also an attractive therapeutic target because of its association with stroke and other vascular diseases, and the availability and long experience with immunosuppressive agents that target anti-ADAMTS13 antibodies and can help increase ADAMTS13 activity levels. Current iTTP management strategies use pre-emptive rituximab during ADAMTS13 relapse to target ADAMTS13 activity > 10–20% to prevent relapse [75]. However, higher ADAMTS13-target activity might mitigate iTTP-related cardiovascular morbidity, which needs to be studied and the optimal ADAMTS13 target needs to be established. Antiplatelet or antithrombotic therapy are also attractive approaches to reduce cardiovascular morbidity but have not been specifically studied in iTTP. Until more data on these approaches are available, it is reasonable to screen for and modify any cardiovascular risk factors.

Table 1. Summary of studies reporting cardiovascular outcomes in iTTP in clinical remission.

Study	Site (s)	N	Female Sex	Race	Median Age (Years)	Median Follow-Up	Cardiovascular Outcomes
Deford 2013 [6]	Oklahoma Registry	57	79%	White: 63% Black: 37%	39 (range 9–71)	7.8 years	19% mortality
Upreti 2019 [15]	Johns Hopkins Registry	137	67.9%	White: 38% Black: 62%	48.8 (IQR 35.3, 60.3)	3.08 years	Stroke during remission in 13.1%
Brodsky 2021 [14]	Ohio State University and Johns Hopkins Registries	181	71.3%	White: 45.9% Black: 53% Other: 1.1%	39 (IQR 27–51)	7.6 years	23.7% MACE rate in clinical remission.
Sukumar 2022 [12]	Ohio State University and Johns Hopkins Registries	222	70.3%	White: 46.8% Black: 50.5% Other: 2.7%	42 (IQR 29–55)	4.5 years	Mortality 222.8 per 100 patient-years (1.8 times higher than age and sex-matched control cohort). Cardiovascular disease and iTTP relapse (27.6% each) were leading causes of death.
Chaturvedi 2023 [35]	Neurologic Sequelae of iTTP (NeST) Study, Johns Hopkins	36	64.3%	White: 14.3% Black: 66.7% Other: 4.8%	48 (IQR 34–56)	5.5 (IQR 1.5–9.3)	50% had silent cerebral infarction on brain MRI

TTP—thrombotic thrombocytopenic purpura. MACE—Major adverse cardiovascular events (any myocardial infarction, stroke, cardiac revascularization). SCI—silent cerebral infarction.

Our current clinical practice is to pursue aggressive cardiovascular risk factor management by (1) screening for and optimizing management of common risk factors like hypertension and hyperlipidemia, including referral to the appropriate specialists as needed, (2) starting aspirin in patients with low bleeding risk who have known coronary artery disease or peripheral vascular disease, history of stroke (including stroke during acute iTTP), are active smokers, have diabetes mellitus, lupus, or a >10% estimated risk of cardiovascular disease at 10 years, though traditional risk calculators may underestimate risk in iTTP. There are currently no data to guide whether all patients with iTTP should undergo additional tests such as cardiac echocardiography, MRI, or brain MRI in clinical remission, and our practice is to do these studies only when clinically indicated or in the research setting. Ultimately, additional research is required to establish the risk factors and mechanisms underlying long-term cardiovascular complications in iTTP and to establish optimal screening strategies and interventions to improve outcomes that can be tested in clinical trials. Future clinical trials of novel agents for iTTP should also evaluate short- and long-term organ damage that is clinically relevant. Given the rarity of iTTP, this will require multicenter studies, with national and international collaboration, and the support and collaboration of patient advocacy groups.

Author Contributions: S.S. and S.C. wrote the paper; M.A.M. critically reviewed the manuscript. All authors have read and agreed to the published version of the manuscript.

Funding: This work was supported by the National Institutes of Health (NIH), Heart, Lung, and Blood Institute grant K99HL150594 (S.C.) and an ASH Scholar Award (S.C.).

Institutional Review Board Statement: Institutional review board was not required for a review paper.

Informed Consent Statement: No enrollment of participants for the purposes of this paper so informed consent is not applicable.

Data Availability Statement: No primary data were generated for this manuscript.

Conflicts of Interest: S.S. has served on advisory boards for Sanofi-Genzyme. S.C. has served on advisory boards and as a consultant for Alexion, Sanofi-Genzyme, and Takeda.

References

1. Moschcowitz, E. An acute febrile pleiochromic anemia with hyaline thrombosis of the terminal arterioles and capillaries: An undescribed disease. 1925. *Mt. Sinai J. Med.* **2003**, *70*, 352–355. [PubMed]
2. Joly, B.S.; Coppo, P.; Veyradier, A. Thrombotic thrombocytopenic purpura. *Blood* **2017**, *129*, 2836–2846. [CrossRef] [PubMed]
3. Bell, W.R.; Braine, H.G.; Ness, P.M.; Kickler, T.S. Improved survival in thrombotic thrombocytopenic purpura–hemolytic uremic syndrome. Clinical experience in 108 patients. *N. Engl. J. Med.* **1991**, *325*, 398–403. [CrossRef] [PubMed]
4. Rock, G.A.; Shumak, K.H.; Buskard, N.A.; Blanchette, V.S.; Kelton, J.G.; Nair, R.C.; Spasoff, R.A.; Canadian Apheresis Study Group. Comparison of plasma exchange with plasma infusion in the treatment of thrombotic thrombocytopenic purpura. Canadian Apheresis Study Group. *N. Engl. J. Med.* **1991**, *325*, 393–397. [CrossRef] [PubMed]
5. Chaturvedi, S.; Abbas, H.; McCrae, K.R. Increased morbidity during long-term follow-up of survivors of thrombotic thrombocytopenic purpura. *Am. J. Hematol.* **2015**, *90*, E208. [CrossRef] [PubMed]
6. Deford, C.C.; Reese, J.A.; Schwartz, L.H.; Perdue, J.J.; Hovinga, J.A.K.; Lämmle, B.; Terrell, D.R.; Vesely, S.K.; George, J.N. Multiple major morbidities and increased mortality during long-term follow-up after recovery from thrombotic thrombocytopenic purpura. *Blood* **2013**, *122*, 2023–2029, quiz 2142. [CrossRef] [PubMed]
7. Page, E.E.; Hovinga, J.A.K.; Terrell, D.R.; Vesely, S.K.; George, J.N. Thrombotic thrombocytopenic purpura: Diagnostic criteria, clinical features, and long-term outcomes from 1995 through 2015. *Blood Adv.* **2017**, *1*, 590–600. [CrossRef]
8. Selvakumar, S.; Liu, A.; Chaturvedi, S. Immune thrombotic thrombocytopenic purpura: Spotlight on long-term outcomes and survivorship. *Front. Med.* **2023**, *10*, 1137019. [CrossRef]
9. Nichols, L.; Berg, A.; Rollins-Raval, M.A.; Raval, J.S. Cardiac injury is a common postmortem finding in thrombotic thrombocytopenic purpura patients: Is empiric cardiac monitoring and protection needed? *Ther. Apher. Dial.* **2015**, *19*, 87–92. [CrossRef]
10. Wiernek, S.L.; Jiang, B.; Gustafson, G.M.; Dai, X. Cardiac implications of thrombotic thrombocytopenic purpura. *World J. Cardiol.* **2018**, *10*, 254–266. [CrossRef]
11. George, J.N. TTP: Long-term outcomes following recovery. *Hematol. Am. Soc. Hematol. Educ. Program* **2018**, *2018*, 548–552. [CrossRef] [PubMed]

12. Sukumar, S.; Brodsky, M.A.; Hussain, S.; Yanek, L.R.; Moliterno, A.R.; Brodsky, R.A.; Cataland, S.R.; Chaturvedi, S. Cardiovascular disease is a leading cause of mortality among TTP survivors in clinical remission. *Blood Adv.* **2022**, *6*, 1264–1270. [CrossRef] [PubMed]
13. Borogovac, A.; George, J.N. Stroke and myocardial infarction in hereditary thrombotic thrombocytopenic purpura: Similarities to sickle cell anemia. *Blood Adv.* **2019**, *3*, 3973–3976. [CrossRef] [PubMed]
14. Brodsky, M.A.; Sukumar, S.; Selvakumar, S.; Yanek, L.; Hussain, S.; Mazepa, M.A.; Braunstein, E.M.; Moliterno, A.R.; Kickler, T.S.; Brodsky, R.A.; et al. Major adverse cardiovascular events in survivors of immune-mediated thrombotic thrombocytopenic purpura. *Am. J. Hematol.* **2021**, *96*, 1587–1594. [CrossRef] [PubMed]
15. Upreti, H.; Kasmani, J.; Dane, K.; Braunstein, E.M.; Streiff, M.B.; Shanbhag, S.; Moliterno, A.R.; Sperati, C.J.; Gottesman, R.F.; Brodsky, R.A.; et al. Reduced ADAMTS13 activity during TTP remission is associated with stroke in TTP survivors. *Blood* **2019**, *134*, 1037–1045. [CrossRef] [PubMed]
16. Alwan, F.; Vendramin, C.; Liesner, R.; Clark, A.; Lester, W.; Dutt, T.; Thomas, W.; Gooding, R.; Biss, T.; Watson, H.G.; et al. Characterization and treatment of congenital thrombotic thrombocytopenic purpura. *Blood* **2019**, *133*, 1644–1651. [CrossRef] [PubMed]
17. van Dorland, H.A.; Taleghani, M.M.; Sakai, K.; Friedman, K.D.; George, J.N.; Hrachovinova, I.; Knöbl, P.N.; von Krogh, A.S.; Schneppenheim, R.; Aebi-Huber, I.; et al. The International Hereditary Thrombotic Thrombocytopenic Purpura Registry: Key findings at enrollment until 2017. *Haematologica* **2019**, *104*, 2107–2115. [CrossRef]
18. Morici, N.; Cantoni, S.; Panzeri, F.; Sacco, A.; Rusconi, C.; Stucchi, M.; Oliva, F.; Cattaneo, M. von Willebrand factor and its cleaving protease ADAMTS13 balance in coronary artery vessels: Lessons learned from thrombotic thrombocytopenic purpura. A narrative review. *Thromb. Res.* **2017**, *155*, 78–85. [CrossRef]
19. Hawkins, B.M.; Abu-Fadel, M.; Vesely, S.K.; George, J.N. Clinical cardiac involvement in thrombotic thrombocytopenic purpura: A systematic review. *Transfusion* **2008**, *48*, 382–392. [CrossRef]
20. Wahla, A.S.; Ruiz, J.; Noureddine, N.; Upadhya, B.; Sane, D.C.; Owen, J. Myocardial infarction in thrombotic thrombocytopenic purpura: A single-center experience and literature review. *Eur. J. Haematol.* **2008**, *81*, 311–316. [CrossRef]
21. Balasubramaniyam, N.; Kolte, D.; Palaniswamy, C.; Yalamanchili, K.; Aronow, W.S.; McClung, J.A.; Khera, S.; Sule, S.; Peterson, S.J.; Frishman, W.H. Predictors of in-hospital mortality and acute myocardial infarction in thrombotic thrombocytopenic purpura. *Am. J. Med.* **2013**, *126*, 1016.e1–1016.e7. [CrossRef] [PubMed]
22. Balasubramaniyam, N.; Yandrapalli, S.; Kolte, D.; Pemmasani, G.; Janakiram, M.; Frishman, W.H. Cardiovascular Complications and Their Association with Mortality in Patients with Thrombotic Thrombocytopenic Purpura. *Am. J. Med.* **2020**, *134*, e89–e97. [CrossRef] [PubMed]
23. Hughes, C.; McEwan, J.R.; Longair, I.; Hughes, S.; Cohen, H.; Machin, S.; Scully, M. Cardiac involvement in acute thrombotic thrombocytopenic purpura: Association with troponin T and IgG antibodies to ADAMTS 13. *J. Thromb. Haemost.* **2009**, *7*, 529–536. [CrossRef] [PubMed]
24. Benhamou, Y.; Boelle, P.Y.; Baudin, B.; Ederhy, S.; Gras, J.; Galicier, L.; Patricia, Z. Cardiac troponin-I on diagnosis predicts early death and refractoriness in acquired thrombotic thrombocytopenic purpura. Experience of the French Thrombotic Microangiopathies Reference Center. *J. Thromb. Haemost.* **2015**, *13*, 293–302. [CrossRef] [PubMed]
25. Goel, R.; King, K.E.; Takemoto, C.M.; Ness, P.M.; Tobian, A.A. Prognostic risk-stratified score for predicting mortality in hospitalized patients with thrombotic thrombocytopenic purpura: Nationally representative data from 2007 to 2012. *Transfusion* **2016**, *56*, 1451–1458. [CrossRef] [PubMed]
26. American College of Cardiology Foundation Appropriate Use Criteria Task Force; American Society of Echocardiography; American Heart Association; American Society of Nuclear Cardiology; Heart Failure Society of America; Heart Rhythm Society; Society for Cardiovascular Angiography and Interventions; Society of Critical Care Medicine; Society of Cardiovascular Computed Tomography; Society for Cardiovascular Magnetic Resonance; et al. ACCF/ASE/AHA/ASNC/HFSA/HRS/SCAI/SCCM/SCCT/SCMR 2011 Appropriate Use Criteria for Echocardiography. A Report of the American College of Cardiology Foundation Appropriate Use Criteria Task Force, American Society of Echocardiography, American Heart Association, American Society of Nuclear Cardiology, Heart Failure Society of America, Heart Rhythm Society, Society for Cardiovascular Angiography and Interventions, Society of Critical Care Medicine, Society of Cardiovascular Computed Tomography, Society for Cardiovascular Magnetic Resonance American College of Chest Physicians. *J. Am. Soc. Echocardiogr.* **2011**, *24*, 229–267.
27. Elverdi, T.; Ozer Cerme, M.D.; Aydin, T.; Eskazan, A.E. Do patients with immune-mediated thrombotic thrombocytopenic purpura receiving caplacizumab need antithrombotic therapy? *Expert. Rev. Clin. Pharmacol.* **2021**, *14*, 1183–1188. [CrossRef]
28. Ho, H.H.; Minutello, R.; Juliano, N.; Wong, S.C. A rare cause of acute myocardial infarction: Thrombotic thrombocytopenic purpura. *Int. J. Cardiol.* **2009**, *133*, e1–e2. [CrossRef]
29. Scully, M.; Yarranton, H.; Liesner, R.; Cavenagh, J.; Hunt, B.; Benjamin, S.; Bevan, D.; Mackie, I.; Machin, S. Regional UK TTP registry: Correlation with laboratory ADAMTS 13 analysis and clinical features. *Br. J. Haematol.* **2008**, *142*, 819–826. [CrossRef]
30. Tomich, C.; Debruxelles, S.; Delmas, Y.; Sagnier, S.; Poli, M.; Olindo, S.; Renou, P.; Rouanet, F.; Sibon, I. Immune-Thrombotic Thrombocytopenic Purpura is a Rare Cause of Ischemic Stroke in Young Adults: Case Reports and Literature Review. *J. Stroke Cerebrovasc. Dis.* **2018**, *27*, 3163–3171. [CrossRef]

31. Prevel, R.; Roubaud-Baudron, C.; Gourlain, S.; Jamme, M.; Peres, K.; Benhamou, Y.; Galicier, L.; Azoulay, E.; Poullin, P.; Provôt, F.; et al. Immune thrombotic thrombocytopenic purpura in older patients: Prognosis and long-term survival. *Blood* **2019**, *134*, 2209–2217. [CrossRef] [PubMed]
32. Berger, A.; Simpson, A.; Bhagnani, T.; Leeper, N.J.; Murphy, B.; Nordstrom, B.; Ting, W.; Zhao, Q.; Berger, J.S. Incidence and Cost of Major Adverse Cardiovascular Events and Major Adverse Limb Events in Patients with Chronic Coronary Artery Disease or Peripheral Artery Disease. *Am. J. Cardiol.* **2019**, *123*, 1893–1899. [CrossRef] [PubMed]
33. Choi, B.G.; Rha, S.; Yoon, S.G.; Choi, C.U.; Lee, M.W.; Kim, S.W. Association of Major Adverse Cardiac Events up to 5 Years in Patients with Chest Pain Without Significant Coronary Artery Disease in the Korean Population. *J. Am. Heart Assoc.* **2019**, *8*, e010541. [CrossRef] [PubMed]
34. Virani, S.S.; Alonso, A.; Aparicio, H.J.; Benjamin, E.J.; Bittencourt, M.S.; Callaway, C.W.; Tsao, C.W. Heart Disease and Stroke Statistics—2021 Update: A Report from the American Heart Association. *Circulation* **2021**, *143*, CIR0000000000000950. [CrossRef] [PubMed]
35. Chaturvedi, S.; Yu, J.; Brown, J.; Wei, A.; Gerber, G.; Pan, X.Z.; Chaturvedi, S. Silent cerebral infarction during immune TTP remission—prevalence, predictors, and impact on cognition. *Blood* **2023**, *140* (Suppl. S1), 338–340. [CrossRef] [PubMed]
36. Sigurdsson, S.; Aspelund, T.; Kjartansson, O.; Gudmundsson, E.F.; Jonsdottir, M.K.; Eiriksdottir, G.; Launer, L.J. Incidence of Brain Infarcts, Cognitive Change, and Risk of Dementia in the General Population: The AGES-Reykjavik Study (Age Gene/Environment Susceptibility-Reykjavik Study). *Stroke* **2017**, *48*, 2353–2360. [CrossRef] [PubMed]
37. Gupta, A.; Giambrone, A.; Gialdini, G.; Finn, C.B.; Delgado, D.; Gutierrez, J.; Wright, C.; Beiser, A.B.; Seshadri, S.; Pandya, A.; et al. Abstract WP165: Silent Brain Infarction and Risk of Future Stroke: A Systematic Review and Meta-Analysis. *Stroke* **2016**, *47*, 719–725. [CrossRef]
38. Howard, M.A.; Duvall, D.; Terrell, D.R.; Christopher, A.T.; Thomas, I.; Holloway, N.; Vesely, S.K.; George, J.N. A support group for patients who have recovered from thrombotic thrombocytopenic purpura-hemolytic uremic syndrome (TTP-HUS): The six-year experience of the Oklahoma TTP-HUS Study Group. *J. Clin. Apher.* **2003**, *18*, 16–20. [CrossRef]
39. George, J.N.; Terrell, D.R.; Swisher, K.K.; Vesely, S.K. Lessons learned from the oklahoma thrombotic thrombocytopenic purpura-hemolytic uremic syndrome registry. *J. Clin. Apher.* **2008**, *23*, 129–137. [CrossRef]
40. Kennedy, A.S.; Lewis, Q.F.; Scott, J.G.; Hovinga, J.A.K.; Lämmle, B.; Terrell, D.R.; Vesely, S.K.; George, J.N. Cognitive deficits after recovery from thrombotic thrombocytopenic purpura. *Transfusion* **2009**, *49*, 1092–1101. [CrossRef]
41. Cataland, S.R.; Scully, M.A.; Paskavitz, J.; Maruff, P.; Witkoff, L.; Jin, M.; Wu, H.M. Evidence of persistent neurologic injury following thrombotic thrombocytopenic purpura. *Am. J. Hematol.* **2011**, *86*, 87–89. [CrossRef] [PubMed]
42. Falter, T.; Schmitt, V.; Herold, S.; Weyer, V.; von Auer, C.; Wagner, S.; Hefner, G.; Beutel, M.; Lackner, K.; Lämmle, B.; et al. Depression and cognitive deficits as long-term consequences of thrombotic thrombocytopenic purpura. *Transfusion* **2017**, *57*, 1152–1162. [CrossRef] [PubMed]
43. Vermeer, S.E.; Koudstaal, P.J.; Oudkerk, M.; Hofman, A.; Breteler, M.M. Prevalence and risk factors of silent brain infarcts in the population-based rotterdam scan study. *Stroke* **2002**, *33*, 21–25. [CrossRef] [PubMed]
44. Schmidt, R.; Schmidt, H.; Pichler, M.; Enzinger, C.; Petrovic, K.; Niederkorn, K.; Fazekas, F. C-reactive protein, carotid atherosclerosis, and cerebral small-vessel disease: Results of the Austrian Stroke Prevention Study. *Stroke* **2006**, *37*, 2910–2916. [CrossRef] [PubMed]
45. Price, T.R.; Manolio, T.A.; Kronmal, R.A.; Kittner, S.J.; Yue, N.C.; Robbins, J.; Anton-Culver, H.; O'leary, D.H. Silent brain infarction on magnetic resonance imaging and neurological abnormalities in community-dwelling older adults. The Cardiovascular Health Study. CHS Collaborative Research Group. *Stroke* **1997**, *28*, 1158–1164. [CrossRef] [PubMed]
46. Howard, G.; Wagenknecht, L.E.; Cai, J.; Cooper, L.; Kraut, M.A.; Toole, J.F. Cigarette smoking and other risk factors for silent cerebral infarction in the general population. *Stroke* **1998**, *29*, 913–917. [CrossRef] [PubMed]
47. DeCarli, C.; Massaro, J.; Harvey, D.; Hald, J.; Tullberg, M.; Au, R.; Beiser, A.; D'agostino, R.; Wolf, P.A. Measures of brain morphology and infarction in the framingham heart study: Establishing what is normal. *Neurobiol. Aging* **2005**, *26*, 491–510. [CrossRef]
48. Das, R.R.; Seshadri, S.; Beiser, A.S.; Kelly-Hayes, M.; Au, R.; Himali, J.J.; Kase, C.S.; Benjamin, E.J.; Polak, J.F.; O'Donnell, C.J.; et al. Prevalence and correlates of silent cerebral infarcts in the framingham offspring study. *Stroke* **2008**, *39*, 2929–2935. [CrossRef]
49. Fanning, J.P.; Wong, A.A.; Fraser, J.F. The epidemiology of silent brain infarction: A systematic review of population-based cohorts. *BMC Med.* **2014**, *12*, 119. [CrossRef]
50. Vermeer, S.E.; Hollander, M.; van Dijk, E.J.; Hofman, A.; Koudstaal, P.J.; Breteler, M.M. Silent brain infarcts and white matter lesions increase stroke risk in the general population: The Rotterdam Scan Study. *Stroke* **2003**, *34*, 1126–1129. [CrossRef]
51. Pegelow, C.H.; Macklin, E.A.; Moser, F.G.; Wang, W.C.; Bello, J.A.; Miller, S.T.; Vichinsky, E.P.; DeBaun, M.R.; Guarini, L.; Zimmerman, R.A.; et al. Longitudinal changes in brain magnetic resonance imaging findings in children with sickle cell disease. *Blood* **2002**, *99*, 3014–3018. [CrossRef] [PubMed]
52. Abdelaal, M.; le Roux, C.W.; Docherty, N.G. Morbidity and mortality associated with obesity. *Ann. Transl. Med.* **2017**, *5*, 161. [CrossRef] [PubMed]
53. Luppino, F.S.; de Wit, L.M.; Bouvy, P.F. Overweight, obesity, and depression: A systematic review and meta-analysis of longitudinal studies. *Arch. Gen. Psychiatry* **2010**, *67*, 220–229. [CrossRef] [PubMed]

54. Hare, D.L.; Toukhsati, S.R.; Johansson, P.; Jaarsma, T. Depression and cardiovascular disease: A clinical review. *Eur. Heart J.* **2014**, *35*, 1365–1372. [CrossRef] [PubMed]
55. Prospective Studies Collaboration; Whitlock, G.; Lewington, S. Body-mass index and cause-specific mortality in 900 000 adults: Collaborative analyses of 57 prospective studies. *Lancet* **2009**, *373*, 1083–1096. [CrossRef] [PubMed]
56. Flegal, K.M.; Kit, B.K.; Orpana, H.; Graubard, B.I. Association of all-cause mortality with overweight and obesity using standard body mass index categories: A systematic review and meta-analysis. *JAMA* **2013**, *309*, 71–82. [CrossRef]
57. Martino, S.; Jamme, M.; Deligny, C.; Busson, M.; Loiseau, P.; Azoulay, E.; Galicier, L.; Pène, F.; Provôt, F.; Dossier, A.; et al. Thrombotic Thrombocytopenic Purpura in Black People: Impact of Ethnicity on Survival and Genetic Risk Factors. *PLoS ONE* **2016**, *11*, e0156679. [CrossRef]
58. Feldman, C.H.; Hiraki, L.T.; Liu, J.; Fischer, M.A.; Solomon, D.H.; Alarcón, G.S.; Winkelmayer, W.C.; Costenbader, K.H. Epidemiology and sociodemographics of systemic lupus erythematosus and lupus nephritis among US adults with Medicaid coverage, 2000–2004. *Arthritis Rheum.* **2013**, *65*, 753–763. [CrossRef]
59. Javed, Z.; Maqsood, M.H.; Yahya, T.; Amin, Z.; Acquah, I.; Valero-Elizondo, J.; Andrieni, J.; Dubey, P.; Jackson, R.K.; Daffin, M.A.; et al. Race, Racism, and Cardiovascular Health: Applying a Social Determinants of Health Framework to Racial/Ethnic Disparities in Cardiovascular Disease. *Circ. Cardiovasc. Qual. Outcomes* **2022**, *15*, e007917. [CrossRef]
60. Devareddy, A.; Sarraju, A.; Rodriguez, F. Health Disparities Across the Continuum of ASCVD Risk. *Curr. Cardiol. Rep.* **2022**, *24*, 1129–1137. [CrossRef]
61. Mariotti, A.; MacLeod, R.; Hillert, E.-K.; Cameron, R.T.; Baillie, G.S.; Moscato, P.; Lustig, L.C.; Ponzielli, R.; Tang, P.S.; Sathiamoorthy, S.; et al. The effects of chronic stress on health: New insights into the molecular mechanisms of brain–body communication. *Futur. Sci. OA* **2015**, *1*, FSO23. [CrossRef] [PubMed]
62. Surachman, A.; Jenkins, A.I.; Santos, A.R.; Almeida, D.M. Socioeconomic status trajectories across the life course, daily discrimination, and inflammation among Black and white adults. *Psychoneuroendocrinology* **2021**, *127*, 105193. [CrossRef] [PubMed]
63. McClendon, J.; Chang, K.; Boudreaux, M.J.; Oltmanns, T.F.; Bogdan, R. Black-White racial health disparities in inflammation and physical health: Cumulative stress, social isolation, and health behaviors. *Psychoneuroendocrinology* **2021**, *131*, 105251. [CrossRef] [PubMed]
64. Sonneveld, M.A.H.; de Maat, M.P.M.; Portegies, M.L.P.; Kavousi, M.; Hofman, A.; Turecek, P.L.; Rottensteiner, H.; Scheiflinger, F.; Koudstaal, P.J.; Ikram, M.A.; et al. Low ADAMTS13 activity is associated with an increased risk of ischemic stroke. *Blood* **2015**, *126*, 2739–2746. [CrossRef] [PubMed]
65. Sonneveld, M.A.H.; Kavousi, M.; Ikram, M.A.; Hofman, A.; Ochoa, O.L.R.; Turecek, P.L.; Franco, O.H.; Leebeek, F.W.G.; de Maat, M.P.M. Low ADAMTS-13 activity and the risk of coronary heart disease—A prospective cohort study: The Rotterdam Study. *J. Thromb. Haemost.* **2016**, *14*, 2114–2120. [CrossRef] [PubMed]
66. Sonneveld, M.A.; Franco, O.H.; Ikram, M.A. Von Willebrand Factor, ADAMTS13, and the Risk of Mortality: The Rotterdam Study. *Arterioscler. Thromb. Vasc. Biol.* **2016**, *36*, 2446–2451. [CrossRef] [PubMed]
67. Federici, A.B.; Bader, R.; Pagani, S.; Colibretti, M.L.; Marco, L.; Mannucci, P.M. Binding of von Willebrand factor to glycoproteins Ib and IIb/IIIa complex: Affinity is related to multimeric size. *Br. J. Haematol.* **1989**, *73*, 93–99. [CrossRef]
68. Noone, D.G.; Riedl, M.; Pluthero, F.G.; Bowman, M.L.; Liszewski, M.K.; Lu, L.; Quan, Y.; Balgobin, S.; Schneppenheim, R.; Schneppenheim, S.; et al. Von Willebrand factor regulates complement on endothelial cells. *Kidney Int.* **2016**, *90*, 123–134. [CrossRef]
69. Turner, N.; Nolasco, L.; Nolasco, J.; Sartain, S.; Moake, J. Thrombotic microangiopathies and the linkage between von willebrand factor and the alternative complement pathway. *Semin. Thromb. Hemost.* **2014**, *40*, 544–550. [CrossRef]
70. Jin, S.-Y.; Tohyama, J.; Bauer, R.C.; Cao, N.N.; Rader, D.J.; Zheng, X.L. Genetic ablation of *adamts13* gene dramatically accelerates the formation of early atherosclerosis in a murine model. *Arter. Thromb. Vasc. Biol.* **2012**, *32*, 1817–1823. [CrossRef]
71. Gandhi, C.; Khan, M.M.; Lentz, S.R.; Chauhan, A.K. ADAMTS13 reduces vascular inflammation and the development of early atherosclerosis in mice. *Blood* **2012**, *119*, 2385–2391. [CrossRef]
72. Cuker, A.; Cataland, S.R.; Coppo, P.; de la Rubia, J.; Friedman, K.D.; George, J.N.; Knoebl, P.N.; Kremer Hovinga, J.A.; Lämmle, B.; Matsumoto, M.; et al. Redefining outcomes in immune TTP: An international working group consensus report. *Blood* **2021**, *137*, 1855–1861. [CrossRef]
73. Scully, M.; Cataland, S.R.; Peyvandi, F.; Coppo, P.; Knöbl, P.; Kremer Hovinga, J.A.; Zeldin, R.K. Caplacizumab Treatment for Acquired Thrombotic Thrombocytopenic Purpura. *N. Engl. J. Med.* **2019**, *380*, 335–346. [CrossRef]
74. de Maat, S.; Clark, C.C.; Barendrecht, A.D.; Smits, S.; van Kleef, N.D.; El Otmani, H.; Waning, M.; van Moorsel, M.V.A.; Szardenings, M.; Delaroque, N.; et al. Microlyse: A thrombolytic agent that targets VWF for clearance of microvascular thrombosis. *Blood* **2022**, *139*, 597–607. [CrossRef]
75. Hie, M.; Gay, J.; Galicier, L.; Provôt, F.; Presne, C.; Poullin, P.; Bonmarchand, G.; Wynckel, A.; Benhamou, Y.; Vanhille, P.; et al. Preemptive rituximab infusions after remission efficiently prevent relapses in acquired thrombotic thrombocytopenic purpura. *Blood* **2014**, *124*, 204–210. [CrossRef] [PubMed]

Disclaimer/Publisher's Note: The statements, opinions and data contained in all publications are solely those of the individual author(s) and contributor(s) and not of MDPI and/or the editor(s). MDPI and/or the editor(s) disclaim responsibility for any injury to people or property resulting from any ideas, methods, instructions or products referred to in the content.

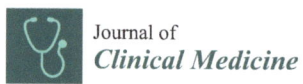

Review

The Highs and Lows of ADAMTS13 Activity

Rebecca J. Shaw [1,2], Simon T. Abrams [2,*], Samuel Badu [1], Cheng-Hock Toh [1,2] and Tina Dutt [1]

1. Liverpool University Hospitals NHS Foundation Trust, Liverpool L7 8YE, UK; r.shaw3@nhs.net (R.J.S.); samuel.badu@liverpoolftt.nhs.uk (S.B.); toh@liverpool.ac.uk (C.-H.T.); tina.dutt@liverpoolft.nhs.uk (T.D.)
2. Clinical Infection, Microbiology and Immunology, Institute of Infection, Veterinary & Ecological Sciences, University of Liverpool, Ronald Ross Building, 8 West Derby Street, Liverpool L69 7BE, UK
* Correspondence: stabrams@liverpool.ac.uk; Tel.: +44-(0)151-795-1327

Abstract: Severe deficiency of ADAMTS13 (<10 iu/dL) is diagnostic of thrombotic thrombocytopenic purpura (TTP) and leads to accumulation of ultra-large vWF multimers, platelet aggregation, and widespread microthrombi, which can be life-threatening. However, the clinical implications of a low ADAMTS13 activity level are not only important in an acute episode of TTP. In this article, we discuss the effects of low ADAMTS13 activity in congenital and immune-mediated TTP patients not only at presentation but once in a clinical remission. Evidence is emerging of the clinical effects of low ADAMTS13 activity in other disease areas outside of TTP, and here, we explore the wider impact of low ADAMTS13 activity on the vascular endothelium and the potential for recombinant ADAMTS13 therapy in other thrombotic disease states.

Keywords: ADAMTS13; TTP; vWF; recombinant

Citation: Shaw, R.J.; Abrams, S.T.; Badu, S.; Toh, C.-H.; Dutt, T. The Highs and Lows of ADAMTS13 Activity. *J. Clin. Med.* **2024**, *13*, 5152. https://doi.org/10.3390/jcm13175152

Academic Editor: Deirdra R. Terrell

Received: 18 June 2024
Revised: 20 August 2024
Accepted: 28 August 2024
Published: 30 August 2024

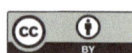

Copyright: © 2024 by the authors. Licensee MDPI, Basel, Switzerland. This article is an open access article distributed under the terms and conditions of the Creative Commons Attribution (CC BY) license (https://creativecommons.org/licenses/by/4.0/).

1. Introduction

The year 2024 marks the passing of a century from the time when Eli Moschowitz described the initial clinical phenotype of thrombotic thrombocytopenic purpura (TTP) in a 16-year-old girl with fever, neurological symptoms, microangiopathic haemolytic anaemia, and thrombocytopenia [1]. The post-mortem histology for this index case confirmed widespread microvascular thrombotic occlusion, compromising the function of multiple vital organs and leading to death. After a series of similar cases in 1947, Singer named the distinct clinical entity "TTP" [2], however, apart from clinical manifestations and significant mortality, little more was known about the underlying pathophysiology of the condition at the time.

Despite early observations linked to the presumed existence of "A disintegrin and metalloproteinase with thrombospondin type 1 motif, member 13" (ADAMTS13), the identity of the enzyme, key to the diagnosis of TTP, remained elusive for many years. In the 1980s, Moake et al. observed the occurrence of platelet attractive ultra-large vWF (ULvWF) multimers in the plasma of relapsing TTP patients, prompting the hypothesis that patients with TTP likely lacked a depolymerase-like enzyme, that if present, would restrict the length of circulating ULvWF [3]. By 1996, Furlan et al. had purified and characterised ADAMTS13 as the metalloprotease responsible for this physiological cleavage of vWF, without which the life-threatening clinical disease TTP would ensue with inevitable morbidity and mortality unless promptly treated [4]. Effective treatment with plasma infusion and later plasma exchange had already been recognised in TTP, and identification of this critical enzyme within plasma was a key discovery representing the missing link [5].

2. The ADAMTS13–VWF Axis

The relationship between vWF and ADAMTS13 is sometimes referred to as the ADAMTS13-vWF axis or the ADAMTS13/vWF ratio, where the relative levels of both in the normal state can be expressed as a percentage of normal, approximately 100% or close to 1.0.

ADAMTS13 is synthesized in hepatic stellate cells and composed of an N-terminal reprolysin-type metalloprotease domain (M), followed by a disintegrin domain (D), a thrombospondin-1–like domain (T), a cysteine-rich domain (C) that contains an arginine-glycine-aspartate sequence, a spacer domain (S), seven additional thrombospondin-1-like domains (T2-8), and two nonidentical CUB-type domains (CUB1-2) at the C-terminal end of the molecule. Circulating in a "closed" formation prevents ADAMTS13 from proteolyzing unselected substrates and reduces susceptibility to inhibitors.

Under conditions of shear stress, vWF unravels from a resting globular state to expose A1 and A2 domains, hosting platelet and ADAMTS13 binding sites respectively. Exposure of the ADAMTS13 binding sites allows for a sequence of domain binding that results in the physiological actions of ADAMTS13. This commences with the induction of an "open" ADAMTS13 conformation by binding CUB1-2 with vWF D4-CK domains, triggering a sequence of binding that results in proteolysis [6]. It is this function that controls platelet-thrombogenic potential under normal conditions and explains the propensity towards microvascular thrombosis if left unchecked.

3. Low ADAMTS13 and Acute TTP

ADAMTS13 is today most well-known for its association with the acute diagnosis of TTP; ADAMTS13 activity <10% is pathognomonic of TTP. Reduced ADAMTS13 activity in TTP is caused by genetic mutations or inhibitory autoantibodies, leading to congenital (cTTP) or immune-mediated (iTTP), respectively [7,8]. Around 95% of patients diagnosed with TTP have immune-mediated disease [9], whilst <5% of cases are congenital [10].

Severe ADAMTS13 deficiency and the presence of inhibitory antibodies to ADAMTS13 is essential for the diagnosis of iTTP, and to differentiate it from other thrombotic microangiopathies (TMAs) [11,12]. Regular monitoring of ADAMTS13 levels during acute treatment can help evaluate clinical response to therapy and guide treatment decisions. Current treatment for acute iTTP includes ADAMTS13 replacement with therapeutic plasma exchange, immune suppression with rituximab (monoclonal anti-CD20), high-dose corticosteroids, plus inhibition of vWF-mediated platelet adhesion with the nanobody caplacizumab [13–15].

The measurement of ADAMTS13 activity in conjunction with genetic analysis is critical in the diagnosis and appropriate management of cTTP [16,17]. In cTTP, various mutations in the ADAMTS13 gene result in either deficient or dysfunctional ADAMTS13, and subsequent impaired cleavage of vWF multimers [16]. cTTP can present at any age; although cTTP patients have a persistently low ADAMTS13 from birth, they may remain asymptomatic until a further triggering event occurs such as pregnancy [18].

Treatment of cTTP has, until recently, focused on ADAMTS13 replacement using plasma infusion (solvent–detergent fresh frozen plasma) or factor VIII concentrates containing ADAMTS13 (BPL 8Y) [10,16,19]. These therapies are effective in the prophylactic and symptomatic management of cTTP, with treatment usually being administered every 1–3 weeks [19]. Congenital TTP patients receiving treatment with regular prophylactic donor plasma infusions to replace ADAMTS13 report symptomatic relief with commencement of prophylaxis and also have a significantly reduced incidence of stroke (2% vs. 17%) compared to those not receiving prophylaxis [17].

4. ADAMTS13 and TTP in Remission

ADAMTS13 activity is known to be a prognostic marker not only in the acute presentation of TTP but also in remission, with persistent undetectable levels in recovering patients associated with an increased risk of disease exacerbation or recurrence [20]. This cohort of TTP patients warrant closer monitoring for the earliest detection of an acute clinical relapse.

The ADAMTS13 activity level in remission TTP is a subject of growing interest. In particular, the population of patients achieving a clinical remission whose ADAMTS13 activity resides in the intermediate zone between low normal and severely deficient levels. George et al. described the heterogeneity of ADAMTS13 activity levels in patients classed as in a remission [21]. The group reported annual evaluations of ADAMTS13 levels between 1995 and 2014 (during a time when regular follow up and interventions were not standard practice) demonstrating natural variations in ADAMST13 activity. Authors divided patients into three categories related to their remission ADAMTS13 activity: (1) A group where remission ADAMTS13 activity was always normal (≥60%) and patients did not incur a relapse, (2) a group where remission ADAMTS13 activity was not always normal but >10%, and (3) a final group in which the ADAMTS13 activity remained 5–15%. For the latter two groups, a proportion of patients relapsed but there were also individuals who avoided acute relapse or spontaneously recovered without any intervention. The authors concluded that ADAMTS13 deficiency during remission was associated with relapse however individual profiles of ADAMTS13 activity were unpredictable and variable. Sustained ADAMTS13 deficiency may be seen without an acute TTP episode, but the potential consequences of chronic sub-normal ADAMTS13 activity levels on longer term health and risk are not clear.

Upreti et al. concluded that TTP patients in remission exhibiting a lower baseline ADAMTS13 level appear to have an increased risk of ischaemic stroke (13.1% TTP in remission versus 2.6% in the general population). In this group, further associations have been made stratifying ADAMTS13 activity in remission, specifically >70%, 40–70%, 10–39%, and <10%. These strata correlate with a 0% incidence of stroke in those with ADAMTS13 over 70% versus 27.6% for those with levels below 70% [22].

Whilst the literature often classifies TTP patients as being in "remission", we are beginning to observe an increasing number of reports detecting subclinical biomarkers for patients whose ADAMTS13 falls below the threshold of 70% and, in some cases, <10% in the presence of normal full blood count indices. Interestingly, a recent longitudinal study by Prasannan et al. demonstrates the importance of ADAMTS13 conformation in determining risk of relapse, with an open conformation often preceding relapse. At their peak ADAMTS13 activity, patients with a closed ADAMTS13 conformation had an eight-fold lower relapse rate within 1 year (9% vs. 46%) and a five-fold lower relapse rate within 2 years (23% vs. 62%) compared to patients with an open ADAMTS13 conformation [23].

A series of recent publications has highlighted the possible connection between white matter changes on MRI, impaired neurocognitive and ADAMTS13 level in patients with TTP [24,25]. In a report by Hannan et al., of the iTTP patients defined as in "remission", half had an ADAMTS13 activity level <70%, and one fifth had a level <10% [26]. Alwan et al. found lower than average ADAMTS13 activity levels in patients with silent cerebral infarction (half the patients studied) versus those without, and higher rates of cognitive impairment [24]. There is an increasing suggestion that patients in a clinical remission with lower-than-average ADAMTS13 activity levels may warrant earlier intervention. This is aimed at restoring ADAMTS13 activity to optimise vascular integrity to potentially retard the rate of sub-clinical cerebrovascular disease. This concept is challenging the way TTP is regarded as a condition characterised by either a distinct acute or remission state [25].

5. ADAMTS13 and Other Disease

The normal reference range for ADAMTS13 varies depending on the assay methodology, age, gender and genetic variants in different ethnic populations, and is usually described with a range between 40–140% of healthy adults. In TTP specialist centres, different thresholds are accepted when monitoring the progress of their patients with TTP. For example, in the UK and Europe, this is usually > 40%, compared to some U.S. centres using > 70%.

Polymorphisms found at higher prevalence in certain populations can also influence normal range limits, for example, the P.Pro475Ser polymorphism known to be heterozygous in approximately 10% of the Japanese population is associated with a reduction in ADAMTS13 activity level [27].

A low ADAMTS13 activity appears to have important clinical implications outside of the field of TTP, particularly in those conditions which are recognised as being pro-thrombotic. This is in keeping with the known antithrombotic action of ADAMTS13, cleaving highly active ultra-large vWF multimers in the circulation [4]. Although extreme deficiency of ADAMTS13 is highly specific for a diagnosis of TTP, lesser reductions are observed in other thrombotic microangiopathies including haemolytic uraemic syndrome, sepsis and malignancy [28].

5.1. Cerebral Ischaemia

In a large study of almost 6000 participants aged ≥ 55 years in the Netherlands, Sonneveld et al. determined that a low ADAMTS13 activity was associated with increased risk of ischaemic stroke in the general population [29]. A low ADAMTS13 activity remained a significant risk factor for stroke, even after adjustment for traditional cardiovascular risk factors (including age, gender, smoking status, blood pressure, diabetes, and cholesterol). Those with an ADAMTS13 activity in the lowest quartile had a significantly higher risk of ischemic stroke than those in the highest quartile (absolute risk, 7.3% vs. 3.8% respectively; hazard ratio, 1.65; 95% confidence interval [CI], 1.16–2.32). Authors proposed that lower ADAMTS13 activity levels would lead to increased prevalence of large procoagulant vWF multimers, which could subsequently lead to development of thrombus especially at sites of high shear stress or endothelial damage [29].

With ischaemic stroke being a major cause of morbidity and mortality worldwide [30], and available treatments options being sub-optimal, there is huge potential for using ADAMTS13 as a novel therapeutic target in these patients.

It is of note that within this large study, individuals with an ADAMTS13 activity in the lowest quartile still had an activity level which would be considered to be in the normal range (>50 iu/dL) [31]. Therefore, it appears that ADAMTS13 activity does not have to be severely low, as in patients diagnosed with TTP, to still have pathological implications and potentially clinical consequences.

5.2. Myocardial Ischaemia

Myocardial ischaemia/infarction is a major cause of global morbidity and mortality; a meta-analysis of >3500 participants (with myocardial infarction and healthy controls) showed that ADAMTS13 level below the 5th centile was associated with a moderate increased risk of myocardial infarction (OR 1.89, [95% CI 1.15–3.12]) [32]. The risk was similar between different age groups but appeared more pronounced in women compared to men, although not all confounding factors were accounted for. Unlike in ischaemic stroke, moderately low ADAMTS13 levels were not associated with an increased risk of myocardial infarction (lowest quartile vs. highest quartile, OR 1.28 [95% CI 0.68–2.45]), and there was no trend observed in the intermediate quartiles, with the authors suggesting a clinically relevant "threshold" for ADAMTS13 activity and increased myocardial ischaemia risk rather than a dose-dependent relationship [32].

The pathophysiology of low ADAMTS13 activity being associated with myocardial infarction is not fully understood. Suggested mechanisms include an effect of ADAMTS13 on the initiation and progression of atherosclerotic plaques [33], its effect on acute arterial thrombus formation, and/or the amplification of a developing thrombus [34,35].

5.3. Renal Disease

The effect of ADAMTS13 deficiency on cardiovascular outcome has also been reported in patients with end-stage renal failure on haemodialysis (HD). One study demonstrates significantly reduced ADAMTS13 activity in HD patients compared to normal healthy controls (mean ADAMTS13 $41.0 \pm 22.8\%$ vs. $102.3 \pm 17.7\%$, respectively), which was an independent risk factor for the development of new cardiovascular events in this group of patients. The cause for the low ADAMTS13 activity in this cohort is not known, although it has been hypothesised that there is a potential role for synthesis of ADAMTS13 from the kidneys, which is therefore reduced in chronic kidney disease [36], and it is recognised that renal failure patients often have other comorbidities which may contribute. Ocak et al. showed an increased mortality in 956 dialysis patients with higher levels of vWF and reduced ADAMTS13 activity; specifically, those dialysis patients in the highest quartile of vWF had a 1.4-fold (95% CI 1.1–1.8) increased mortality risk compared with those in the lowest quartile for vWF, even after adjustment for other risk factors including age, sex, body mass index, cardiovascular disease, smoking, type of dialysis, primary kidney disease, use of antithrombotic medication, blood pressure, albumin levels, CRP levels and baseline eGFR [37]. The lowest quartile of ADAMTS13 activity (mean level 16.7%) was associated with a 1.3-fold (95% CI 1.0–1.7) increased mortality risk after adjustment, compared with the highest quartile of ADAMTS13 activity (mean level 68.1%). Different causes for mortality in these patients were explored, and overall high vWF levels and low ADAMTS13 activity were associated with a 1.8-fold (95% CI 1.0–3.2) increased cardiovascular mortality risk and a 2.1-fold (95% CI 1.2–3.7) increased non-cardiovascular mortality risk [37], with the increased mortality speculated to be likely due to an increased prothrombotic tendency.

5.4. COVID-19 Infection

The COVID-19 pandemic has had a hugely significant global impact since 2020 [38]. While little was known early on about this novel virus, reports soon emerged of the prothrombotic nature of SARS-CoV-2 infection, with patients at increased risk of developing thromboses acutely and even post-discharge from hospital [39–42].

COVID-19 infection has been shown to be associated with a reduction in activity of ADAMTS13, which was particularly seen in those with severe infection [43]. As expected, a decrease in ADAMTS13 activity leads to an increase in vWF concentration and activity and alteration of the vWF:ADAMTS13 ratio in this carefully balanced axis. Mancini et al. found a moderate reduction in ADAMTS13 activity in the more severe cases of COVID-19 infection; around one-third of patients in critical care presented with ADAMTS13 activity levels of <50 iu/dL. They also observed a 3–7-fold increase in the vWF antigen:ADAMTS13 activity ratio associated with the severity of COVID-19 infection [44]. This study found a slight decrease in high-molecular-weight vWF multimers and a relative increase of intermediate/low-molecular-weight vWF multimers, which was more pronounced in the most severe cases of COVID-19 infection; authors proposed that this may be explained by an early increase of vWF proteolysis by ADAMTS13, as it attempts to overcome the excess release of vWF in response to local hyperinflammation and endothelial activation in COVID-19. The theory is that ADAMTS13 will be "consumed" during this process, tipping the balance in the ADAMTS13-vWF axis and reaching reduced levels in the most critically ill patients. High molecular weight multimers may also be consumed in vWF-platelet aggregates and microthrombi, similar to the pathophysiology seen in the acute presentation of TTP.

As well as an association with severity of infection, ADAMTS13 activity has been shown in several studies to be associated with mortality in COVID-19. A study of 88 PCR-proven COVID-19 patients demonstrated that COVID-19 non-survivors had significantly lower levels of ADAMTS-13 activity (32.2 iu/dL vs. 50.6 iu/dL, $p = 0.035$) and higher levels of vWF (395.5 iu/dL vs. 295.5 iu/dL, $p = 0.033$) when compared to patients who survived [45]. Looking at ratios, a vWF:RCo/ADAMTS13:activity ratio of >5.7 was associated with ICU admission, and a ratio >6.5 was associated with increased patient mortality [46] in COVID-19 infection.

The implications of low ADAMTS13 activity in COVID-19 have also been shown in pregnancy, with an increased vWF RiCof:ADAMTS13 activity ratio being significantly associated with a higher risk of pregnancy-related complications including pre-term delivery (OR 1.9, 95% CI 1.1–3.5). The placentae of women with COVID-19 infection show inflammatory histological features, with increased vWF expression in the endothelium, particularly in severe cases [47].

Studies suggest ADAMTS13 deficiency may also play a role in the long-term complications of COVID-19 or "Long COVID", which is estimated to affect 30–40% of individuals after infection with SARS-CoV-2. Prasannan et al. found an abnormal vWF:ADAMTS13 ratio > 1.5 correlated with patients with long COVID and impaired exercise capacity [48]

(OR 4). Additionally, a study of 50 patients at least 6 weeks post-infection with COVID-19 showed plasma ADAMTS13 levels were significantly reduced when compared to healthy controls (Lower limit of normal local reference for the study 399 ng/mL [Median 598 ng/mL vs. 630 ng/mL, $p = 0.009$]) [49]. ADAMTS13 levels were also significantly lower in convalescent patients who had required hospitalisation when compared to those who had been managed as outpatients ($p = 0.04$) [49]. Reduced ADAMTS13 levels were seen alongside elevated vWF antigen levels in the convalescent patients, leading to an increased vWF:ADAMTS13 ratio [49] and axis imbalance.

5.5. Sepsis

As microangiopathic changes are not uncommon in patients with sepsis, it is unsurprising to find several studies confirming the finding of low ADAMTS13 levels [50–52]. Low ADAMTS13 activity is a clinically relevant finding as the magnitude of the decrease in ADAMTS13 is strongly correlated with adverse outcomes in sepsis; approximately a third of patients with sepsis have ADAMTS13 activity levels that are less than 50% of normal [52–54]. Furthermore, sepsis patients with such low levels have an ~10% higher risk of death compared with patients who present with no/mild reductions in ADAMTS13 activity levels [55]. Notably, the level of ultra-large vWF multimers in patients with sepsis is inversely correlated with the ADAMTS13 level [51]. These findings may be from a combination of increased consumption of ADAMTS13, its reduced synthesis, proteolytic clearance by thrombin, plasmin and/or leucocyte elastase, or the presence of proinflammatory cytokines that inhibit ADAMTS13, e.g., IL6.

5.6. Heparin-Induced Thrombocytopenia (HIT)

ADAMTS13 deficiency has also been associated with other thrombotic disease processes. HIT is a potentially life-threatening thrombotic complication that can occur after administration of heparin, or rarely, as an autoimmune phenomenon. It is driven by the formation of antibodies against platelet factor 4 (PF4)- heparin complexes [56,57]. Chan et al. analysed 261 patients with suspected HIT, of which one-third were confirmed positive for HIT antibodies by enzyme immunoassay [58]. They found a significant difference in ADAMTS13 activity between healthy volunteers and those with confirmed HIT, there was also a significantly lower ADAMTS13:vWF antigen ratio in the patients with HIT. In terms of clinical relevance, a multivariate analysis demonstrated that an ADAMTS13 activity of <50 iu/dL was associated with an increased risk of 90-day mortality in all patients with suspected HIT, regardless of the HIT antibody results, however the predictive value was better in those with confirmed positive antibody testing [58].

5.7. Sickle Cell Disease

Sickle cell disease is a haemoglobinopathy resulting from a single amino-acid mutation of the beta-globin chain of haemoglobin and can be complicated by vaso-occlusive crises, acute chest syndrome and multi-organ failure. Thrombotic complications can also include venous thrombosis and stroke. Although Demagny et al. did not find any significant reduction in ADAMTS13 antigen in patients with sickle cell compared to healthy controls, nor any difference in ADAMTS13 antigen between sickle cell patients in chronic steady state vs. those with veno-occlusive crises/acute chest syndrome [59], significant differences have been seen in vWF antigen, with increased levels in patients presenting with vaso-occlusive crisis [59–61] and elevated levels in more severe genotypes (HbSS or HBSβ0) [62], suggesting dysregulation of ADAMTS13-vWF axis. Fogarty et al. demonstrate that despite treatment with hydroxycarbamide or blood transfusion, a proportion of children with sickle cell disease (HbSS) had persistently elevated vWF antigen and activity, as well as elevated vWF propeptide consistent with acute endothelial cell activation [63]. Sickle cell disease mice models appear to show a benefit of recombinant ADAMTS13; administering recombinant ADAMTS13 to these mice reduced hypoxia-reoxygenation induced haemolysis as well as systemic/local inflammation in lungs and kidneys. Colombatti et al. demonstrate that patients with sickle cell disease and silent cerebral infarcts, have a significant decrease in ADAMTS13 antigen levels [64]. Together, this suggests that recombinant ADAMTS13 may be an effective novel therapy for sickle cell-related acute events and reducing organ damage [65].

5.8. Solid Organ Transplant

Reduced ADAMTS13 activity (hence reduced cleavage of vWF) has been implicated in both liver and lung transplant failures [66,67]. Furthermore, recombinant human ADAMTS13 therapy has been shown to significantly improve duration of skin allograft survival in mice models [68]. Although the mechanism by which recombinant ADAMTS13 therapy had effect was not determined, authors postulated this could be due to disruption of neutrophil extracellular traps (NETs) within the graft or reduction in NETs formation due to lack of ULvWF. The role of NETs within the ADAMTS13-vWF axis and relevance within other prothrombotic diseases is an evolving field.

6. Recombinant ADAMTS13 Therapy

Hypothetically, restoring ADAMTS13 levels and/or reducing ULvWF multimer levels may be effective treatment in a variety of disease states.

Recombinant human ADAMTS13 (rhADAMTS13) has been evaluated in animal models of thrombotic microangiopathy. Mouse, rat and baboon models were originally utilised to determine the pathophysiology of TTP [69,70]. As well as providing a deeper understanding of TTP, these animal models have proven invaluable in the development and evaluation of recent novel therapies, including recombinant human ADAMTS13 [71]. ADAMTS13-deficient (ADAMTS13$-/-$) mice have been developed by several research groups by gene targeting using a mixed-strain C57BL/6J-129X1/SvJ genetic background. ADAMTS13 knock-out mice do not spontaneously develop clinical evidence of TTP and have a comparable life expectancy compared to wild-type mice [72,73].

Recombinant human ADAMTS-13 has been tested in mice models of TTP. ADAMTS13 $-/-$ mice were challenged with a high dose of recombinant human vWF (2000 units/kg). Animals rapidly developed severe thrombocytopenia and clinical symptoms of TTP. Prophylactic infusion (200 U/kg) or therapeutic infusion (320 U/kg; up to 180 min post vWF challenge) reduced disease severity [71]. Specifically, when ADAMTS13 $-/-$ were treated with prophylactic rhADAMTS13 prior to vWF administration, no mice showed clinical, hematologic, or pathologic signs of TTP. However, therapeutic infusion of rhADAMTS13 demonstrated differing pathologic clinical and in histopathologic improvements, with the most favourable being observed at earlier time points of administration (15 min). These data highlight the benefit of early administration of rhADAMTS13 in mice models of TTP.

Tersteeg et al. developed a rat model by injecting polyclonal anti-ADAMTS13 antibodies, additional infusion of recombinant vWF was required to induce the clinical syndrome of TTP. In addition, the TTP syndrome was short-lasting, and rats began to recover after 24 h. Recombinant ADAMTS13 at doses between 400–1600 U/kg (injected into the rats 15 min after TTP symptoms were triggered) prevented cytopenias and the rise in LDH and reduced microthrombi in organs compared to control rats [74].

The most advanced evidence is in patients with congenital TTP (cTTP). A Phase III trial evaluating recombinant ADAMTS13 (TAK-755) replacement therapy for cTTP facilitated a five-fold increase in ADAMTS13 activity levels compared to patients receiving plasma-based therapy [75]. The incidence of thrombocytopenia was reduced by 60 percent in recipients of recombinant human ADAMTS13 (rhADAMTS13) and the drug was found to be safe, non-immunogenic and well tolerated. Recombinant ADAMTS13 was FDA approved in November 2023 for prophylaxis and on-demand treatment of adult and pediatric patients with cTTP. There is now considerable interest on its potential for improving outcomes in acquired deficiency states, as described above. In particular, trials assessing whether recombinant ADAMTS13 may have a role in the acute presentation of iTTP and affect the need for plasma exchange are currently being investigated. There is also an ongoing clinical trial investigating the benefit of recombinant ADAMTS13 therapy in sickle cell disease, which showed no safety signals or dose-limiting toxicities, such as bleeding events, in the Phase I placebo-controlled study [76].

7. Conclusions

The role of ADAMT13 in disease states, not least TTP, has entered a new era. We not only seek to confirm a severe deficiency of ADAMTS13 activity level in suspected acute presentations but now also regularly monitor levels life-long to predict relapse. The clinical phenotype of TTP is no longer perceived as two ends of a spectrum represented by distinct acute and remission states, but a disease where resting ADAMTS13 levels may predict vascular health in the mid-long term for patients with congenital and immune-mediated TTP. The evolving literature of the role of ADAMTS13 in other prothrombotic health conditions, affecting larger numbers of the population experiencing myocardial ischaemia, cerebrovascular disease and infections such as COVID-19, confirm the importance of this enzyme in regulating haemostasis, and its value as a target for novel therapies. Recombinant ADAMTS13 therapy is set to become an integrated component of management for cTTP and potentially iTTP in the near future, with potential benefits for both patient outcome and quality of life. With increasing scrutiny of the effects of fluctuating ADAMTS13 activity levels, the value of recombinant ADAMTS13 therapy may extend to the group of patients who experience sub-optimal ADAMTS13 level recovery. The role of ADAMTS13 outside the traditional context of rare disease is increasingly being characterised, broadening the scope for novel therapies to provide health benefits to larger disease populations at risk of microvascular thrombosis.

Author Contributions: S.T.A., S.B. and C.-H.T. wrote the manuscript. R.J.S. and T.D. wrote and critically reviewed the manuscript. All authors have read and agreed to the published version of the manuscript.

Funding: No specific funding was received for this work.

Conflicts of Interest: All authors have completed ICMJE conflict of interest disclosures forms; there are no relevant conflicts of interest to declare.

References

1. Moschcowitz, E. An acute febrile pleiochromic anemia with hyaline thrombosis of the terminal arterioles and capillaries: An undescribed disease. *Am. J. Med.* **1952**, *13*, 567–569. [CrossRef] [PubMed]
2. Singer, K.; Bornstein, F.P.; Wile, S.A. Thrombotic thrombocytopenic purpura; hemorrhagic diathesis with generalized platelet thromboses. *Blood* **1947**, *2*, 542–554. [CrossRef] [PubMed]
3. Moake, J.L.; Rudy, C.K.; Troll, J.H.; Weinstein, M.J.; Colannino, N.M.; Azocar, J.; Seder, R.H.; Hong, S.L.; Deykin, D. Unusually large plasma factor VIII:von Willebrand factor multimers in chronic relapsing thrombotic thrombocytopenic purpura. *N. Engl. J. Med.* **1982**, *307*, 1432–1435. [CrossRef] [PubMed]
4. Furlan, M.; Robles, R.; Lämmle, B. Partial purification and characterization of a protease from human plasma cleaving von Willebrand factor to fragments produced by in vivo proteolysis. *Blood* **1996**, *87*, 4223–4234. [CrossRef]
5. Rock, G.A.; Shumak, K.H.; Buskard, N.A.; Blanchette, V.S.; Kelton, J.G.; Nair, R.C.; Spasoff, R.A. Comparison of Plasma Exchange with Plasma Infusion in the Treatment of Thrombotic Thrombocytopenic Purpura. *N. Engl. J. Med.* **1991**, *325*, 393–397. [CrossRef]
6. Petri, A.; Kim, H.J.; Xu, Y.; de Groot, R.; Li, C.; Vandenbulcke, A.; Vanhoorelbeke, K.; Emsley, J.; Crawley, J.T.B. Crystal structure and substrate-induced activation of ADAMTS13. *Nat. Commun.* **2019**, *10*, 3781. [CrossRef]
7. Bonnez, Q.; Sakai, K.; Vanhoorelbeke, K. ADAMTS13 and Non-ADAMTS13 Biomarkers in Immune-Mediated Thrombotic Thrombocytopenic Purpura. *J. Clin. Med.* **2023**, *12*, 6169. [CrossRef]
8. Levy, G.G.; Nichols, W.C.; Lian, E.C.; Foroud, T.; McClintick, J.N.; McGee, B.M.; Yang, A.Y.; Siemieniak, D.R.; Stark, K.R.; Gruppo, R.; et al. Mutations in a member of the ADAMTS gene family cause thrombotic thrombocytopenic purpura. *Nature* **2001**, *413*, 488–494. [CrossRef]
9. Scully, M.; Yarranton, H.; Liesner, R.; Cavenagh, J.; Hunt, B.; Benjamin, S.; Bevan, D.; Mackie, I.; Machin, S. Regional UK TTP Registry: Correlation with laboratory ADAMTS 13 analysis and clinical features. *Br. J. Haematol.* **2008**, *142*, 819–826. [CrossRef]
10. Scully, M.; Hunt, B.J.; Benjamin, S.; Liesner, R.; Rose, P.; Peyvandi, F.; Cheung, B.; Machin, S.J. Guidelines on the diagnosis and management of thrombotic thrombocytopenic purpura and other thrombotic microangiopathies. *Br. J. Haematol.* **2012**, *158*, 323–335. [CrossRef]

11. Thomas, M.R.; de Groot, R.; Scully, M.A.; Crawley, J.T. Pathogenicity of Anti-ADAMTS13 Autoantibodies in Acquired Thrombotic Thrombocytopenic Purpura. *EBioMedicine* **2015**, *2*, 942–952. [CrossRef] [PubMed]
12. Tersteeg, C.; Verhenne, S.; Roose, E.; Schelpe, A.S.; Deckmyn, H.; De Meyer, S.F.; Vanhoorelbeke, K. ADAMTS13 and anti-ADAMTS13 autoantibodies in thrombotic thrombocytopenic purpura—Current perspectives and new treatment strategies. *Expert. Rev. Hematol.* **2016**, *9*, 209–221. [CrossRef]
13. Zheng, X.L.; Vesely, S.K.; Cataland, S.R.; Coppo, P.; Geldziler, B.; Iorio, A.; Matsumoto, M.; Mustafa, R.A.; Pai, M.; Rock, G.; et al. ISTH guidelines for treatment of thrombotic thrombocytopenic purpura. *J. Thromb. Haemost.* **2020**, *18*, 2496–2502. [CrossRef]
14. Coppo, P.; Cuker, A.; George, J.N. Thrombotic thrombocytopenic purpura: Toward targeted therapy and precision medicine. *Res. Pract. Thromb. Haemost.* **2018**, *3*, 26–37. [CrossRef] [PubMed]
15. Bresin, E.; Gastoldi, S.; Daina, E.; Belotti, D.; Pogliani, E.; Perseghin, P.; Scalzulli, P.R.; Paolini, R.; Marceno, R.; Remuzzi, G.; et al. Rituximab as pre-emptive treatment in patients with thrombotic thrombocytopenic purpura and evidence of anti-ADAMTS13 autoantibodies. *Thromb. Haemost.* **2009**, *101*, 233–238. [PubMed]
16. Hovinga, J.A.K.; George, J.N. Hereditary Thrombotic Thrombocytopenic Purpura. *N. Engl. J. Med.* **2019**, *381*, 1653–1662. [CrossRef]
17. Alwan, F.; Vendramin, C.; Liesner, R.; Clark, A.; Lester, W.; Dutt, T.; Thomas, W.; Gooding, R.; Biss, T.; Watson, H.G.; et al. Characterization and treatment of congenital thrombotic thrombocytopenic purpura. *Blood* **2019**, *133*, 1644–1651. [CrossRef]
18. Fujimura, Y.; Matsumoto, M.; Kokame, K.; Isonishi, A.; Soejima, K.; Akiyama, N.; Tomiyama, J.; Natori, K.; Kuranishi, Y.; Imamura, Y.; et al. Pregnancy-induced thrombocytopenia and TTP, and the risk of fetal death, in Upshaw-Schulman syndrome: A series of 15 pregnancies in 9 genotyped patients. *Br. J. Haematol.* **2009**, *144*, 742–754. [CrossRef]
19. Sakai, K.; Hamada, E.; Kokame, K.; Matsumoto, M. Congenital thrombotic thrombocytopenic purpura: Genetics and emerging therapies. *Ann. Blood* **2022**, *8*. [CrossRef]
20. Ferrari, S.; Scheiflinger, F.; Rieger, M.; Mudde, G.; Wolf, M.; Coppo, P.; Girma, J.P.; Azoulay, E.; Brun-Buisson, C.; Fakhouri, F.; et al. Prognostic value of anti-ADAMTS 13 antibody features (Ig isotype, titer, and inhibitory effect) in a cohort of 35 adult French patients undergoing a first episode of thrombotic microangiopathy with undetectable ADAMTS 13 activity. *Blood* **2007**, *109*, 2815–2822. [CrossRef]
21. Page, E.E.; Kremer Hovinga, J.A.; Terrell, D.R.; Vesely, S.K.; George, J.N. Clinical importance of ADAMTS13 activity during remission in patients with acquired thrombotic thrombocytopenic purpura. *Blood* **2016**, *128*, 2175–2178. [CrossRef]
22. Upreti, H.; Kasmani, J.; Dane, K.; Braunstein, E.M.; Streiff, M.B.; Shanbhag, S.; Moliterno, A.R.; Sperati, C.J.; Gottesman, R.F.; Brodsky, R.A.; et al. Reduced ADAMTS13 activity during TTP remission is associated with stroke in TTP survivors. *Blood* **2019**, *134*, 1037–1045. [CrossRef]
23. Prasannan, N.; Dragunaite, B.; Subhan, M.; Thomas, M.; de Groot, R.; Singh, D.; Vanhoorelbeke, K.; Scully, M. Peak ADAMTS13 activity to assess ADAMTS13 conformation and risk of relapse in immune-mediated thrombotic thrombocytopenic purpura. *Blood* **2024**, *143*, 2644–2653. [CrossRef]
24. Alwan, F.; Mahdi, D.; Tayabali, S.; Cipolotti, L.; Lakey, G.; Hyare, H.; Scully, M. Cerebral MRI findings predict the risk of cognitive impairment in thrombotic thrombocytopenic purpura. *Br. J. Haematol.* **2020**, *191*, 868–874. [CrossRef] [PubMed]
25. Dutt, T.; Toh, C.-H. Shades of Grey—The brain in TTP. *Br. J. Haematol.* **2024**, *204*, 757–758. [CrossRef]
26. Hannan, F.; Hamilton, J.; Patriquin, C.J.; Pavenski, K.; Jurkiewicz, M.T.; Tristao, L.; Owen, A.M.; Kosalka, P.K.; Deoni, S.C.L.; Théberge, J.; et al. Cognitive decline in thrombotic thrombocytopenic purpura survivors: The role of white matter health as assessed by MRI. *Br. J. Haematol.* **2024**, *204*, 1005–1016. [CrossRef] [PubMed]
27. Miyata, T.; Kokame, K.; Matsumoto, M.; Fujimura, Y. ADAMTS13 activity and genetic mutations in Japan. *Hamostaseologie* **2013**, *33*, 131–137. [CrossRef] [PubMed]
28. Favaloro, E.J.; Henry, B.M.; Lippi, G. Increased VWF and Decreased ADAMTS-13 in COVID-19: Creating a Milieu for (Micro)Thrombosis. *Semin. Thromb. Hemost.* **2021**, *47*, 400–418. [CrossRef]
29. Sonneveld, M.A.H.; de Maat, M.P.M.; Portegies, M.L.P.; Kavousi, M.; Hofman, A.; Turecek, P.L.; Rottensteiner, H.; Scheiflinger, F.; Koudstaal, P.J.; Ikram, M.A.; et al. Low ADAMTS13 activity is associated with an increased risk of ischemic stroke. *Blood* **2015**, *126*, 2739–2746. [CrossRef]
30. Feigin, V.L.; Forouzanfar, M.H.; Krishnamurthi, R.; Mensah, G.A.; Connor, M.; Bennett, D.A.; Moran, A.E.; Sacco, R.L.; Anderson, L.; Truelsen, T.; et al. Global and regional burden of stroke during 1990–2010: Findings from the Global Burden of Disease Study 2010. *Lancet* **2014**, *383*, 245–254. [CrossRef]
31. Gerritsen, H.E.; Turecek, P.L.; Schwarz, H.P.; Lämmle, B.; Furlan, M. Assay of von Willebrand factor (vWF)-cleaving protease based on decreased collagen binding affinity of degraded vWF: A tool for the diagnosis of thrombotic thrombocytopenic purpura (TTP). *Thromb. Haemost.* **1999**, *82*, 1386–1389. [CrossRef]
32. Maino, A.; Siegerink, B.; Lotta, L.A.; Crawley, J.T.B.; le Cessie, S.; Leebeek, F.W.G.; Lane, D.A.; Lowe, G.D.O.; Peyvandi, F.; Rosendaal, F.R. Plasma ADAMTS-13 levels and the risk of myocardial infarction: An individual patient data meta-analysis. *J. Thromb. Haemost.* **2015**, *13*, 1396–1404. [CrossRef] [PubMed]
33. Jin, S.Y.; Tohyama, J.; Bauer, R.C.; Cao, N.N.; Rader, D.J.; Zheng, X.L. Genetic ablation of Adamts13 gene dramatically accelerates the formation of early atherosclerosis in a murine model. *Arterioscler. Thromb. Vasc. Biol.* **2012**, *32*, 1817–1823. [CrossRef]

34. Xiao, J.; Jin, S.Y.; Xue, J.; Sorvillo, N.; Voorberg, J.; Zheng, X.L. Essential domains of a disintegrin and metalloprotease with thrombospondin type 1 repeats-13 metalloprotease required for modulation of arterial thrombosis. *Arterioscler. Thromb. Vasc. Biol.* **2011**, *31*, 2261–2269. [CrossRef]
35. Fujioka, M.; Hayakawa, K.; Mishima, K.; Kunizawa, A.; Irie, K.; Higuchi, S.; Nakano, T.; Muroi, C.; Fukushima, H.; Sugimoto, M.; et al. ADAMTS13 gene deletion aggravates ischemic brain damage: A possible neuroprotective role of ADAMTS13 by ameliorating postischemic hypoperfusion. *Blood* **2010**, *115*, 1650–1653. [CrossRef]
36. Hung, S.-Y.; Lin, T.-M.; Liou, H.-H.; Chen, C.-Y.; Liao, W.-T.; Wang, H.-H.; Ho, L.-C.; Wu, C.-F.; Lee, Y.-C.; Chang, M.-Y. Association between ADAMTS13 deficiency and cardiovascular events in chronic hemodialysis patients. *Sci. Rep.* **2021**, *11*, 22816. [CrossRef]
37. Ocak, G.; Roest, M.; Verhaar, M.C.; Rookmaaker, M.B.; Blankestijn, P.J.; Bos, W.J.W.; Fijnheer, R.; Péquériaux, N.C.; Dekker, F.W. Von Willebrand factor, ADAMTS13 and mortality in dialysis patients. *BMC Nephrol.* **2021**, *22*, 222. [CrossRef]
38. WHO. Coronavirus Disease (COVID-19) Dashboard. Available online: https://covid19.who.int/ (accessed on 18 September 2023).
39. Bilaloglu, S.; Aphinyanaphongs, Y.; Jones, S.; Iturrate, E.; Hochman, J.; Berger, J.S. Thrombosis in Hospitalized Patients With COVID-19 in a New York City Health System. *JAMA* **2020**, *324*, 799–801. [CrossRef] [PubMed]
40. Klok, F.A.; Kruip, M.J.H.A.; van der Meer, N.J.M.; Arbous, M.S.; Gommers, D.A.M.P.J.; Kant, K.M.; Kaptein, F.H.J.; van Paassen, J.; Stals, M.A.M.; Huisman, M.V.; et al. Incidence of thrombotic complications in critically ill ICU patients with COVID-19. *Thromb. Res.* **2020**, *191*, 145–147. [CrossRef] [PubMed]
41. Lodigiani, C.; Iapichino, G.; Carenzo, L.; Cecconi, M.; Ferrazzi, P.; Sebastian, T.; Kucher, N.; Studt, J.-D.; Sacco, C.; Alexia, B.; et al. Venous and arterial thromboembolic complications in COVID-19 patients admitted to an academic hospital in Milan, Italy. *Thromb. Res.* **2020**, *191*, 9–14. [CrossRef] [PubMed]
42. Richardson, S.; Hirsch, J.S.; Narasimhan, M.; Crawford, J.M.; McGinn, T.; Davidson, K.W. Consortium atNC-R. Presenting Characteristics, Comorbidities, and Outcomes Among 5700 Patients Hospitalized With COVID-19 in the New York City Area. *JAMA* **2020**, *323*, 2052–2059. [CrossRef]
43. Dolgushina, N.; Gorodnova, E.; Beznoshenco, O.; Romanov, A.; Menzhinskaya, I.; Krechetova, L.; Sukhikh, G. Von Willebrand Factor and ADAMTS-13 Are Associated with the Severity of COVID-19 Disease. *J. Clin. Med.* **2022**, *11*, 4006. [CrossRef]
44. Mancini, I.; Baronciani, L.; Artoni, A.; Colpani, P.; Biganzoli, M.; Cozzi, G.; Novembrino, C.; Boscolo Anzoletti, M.; De Zan, V.; Pagliari, M.T.; et al. The ADAMTS13-von Willebrand factor axis in COVID-19 patients. *J. Thromb. Haemost.* **2021**, *19*, 513–521. [CrossRef] [PubMed]
45. Bazzan, M.; Montaruli, B.; Sciascia, S.; Cosseddu, D.; Norbiato, C.; Roccatello, D. Low ADAMTS 13 plasma levels are predictors of mortality in COVID-19 patients. *Intern. Emerg. Med.* **2020**, *15*, 861–863. [CrossRef]
46. Tiscia, G.; Favuzzi, G.; De Laurenzo, A.; Cappucci, F.; Fischetti, L.; Colaizzo, D.; Chinni, E.; Florio, L.; Miscio, G.; Piscitelli, A.P.; et al. The Prognostic Value of ADAMTS-13 and von Willebrand Factor in COVID-19 Patients: Prospective Evaluation by Care Setting. *Diagnostics* **2021**, *11*, 1648. [CrossRef] [PubMed]
47. Flores-Pliego, A.; Miranda, J.; Vega-Torreblanca, S.; Valdespino-Vázquez, Y.; Helguera-Repetto, C.; Espejel-Nuñez, A.; Borboa-Olivares, H.; Espino, Y.S.S.; Mateu-Rogell, P.; León-Juárez, M.; et al. Molecular Insights into the Thrombotic and Microvascular Injury in Placental Endothelium of Women with Mild or Severe COVID-19. *Cells* **2021**, *10*, 364. [CrossRef] [PubMed]
48. Prasannan, N.; Heightman, M.; Hillman, T.; Wall, E.; Bell, R.; Kessler, A.; Neave, L.; Doyle, A.; Devaraj, A.; Singh, D.; et al. Impaired exercise capacity in post-COVID-19 syndrome: The role of VWF-ADAMTS13 axis. *Blood Adv.* **2022**, *6*, 4041–4048. [CrossRef]
49. Fogarty, H.; Ward, S.E.; Townsend, L.; Karampini, E.; Elliott, S.; Conlon, N.; Dunne, J.; Kiersey, R.; Naughton, A.; Gardiner, M.; et al. Sustained VWF-ADAMTS-13 axis imbalance and endotheliopathy in long COVID syndrome is related to immune dysfunction. *J. Thromb. Haemost.* **2022**, *20*, 2429–2438. [CrossRef]
50. Bockmeyer, C.L.; Claus, R.A.; Budde, U.; Kentouche, K.; Schneppenheim, R.; Lösche, W.; Reinhart, K.; Brunkhorst, F.M. Inflammation-associated ADAMTS13 deficiency promotes formation of ultra-large von Willebrand factor. *Haematologica* **2008**, *93*, 137–140. [CrossRef]
51. Löwenberg, E.C.; Meijers, J.C.; Levi, M. Platelet-vessel wall interaction in health and disease. *Neth. J. Med.* **2010**, *68*, 242–251.
52. Schwameis, M.; Schörgenhofer, C.; Assinger, A.; Steiner, M.M.; Jilma, B. VWF excess and ADAMTS13 deficiency: A unifying pathomechanism linking inflammation to thrombosis in DIC, malaria, and TTP. *Thromb. Haemost.* **2015**, *113*, 708–718. [CrossRef]
53. Ono, T.; Mimuro, J.; Madoiwa, S.; Soejima, K.; Kashiwakura, Y.; Ishiwata, A.; Takano, K.; Ohmori, T.; Sakata, Y. Severe secondary deficiency of von Willebrand factor-cleaving protease (ADAMTS13) in patients with sepsis-induced disseminated intravascular coagulation: Its correlation with development of renal failure. *Blood* **2006**, *107*, 528–534. [CrossRef]

54. Kremer Hovinga, J.A.; Zeerleder, S.; Kessler, P.; Romani de Wit, T.; van Mourik, J.A.; Hack, C.E.; Ten Cate, H.; Reitsma, P.H.; Wuillemin, W.A.; Lämmle, B. ADAMTS-13, von Willebrand factor and related parameters in severe sepsis and septic shock. *J. Thromb. Haemost.* **2007**, *5*, 2284–2290. [CrossRef] [PubMed]
55. Martin, K.; Borgel, D.; Lerolle, N.; Feys, H.B.; Trinquart, L.; Vanhoorelbeke, K.; Deckmyn, H.; Legendre, P.; Diehl, J.L.; Baruch, D. Decreased ADAMTS-13 (A disintegrin-like and metalloprotease with thrombospondin type 1 repeats) is associated with a poor prognosis in sepsis-induced organ failure. *Crit. Care Med.* **2007**, *35*, 2375–2382. [CrossRef] [PubMed]
56. Amiral, J.; Bridey, F.; Dreyfus, M.; Vissoc, A.M.; Fressinaud, E.; Wolf, M.; Meyer, D. Platelet factor 4 complexed to heparin is the target for antibodies generated in heparin-induced thrombocytopenia. *Thromb. Haemost.* **1992**, *68*, 95–96. [CrossRef] [PubMed]
57. Amiral, J.; Bridey, F.; Wolf, M.; Boyer-Neumann, C.; Fressinaud, E.; Vissac, A.M.; Peynaud-Debayle, E.; Dreyfus, M.; Meyer, D. Antibodies to macromolecular platelet factor 4-heparin complexes in heparin-induced thrombocytopenia: A study of 44 cases. *Thromb. Haemost.* **1995**, *73*, 21–28. [CrossRef]
58. Chan, M.; Zhao, X.; Zheng, X.L. Low ADAMTS-13 predicts adverse outcomes in hospitalized patients with suspected heparin-induced thrombocytopenia. *Res. Pract. Thromb. Haemost.* **2021**, *5*, e12581. [CrossRef]
59. Demagny, J.; Driss, A.; Stepanian, A.; Anguel, N.; Affo, L.; Roux, D.; Habibi, A.; Benghezal, S.; Capdenat, S.; Coppo, P.; et al. ADAMTS13 and von Willebrand factor assessment in steady state and acute vaso-occlusive crisis of sickle cell disease. *Res. Pract. Thromb. Haemost.* **2021**, *5*, 197–203. [CrossRef]
60. Schnog, J.J.; Kremer Hovinga, J.A.; Krieg, S.; Akin, S.; Lämmle, B.; Brandjes, D.P.; Mac Gillavry, M.R.; Muskiet, F.D.; Duits, A.J. ADAMTS13 activity in sickle cell disease. *Am. J. Hematol.* **2006**, *81*, 492–498. [CrossRef]
61. Vital, E.F.; Lam, W.A. Hidden behind thromboinflammation: Revealing the roles of von Willebrand factor in sickle cell disease pathophysiology. *Curr. Opin. Hematol.* **2023**, *30*, 86–92. [CrossRef] [PubMed]
62. Van der Land, V.; Peters, M.; Biemond, B.J.; Heijboer, H.; Harteveld, C.L.; Fijnvandraat, K. Markers of endothelial dysfunction differ between subphenotypes in children with sickle cell disease. *Thromb. Res.* **2013**, *132*, 712–717. [CrossRef] [PubMed]
63. Fogarty, H.; Ahmad, A.; Atiq, F.; Doherty, D.; Ward, S.; Karampini, E.; Rehill, A.; Leon, G.; Byrne, C.; Geoghegan, R.; et al. VWF–ADAMTS13 axis dysfunction in children with sickle cell disease treated with hydroxycarbamide vs blood transfusion. *Blood Adv.* **2023**, *7*, 6974–6989. [CrossRef] [PubMed]
64. Colombatti, R.; De Bon, E.; Bertomoro, A.; Casonato, A.; Pontara, E.; Omenetto, E.; Saggiorato, G.; Steffan, A.; Damian, T.; Cella, G.; et al. Coagulation activation in children with sickle cell disease is associated with cerebral small vessel vasculopathy. *PLoS ONE* **2013**, *8*, e78801. [CrossRef] [PubMed]
65. Rossato, P.; Federti, E.; Matte, A.; Glantschnig, H.; Canneva, F.; Schuster, M.; Coulibaly, S.; Schrenk, G.; Voelkel, D.; Dockal, M.; et al. Evidence of protective effects of recombinant ADAMTS13 in a humanized model of sickle cell disease. *Haematologica* **2022**, *107*, 2650–2660. [CrossRef]
66. Ko, S.; Okano, E.; Kanehiro, H.; Matsumoto, M.; Ishizashi, H.; Uemura, M.; Fujimura, Y.; Tanaka, K.; Nakajima, Y. Plasma ADAMTS13 activity may predict early adverse events in living donor liver transplantation: Observations in 3 cases. *Liver Transpl.* **2006**, *12*, 859–869. [CrossRef]
67. Sayah, D.M.; Mallavia, B.; Liu, F.; Ortiz-Muñoz, G.; Caudrillier, A.; DerHovanessian, A.; Ross, D.J.; Lynch, J.P., 3rd; Saggar, R.; Ardehali, A.; et al. Neutrophil extracellular traps are pathogenic in primary graft dysfunction after lung transplantation. *Am. J. Respir. Crit. Care Med.* **2015**, *191*, 455–463. [CrossRef]
68. Wong, S.L.; Goverman, J.; Staudinger, C.; Wagner, D.D. Recombinant human ADAMTS13 treatment and anti-NET strategies enhance skin allograft survival in mice. *Am. J. Transplant.* **2020**, *20*, 1162–1169. [CrossRef]
69. Vanhoorelbeke, K.; De Meyer, S.F. Animal models for thrombotic thrombocytopenic purpura. *J. Thromb. Haemost.* **2013**, *11*, 2–10. [CrossRef]
70. Feys, H.B.; Roodt, J.; Vandeputte, N.; Pareyn, I.; Lamprecht, S.; van Rensburg, W.J.; Anderson, P.J.; Budde, U.; Louw, V.J.; Badenhorst, P.N.; et al. Thrombotic thrombocytopenic purpura directly linked with ADAMTS13 inhibition in the baboon (*Papio ursinus*). *Blood* **2010**, *116*, 2005–2010. [CrossRef]
71. Schiviz, A.; Wuersch, K.; Piskernik, C.; Dietrich, B.; Hoellriegl, W.; Rottensteiner, H.; Scheiflinger, F.; Schwarz, H.P.; Muchitsch, E.M. A new mouse model mimicking thrombotic thrombocytopenic purpura: Correction of symptoms by recombinant human ADAMTS13. *Blood* **2012**, *119*, 6128–6135. [CrossRef]
72. Motto, D.G.; Chauhan, A.K.; Zhu, G.; Homeister, J.; Lamb, C.B.; Desch, K.C.; Zhang, W.; Tsai, H.-M.; Wagner, D.D.; Ginsburg, D. Shigatoxin triggers thrombotic thrombocytopenic purpura in genetically susceptible ADAMTS13-deficient mice. *J. Clin. Investig.* **2005**, *115*, 2752–2761. [CrossRef] [PubMed]
73. Banno, F.; Kokame, K.; Okuda, T.; Honda, S.; Miyata, S.; Kato, H.; Tomiyama, Y.; Miyata, T. Complete deficiency in ADAMTS13 is prothrombotic, but it alone is not sufficient to cause thrombotic thrombocytopenic purpura. *Blood* **2006**, *107*, 3161–3166. [CrossRef] [PubMed]
74. Tersteeg, C.; Schiviz, A.; De Meyer, S.F.; Plaimauer, B.; Scheiflinger, F.; Rottensteiner, H.; Vanhoorelbeke, K. Potential for Recombinant ADAMTS13 as an Effective Therapy for Acquired Thrombotic Thrombocytopenic Purpura. *Arterioscler. Thromb. Vasc. Biol.* **2015**, *35*, 2336–2342. [CrossRef] [PubMed]

75. Scully, M.; Antun, A.; Cataland, S.R.; Coppo, P.; Dossier, C.; Biebuyck, N.; Hassenpflug, W.-A.; Kentouche, K.; Knöbl, P.; Hovinga, J.A.K.; et al. Recombinant ADAMTS13 in Congenital Thrombotic Thrombocytopenic Purpura. *N. Engl. J. Med.* **2024**, *390*, 1584–1596. [CrossRef]
76. Kanter, J.; Patwari, P.; Desai, P.; Ataga, K.I.; Crary, S.E.; Lanzkron, S.; Field, J.; Chung, Y.-C.; Wang, L.T.; Mellgård, B.; et al. Safety and Pharmacokinetics osf Recombinant ADAMTS13 in Patients with Sickle Cell Disease: A Phase 1 Randomized, Double-Blind, Placebo-Controlled Study. *Blood* **2023**, *142*, 149. [CrossRef]

Disclaimer/Publisher's Note: The statements, opinions and data contained in all publications are solely those of the individual author(s) and contributor(s) and not of MDPI and/or the editor(s). MDPI and/or the editor(s) disclaim responsibility for any injury to people or property resulting from any ideas, methods, instructions or products referred to in the content.

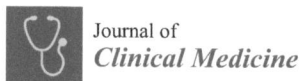

Journal of
Clinical Medicine

Systematic Review

Patient-Reported Outcome Measures in Patients with Thrombotic Thrombocytopenic Purpura: A Systematic Review of the Literature

Alexandre Soares Ferreira Junior [1], Morgana Pinheiro Maux Lessa [1], Samantha Kaplan [2], Theresa M. Coles [3], Deirdra R. Terrell [4] and Oluwatoyosi A. Onwuemene [5,*]

1. Department of Medicine, Faculdade de Medicina de São José do Rio Preto, São José do Rio Preto 15090-000, São Paulo, Brazil
2. Medical Center Library & Archives, Duke University Medical Center, Durham, NC 27710, USA; samantha.kaplan@duke.edu
3. Department of Population Health Sciences, Duke University School of Medicine, Durham, NC 27710, USA; theresa.coles@duke.edu
4. Department of Biostatistics and Epidemiology, Hudson College of Public Health, University of Oklahoma Health Sciences Center, Oklahoma City, OK 73104, USA; dee-terrell@ouhsc.edu
5. Division of Hematology, Department of Medicine, Duke University School of Medicine, Durham, NC 27710, USA
* Correspondence: toyosi.onwuemene@duke.edu; Tel.: +1-(919)-684-5350; Fax: +1-(919)-681-1177

Citation: Soares Ferreira Junior, A.; Pinheiro Maux Lessa, M.; Kaplan, S.; Coles, T.M.; Terrell, D.R.; Onwuemene, O.A. Patient-Reported Outcome Measures in Patients with Thrombotic Thrombocytopenic Purpura: A Systematic Review of the Literature. *J. Clin. Med.* **2023**, *12*, 5155. https://doi.org/10.3390/jcm12155155

Academic Editors: Ilaria Mancini and Andrea Artoni

Received: 14 June 2023
Revised: 31 July 2023
Accepted: 1 August 2023
Published: 7 August 2023

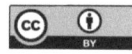

Copyright: © 2023 by the authors. Licensee MDPI, Basel, Switzerland. This article is an open access article distributed under the terms and conditions of the Creative Commons Attribution (CC BY) license (https://creativecommons.org/licenses/by/4.0/).

Abstract: Health-related quality of life (HRQoL) impacts of thrombotic thrombocytopenic purpura (TTP) have been captured in clinical studies using patient-reported outcome (PRO) measures (PROMs) that are validated for other diseases. However, the validity evidence to support the use of existing PROMs in patients with TTP is unknown. In a systematic review of the literature, including studies of adults and children with TTP, we assessed the validity evidence for use of PROMs in clinical research and clinical practice, characterized HRQoL, described the integration of PROMs in clinical practice and evaluated PRO scores for patients with TTP compared with reference populations. From an initial 4518 studies, we identified 14 studies using 16 PROMs to assess general HRQoL domains in patients in remission. No identified studies assessed the validity of PROMs for the context of use of TTP and no studies described PROM integration into TTP clinical practice or evaluated PROMs that were specific for patients with TTP. Moreover, PRO scores were worse in patients with TTP compared with reference populations and other chronic conditions. We conclude that, in patients with TTP, PROMs pick up on important patient experiences not captured by clinical outcomes at present. There is, therefore, a need for studies that assess the validity of existing PROMs in patients with TTP to determine if TTP-specific PROMs specific to patients with TTP should be developed.

Keywords: patient reported outcomes; patient reported outcome measures; health-related quality of life; thrombotic thrombocytopenic purpura

1. Introduction

Thrombotic thrombocytopenic purpura (TTP) is a life-threatening thrombotic disorder with significant impacts on health-related quality of life (HRQoL) [1,2]. While healthcare providers prioritize clinical outcomes, such as platelet counts, lactate dehydrogenase levels, and ADAMTS13 (a disintegrin and metalloproteinase with a thrombospondin type 1 motif, member 13) activity, HRQoL outcomes are most important to patients [3–6]. Significant HRQoL impacts reported by patients in remission from acute TTP include fatigue, headache, depression, and cognitive impairment [2,4,7–9].

HRQoL impacts are best measured using patient reported outcome measures (PROMs). PROMs are self-completed tools that assess one or multiple outcomes from the patient's perspective. PROMs capture HRQoL impacts by direct patient self-report, without interpretation through the lens of a healthcare provider [10]. PROMs can help assess disease burden and evaluate response to therapy [11–13]. PROMs can also help improve the assessment of HRQoL impacts of therapies by patients, clinicians, and researchers. Additionally, if shown to be valid and reliable, PROMs can be used to support FDA approval of candidate therapies in clinical trials [14].

PROMs are increasingly being used in research studies to measure TTP-associated HRQoL impacts. However, it is not known if and how PROMs have been implemented in TTP clinical settings. It is also not known whether PROMs used at present capture TTP-specific HRQoL impacts or how they may change TTP clinical management. Finally, it is also not known what the validity evidence is for using PROMs for the context of use of TTP. Therefore, to define the landscape of PROMs at present and their validity evidence in studies of patients with TTP, we undertook a systematic review of the literature. As an exploratory objective to characterize TTP-related morbidity, we also reported patient-reported outcomes (PROs) scores across studies.

2. Materials and Methods

2.1. Search Strategy and Selection Criteria

This study was a systematic review reported in concordance with PRISMA guidelines (Preferred Reporting Items for Systematic Reviews and Meta-Analyses) [15], and registered with PROSPERO (Registration CRD42022347498) [16].

An electronic search of the literature was conducted using the databases Medline (PubMed), Embase (Elsevier), Scopus (Elsevier), and CINAHL (EBSCO) from inception to 10 June 2022. On 10 October 2022, an updated and more sensitive search was completed, to which was added ClinicalTrials.gov. Search keywords were the following: thrombotic thrombocytopenic purpura, quality of life, anxiety, memory, cognition, outcome, attention, and PROMs (for the detailed search strategy, see supplemental Appendix SA Table SA1–SA9).

Study inclusion criteria were the following: (1) studies of patients with a TTP clinical diagnosis (regardless of ADAMTS13 activity) and (2) studies that reported on the use of PROMs (utilization, development, and testing of measurement properties). PROMs could include known PROMs previously identified in the literature or any other patient self-administered instrument.

Studies were excluded for the following reasons: (1) the population included patients with hereditary TTP alone; (2) PROMs were not evaluated; or (3) PRO results were not reported. Also excluded were case reports (sample size of one patient), reviews, commentaries, studies in non-human subjects, and studies in languages other than English.

The search strategy included a manual review of published article reference lists. We also searched were unpublished studies using gray literature sources (ClinicalTrials.gov and Embase). References were compiled in Endnote and articles were uploaded into Covidence systematic review software (Veritas Health Innovation, Melbourne, Australia) [17]. After deduplication, all titles and abstracts were screened by two independent reviewers (ASFJ and MPML) to determine their suitability for a full-text review. Full-text articles were reviewed by the same independent reviewers (ASFJ and MPML). Conflicts were resolved through a discussion between the two reviewers or by a binding vote from a third independent reviewer (OAO).

2.2. Data Analysis

Study quality was assessed by two independent reviewers (ASFJ and MPML) using the Joanna Briggs Institute Clinical Appraisal Tools checklist for Cross-Sectional, Cohort, and Clinical Trial Studies [18]. Conflicts were resolved through discussions or by a third independent reviewer (OAO).

As an initial template to capture the data, the reviewers used a data abstraction table. Summary data were extracted from published reports and included the following variables:

primary author and year of study; study objective; number of patients; time from last TTP episode; mean time of PROM completion; PROM characteristics (names, number of PROMs used, and domains assessed); PROM clinical practice integration strategies; PROM clinical practice integration impacts; and PRO scores for patients with TTP and the reference population.

As an exploratory objective to characterize TTP-related morbidity across studies, PRO scores comparing patients with TTP to normal controls or the general population were reported. This report assumed that the PROMs were appropriate for patients with TTP within the specified contexts of use. Where applicable, the results of statistical analyses performed within each study are noted.

Finally, in a post hoc analysis, we identified important TTP domains from the patient's perspective that have not yet been assessed by studies evaluating PROMs in the literature.

3. Results

3.1. Included Studies

Following deduplication, the search strategy yielded 4518 studies for screening. Nine additional articles were identified through article reference lists. After the abstract review, 41 articles advanced to a full-text review. Of those 41 articles, 25 studies were excluded (see Figure 1). Studies excluded for using instruments that did not meet criteria for PROMs are summarized in Table S1 (Supplementary Materials) [7,13,19–27]. Therefore, 16 articles were advanced to a quality review. During the quality review, two additional studies were excluded due to the inability to distinguish the results of patients with TTP from those of other diseases [28,29]. Therefore, the final number of studies for analysis was 14, of which five (36%) were cross-sectional studies, eight (57%) were cohort, and one was a clinical trial (7%). These 14 studies covered 16 PROMs in 970 patients with TTP.

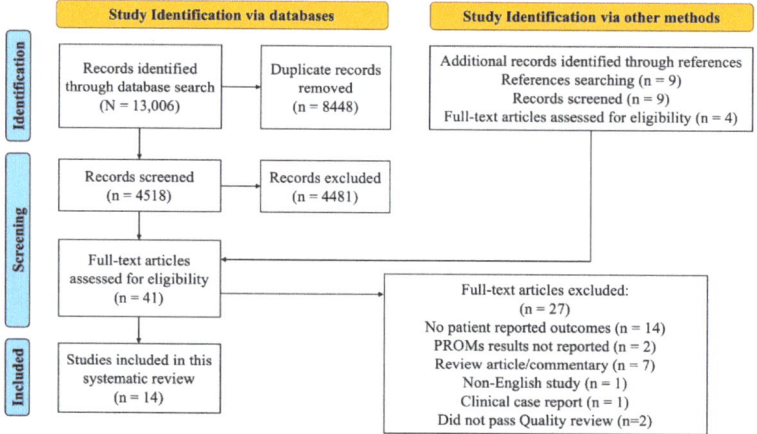

Figure 1. PRISMA flow diagram. There were 13,006 references imported for screening and 8448 duplicates removed. The number of studies screened against title and abstract was 4518. Based on the title and abstract screening, 4481 studies were excluded. Additionally, nine studies were identified manually through references searching. Among those, four studies were assessed for eligibility in the full-text review. Of all full text studies assessed (n = 41), 27 studies were excluded, including 14 with no PROMs, two with no PROMs results, seven review/commentary articles, one clinical case report, and one non-English study. Two studies were also excluded in the quality review. The final number of included studies was 14.

3.2. PROMs in Published Studies

Among the 14 studies assessing 16 PROMs (see Table 1 for detailed PROMs data), none reported the use of TTP-specific PROMs. Additionally, none of the studies assessed either strategies for, or the impact of, PROM integration into TTP clinical practice. Only one study evaluated the ease of understanding and relevancy of TTP-specific questions [5]. Additionally, PROMs were mostly assessed for adult patients (TTP typically occurs in adults). Only one study evaluated PROMs in pediatric patients (minimum age: 13 years old); however; the results specific to pediatric patients were not reported [21].

Table 1. (a) PROMs measuring overall health-related quality of life in patients with thrombotic thrombocytopenic purpura *. (b) PROMs measuring specific domains of health-related quality of life in patients with thrombotic thrombocytopenic purpura.

(a)		
Measure Average Completion Time	Number of Items Recall Period	Domains Evaluated
SF-36 [5,30] ** <15 min [2]	36 4 weeks	Physical Functioning
		Bodily Pain
		General Health
		Vitality
		Role Physical
		Role Emotional
		Social Functioning
		Mental Health
QLQ-C30 [31–33] <9 min [34]	30 1 week	Physical Functioning
		Role Functioning
		Cognitive Functioning
		Emotional Functioning
		Social Functioning
		Global Quality of Life
		Fatigue
		Nausea/Vomiting
		Pain
		Appetite Loss
		Diarrhea
		Dyspnea
		Constipation
		Insomnia
		Financial Impact
HIT-6 [8,35] <2 min [36]	6 4 weeks	Pain
		Role Functioning
		Social Functioning
		Vitality (Energy/Fatigue)
		Cognition
		Emotion Distress

Table 1. Cont.

(b)		
Depression and Anxiety Instruments		
PHQ-8/-9 [12,37] <5 min [37–40]	8 or 9 *** 2 weeks	Depression
BDI-II [5,41] 5–10 min [42]	21 2 weeks	Depression
GAD-7 [12,43] <2 min [44]	7 2 weeks	Anxiety
HADS [5,45] <5 min [45]	14 1 week	Depression
		Anxiety
IDS-SR [46–48] <7 min [49]	30 1 week	Depression
DASS [50] 10 to 20 min [51]	42 1 week	Depression
		Anxiety
		Stress
Post-traumatic Stress Disorder Instrument		
PCL-5 [52,53] 5–10 min [54]	20 1 month	PTSD
Cognitive Function Instruments		
PROMIS CFAS-SF6a [5,55] Time to complete NR	6 1 week	Cognitive Function Abilities
Flei [9,56–58] 10 min [59]	30 6 months	Attention
		Memory
		Executive Functions
Resilience and Life Orientation Instruments		
RS-11 [60,61] Time to complete NR	11 N/A	Mental Resistance
LOT-R [58,62] <3 min [63]	10 N/A	Attitude to Life
Work Activity Instruments		
WPAI-SHP [64,65] Time to complete NR	6 1 week	Absenteeism
		Presenteeism
		Work Productivity Loss
		Activity Impairment

BDI-II = Beck Depression Inventory II; DASS = Depression, Anxiety, and Stress Scale; FLei = German questionnaire for complaints of cognitive disturbances; GAD-7 = Generalized Anxiety Disorder; HADS = Hospital Anxiety and Depression Scale; HIT-6 = Headache Impact Test-6; IDS-SR = Inventory of Depressive Symptomatology Self Report; LOT-R = Life Orientation Test—Revised; N/A = not applicable; PCL-5 = PTSD checklist for Diagnostic and Statistical Manual of Mental Disorders (DSM-5); Patient-Reported Outcomes Measurement Information System (PROMIS)-CFAS-SF6a = PROMIS Cognitive Function Abilities Subset Short Form 6a; PTSD = Post-Traumatic Stress Disorder; PHQ-8 = Patient Health Questionnaire Depression Scale 8; PHQ-9 = Patient Health Questionnaire Depression Scale 9; QLQ-C30 = Quality of Life Questionnaire C30; RS-11 = Resilience Scale; SF-36 = Short-Form Health Survey; WPAI-SHP = Work Productivity Activity Impairment: Specific Health Problem; * = HIT-6 included among HRQoL instruments to facilitate reading; ** = includes both versions 1 and 2 of the SF-36; *** = PHQ-8 includes only 8 questions.

Following recovery from an acute TTP episode, the three most common domains assessed were overall HRQoL, depression, and anxiety. In eight studies (57%), the overall HRQoL was assessed using three different PROMs: Short-Form Health Survey (SF-36) [2,5,13,19,20,66]; Headache Impact Test-6 (HIT-6) [8,13]; and Quality of Life Questionnaire C30 (QLQ-C30) [58]. In eight studies (57%), depression was assessed using six different PROMs: Patient Health Questionnaire Depression Scale 9-item and 8-item instruments (PHQ-9; PHQ-8) [4,21,58,67]; Beck Depression Inventory (BDI-II) [7,52,67]; Inventory of Depressive Symptomatology Self Report (IDS-SR) [9]; Depression, Anxiety and Stress Scale (DASS); [21] and Hospital Anxiety and Depression Scale (HADS) [5,21]. In three studies (21%), anxiety was assessed using three different PROMs: Generalized Anxiety Disorder (GAD-7) [21,58]; Hospital Anxiety and Depression Scale (HADS) [5,21]; and Depression, Anxiety, and Stress Scale (DASS) [21].

Domains less commonly evaluated were post-traumatic stress disorder (PTSD) [52], resilience and life orientation [58], memory [9,58], attention [9,58], executive function [9,58], cognitive function abilities [5], work absenteeism [5], work presenteeism [5], work productivity loss [5], and activity impairment [5] (see Tables S2–S4).

The post hoc analysis identified four qualitative studies reporting important domains from the patient's perspective (see Table 2) [5,67–69]. These findings are summarized in Figure 2.

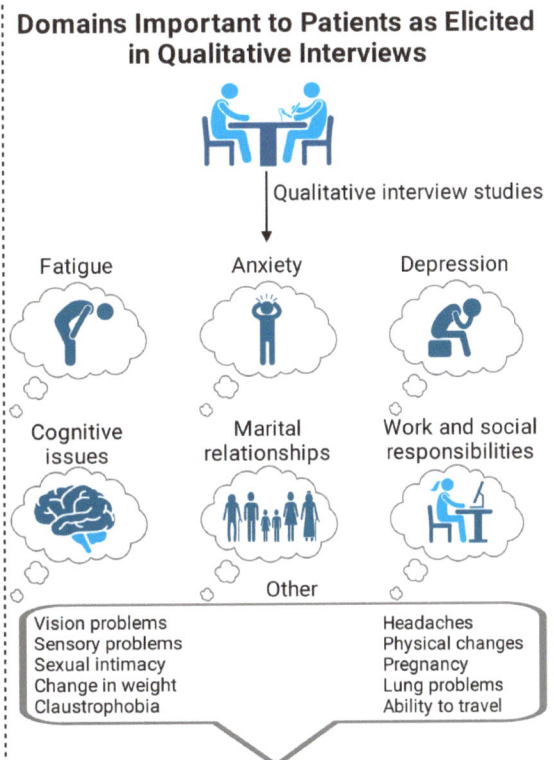

Figure 2. Important domains and impacts from the patient's perspective. Created with BioRender.com accessed on 12 June 2023.

Table 2. Important TTP domains and impacts from the patient's perspective.

Patient-Reported Domains/Impacts	Prior Studies Assessing Patient's Perspective				Administered PROMs in Prior Studies
	Oladapo et al. 2018 [69,70]	Holmes et al. 2005 [5]	Terrell et al. 2019 [6]	Kelley et al. 2022 [68]	
Cognitive issues	N/A	X	X	X	FLei [9,58] PROMIS CFAS-SF6a [5]
Fatigue	X	X	X	X	QLQ-C30 [9]
Depression	N/A	X	X	X	PHQ-8/9 [4,6,21,58] BDI-II [6,7,52] IDS-SR [9] HADS [5,21] DASS [21]
Anxiety (including fear of relapse)	X	X	X	X	HADS [5,21] DASS [21] GAD-7 [9,21]
Impact on relationships/family	N/A	X	X	X	SF-36 [2,13,19,20]
Impact on social activities	N/A	X	X	X	SF-36 [2,13,19,20] QLQ-C30 [9]
Impact on work/career	X	X	X	X	WPAI-SHP [5] SF-36 [2,13,19,20]
Experience of flashbacks	N/A	X	N/A	N/A	Not assessed
PTSD	N/A	X	N/A	N/A	PCL-5 [52]
Lack of independence	N/A	X	N/A	N/A	Not assessed
Pain/Headache	X	N/A	N/A	X	HIT-6 [8,13] SF-36 [2,13,19,20] QLQ-C30 [9]
Bruising	X	N/A	N/A	N/A	Not assessed
Sensory problems	X	N/A	N/A	X	Not assessed
Lung problems	N/A	N/A	N/A	X	Not assessed
Claustrophobia	N/A	N/A	N/A	X	Not assessed

BDI-II = Beck Depression Inventory II; DASS = Depression, Anxiety and Stress Scale; FLei = German questionnaire for complaints of cognitive disturbances; GAD-7 = Generalized Anxiety Disorder; HADS = Hospital Anxiety and Depression Scale; HIT-6 = Headache Impact Test-6; IDS-SR = Inventory of Depressive Symptomatology Self Report; N/A = not applicable; PCL-5 = PTSD checklist for Diagnostic and Statistical Manual of Mental Disorders (DSM-5); Patient-Reported Outcomes Measurement Information System (PROMIS)-CFAS-SF6a = PROMIS Cognitive Function Abilities Subset Short Form 6a; PTSD = Post-Traumatic Stress Disorder; PHQ-8 = Patient Health Questionnaire Depression Scale 8; PHQ-9 = Patient Health Questionnaire Depression Scale 9; QLQ-C30 = Quality of Life Questionnaire C30; SF-36 = Short-Form Health Survey; WPAI-SHP = Work Productivity Activity Impairment: Specific Health Problem; X = Assessed.

3.3. PROMs in Unpublished Studies

Three studies were identified through clinicaltrials.gov and the published results were available for one study: the post-HERCULES trial (included in summaries of published studies above). Published results were not available for two studies: the ConNeCT Study (Neurological Complications of TTP), an observational study, and CAPLAVIE (Efficacy of a Personalized Caplacizumab Regimen Based on ADAMTS13 Activity Monitoring in Adult TTP), a clinical trial [26,27]. While the ConNeCT study assessed depression and overall HRQoL using PHQ-9 and SF-36 [26], the CAPLAVIE trial assessed PTSD symptom severity using the PCL-5 [27].

3.4. PROMs Capturing the Impact of TTP-Related Morbidity

The results of our exploratory analyses, in which HRQoL domains in patients with TTP were compared with a reference population, are shown in Supplementary Tables S2–S4. In general, following recovery from an acute TTP episode, patients had significant HRQoL impacts.

When PROMs were used to assess overall HRQoL, patients with TTP had worse scores than the general US and Italian population (norms). Additionally, patients with TTP had similar or worse scores than patients with other chronic conditions (anemia, cancer, and depression) [2,5,8,13,19,20,58,66].

Similar findings are shown when PROMs are used to assess specific HRQoL domains. Across the studies, there was a statistically higher prevalence of depression and anxiety in patients with TTP when compared with the control groups [4,7,9,58]. Additionally, in patients with TTP, a positive PTSD screen was prevalent (35%) [52]. Patients with TTP also had worse scores than healthy controls in cognitive function (memory, attention, executive function, and cognitive function abilities) [5,9]. Finally, patients with TTP reported significant impacts on work-related quality of life (see Supplementary Tables S2–S4) [5].

3.5. Association between PROMs and TTP Episode Characteristics

Seven studies evaluated the relationship between PROMs and TTP episode characteristics (number of TTP episodes, neurological symptoms, number of therapeutic plasma exchange [TPE] procedures, ADAMTS13 activity during remission, and abnormal magnetic resonance imaging [MRI]). These studies used nine PROMs: SF-36 [2], HIT-6 [8], IDS-SR [9], PHQ-8 or 9 [4,21], HADS [21], DASS [21], GAD-7 [21], BDI-II [7,52], and PCL-5 [52].

Most studies (5/7, 71%) assessed the relationship between TTP episode characteristics and depression and anxiety. In these studies, anxiety and depression were assessed after the TTP episode; however, the time from the TTP episode to administering the PROM was reported by only two studies [7,52]. For these studies, the median time from the TTP episode to administering the PROM was 6.3 and 6.6 years. Depression and anxiety scores were not statistically associated with number of TTP episodes [4,7,9,52], presence of neurological symptoms [4,9,52], number of TPE procedures [4], ADAMTS13 activity during remission [7], and abnormal MRI [21].

One study assessed the relationship between TTP episode characteristics and scores on all SF-36 domains after the initial TTP diagnosis (median time 1.53 years). Scores on all domains were not statistically associated with TTP clinical triggers (idiopathic vs. other), presence of severe ADAMTS13 deficiency, number of TPE procedures, and presence of neurologic symptoms [2].

Additionally, one study assessed the relationship between TTP episode characteristics and HIT-6 scores after the last TTP episode (average time: 3.12 years). Although no statistical analyses were performed, the study suggested that headache severity scores were not associated with the number of TTP episodes, time from last TTP episode, or ADAMTS13 activity level [8].

Finally, one study assessed the relationship between TTP episode characteristics and cognitive deficits using FLei. Cognitive scores were not found to be statistically associated with the number of TTP episodes and the presence of neurological symptoms [9].

4. Discussion

Our systematic review identified 14 studies that used 16 PROMs to assess HRQoL domains in TTP. The five main findings were the following: (1) the small number of studies using PROMs in patients with TTP; (2) the absence of studies assessing psychometric properties of PROMs in patients with TTP; (3) the absence of studies evaluating strategies for, and the impact of, integrating PROMs into TTP clinical practice; (4) the absence of PROMs developed specifically for patients with TTP; and (5) decreased HRQoL in patients with TTP when compared with reference populations and other chronic conditions.

PROMs were originally developed for pharmacological research to assess therapeutic effectiveness [71]. More recently, PROMs have been used to support clinical decision making, prioritize patients for surgical procedures, and improve healthcare quality in clinical practice [71,72]. When integrated into clinical practice, PROMs have been shown to optimize provision of patient-centered healthcare, reduce healthcare services utilization, and enhance patient–clinician communication. PROMs have also been shown to increase patient satisfaction and improve HRQoL outcomes [73,74]. In the clinical care of patients with chronic conditions, PROMs have been shown to both improve disease activity and increase survival [73].

Although PROMs are used in hematological research, little is known about their integration into hematology clinical practice [68,75]. For chronic hematological disorders, integrating PROMs into clinical practice may reduce disease burden through the early identification and management of residual symptoms, such as fatigue, depression and anxiety [68,75]. Despite the growing number of PROMs being applied in hematology, integrating PROMs into clinical practice poses some challenges. First, a standard PROM scoring system does not exist and medical providers find it difficult to make clinical decisions using normative-based scores [76]. Second, the integration of PROMs into healthcare systems may be influenced by structural barriers. These barriers include consultation time, absence of implementation recommendations, and prioritization of laboratory outcomes [75]. Third, successful integration relies on using validated PROMs that have undergone psychometric processes to ensure that the PROM measures what is intended [75]. Although PROMs represent the patient's views of their own health, the outcome assessed may not be important to the patient or to health itself [71]. Therefore, PROMs that are ideal for use in clinical practices are those that both assess important outcomes for patients and providers and are valid, reliable, and specific to the context of use for the disease under study [71].

In other chronic conditions with significant impacts on HRQoL, PROMs have been used for clinical purposes [12,77–79]. In two prior systematic reviews, PROMs were identified to have the potential to be applied to clinical practice in the following five ways: (1) assess HRQoL in a structured and validated way; (2) foster patient–clinician communication; (3) monitor therapeutic impacts on HRQoL; (4) develop personalized management plans; and (5) increase health awareness [12,77]. Similar clinical applications were also suggested by a qualitative study of 44 patients with TTP in remission. In this study, focus groups (7 groups; n = 25) and individual interviews (n = 19) were conducted to assess TTP residual symptoms and patient–hematologist communication [68]. In all 7 (100%) focus groups and 18 (95%) individual interviews, patients reported residual TTP symptoms that were negatively impacting their activities of daily living [68]. Most patients also reported barriers to communicating these residual symptoms to their hematologists. Based on the abovementioned studies and considering TTP-related morbidity, the potential goals for PROM utilization in TTP are summarized in Figure 3.

Despite these potential applications in TTP care, integrating PROMs into clinical practice poses the aforementioned challenges [75,76]. Therefore, future prospective studies are desired to determine the optimal strategies for integrating PROMs into TTP clinical practice and assess other potential applications.

Our post hoc analysis revealed TTP domains that were felt to be important from the patient's perspective but were not evaluated in any of the included studies (see Figure 2). In a qualitative study of 50 patients, Holmes et al. identified domains that were important to patients with TTP. These domains included: (1) fatigue; (2) cognitive domains of attention, concentration, and the ability to use language; (3) ability to travel; (4) fear of relapse; and (5) desire/ability to have sex [5]. Another qualitative study of 44 patients with TTP determined that the most important symptoms impacting activities of daily life were cognitive impairment, fatigue, relapse-related anxiety, and depression [68]. Another study by Oladapo et al. reported that domains previously identified as important to patients with hereditary TTP were also relevant to patients with acquired TTP. These domains included vision problems, bruising, dizziness, numbness, sleep disturbance, and fear of relapse [69,70]. Although these domains may be assessed by PROMs available at present, these PROMs cannot be recommended for use in patients with TTP until studies are conducted to evaluate the content validity (understandability and appropriateness) for the context of use of TTP [80]. Thus, content validity studies are needed to facilitate the interpretation of currently available generic PROMs in patients with TTP.

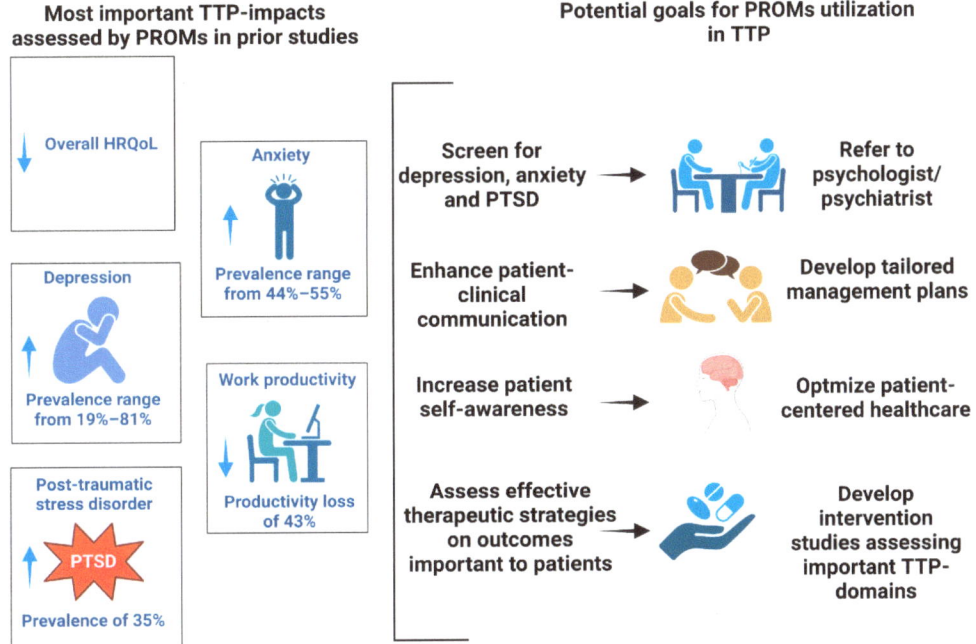

Figure 3. Potential goals for PROM utilization in patients with TTP. Created with BioRender.com accessed on 11 July 2023.

There may be a potential benefit of incorporating PROMs that assess specific domains relevant to patients with TTP [5,68–70]. Disease-specific PROMs are designed to capture elements relevant to a specific population or condition and can be used to identify unmet needs and patients priorities [81–83]. Rather than disease-specific PROMs, TTP studies have used only generic PROMs. Although widely used across different diseases, generic PROMs may not be sensitive enough to pick up certain specific aspects of the disease under study [81]. Therefore, including disease-specific PROMs in clinical studies would illuminate important information about the impacts of TTP and TTP therapies from the patient's perspective [5,69,70]. Nevertheless, to guide the development of TTP-specific PROMs, future studies are needed using validated methodological processes. These would include both quantitative and qualitative studies [84].

The strengths of our study lie in its comprehensive review of the landscape of PROMs used in patients with TTP and summary of TTP-related morbidity based on PRO scores. Our review, however, is limited by the overlap of patients across studies, in which PROMs may have been repeatedly administered to the same population. Additionally, since ADAMTS13 activity was not used as an inclusion criterion, patients with other types of thrombotic microangiopathy may have been included among our cohort. Furthermore, since our review included qualitative studies only in a post hoc analysis, some concepts, such as understandability, could not be assessed. Finally, the heterogeneity in domains assessed by different PROMs prevented effective comparisons across studies. Nevertheless, our systematic review is an important milestone in defining the landscape of PROMs in

TTP and providing data to guide future studies assessing the use of PROMs in patients with TTP.

5. Conclusions

Although PROMs are being used to assess several domains in patients with TTP, studies assessing the psychometric properties of present measures are desired. Additionally desired are qualitative concept elicitation studies. These studies would assess the acceptability of current PROMs for the context of use of patients with TTP. They would also determine whether existing PROMs should be modified for use in patients with TTP or whether there is a need to develop disease-specific PROMs.

Supplementary Materials: The following supporting information can be downloaded at: https://www.mdpi.com/article/10.3390/jcm12155155/s1, Appendix SA: Detailed search strategy (Tables SA1–SA9). Table S1: List of instruments excluded in the full-text review; Table S2: patient-reported outcome measures in patients with TTP assessing physical health; Table S3: patient-reported outcome measures in patients with TTP assessing mental health and cognitive function; Table S4: patient-reported outcome measures in patients with TTP assessing work productivity.

Author Contributions: O.A.O. conceived and designed the systematic review and O.A.O. and A.S.F.J. developed the systematic review protocol with input from T.M.C. and D.R.T., S.K. performed the literature search. A.S.F.J., M.P.M.L. and O.A.O. created the title and abstract screen, full-text review, and finalized the list of studies for inclusion. A.S.F.J. and M.P.M.L. performed the data abstraction. T.M.C. and D.R.T. led the data interpretation. A.S.F.J. wrote the first full manuscript draft. All authors have read and agreed to the published version of the manuscript.

Funding: This work was supported in part by a grant to O.A.O. from the American Society of Hematology/Harold Amos Faculty Development Program Award and a grant to D.R.T. by the National Heart, Lung, and Blood Institute of the National Institutes of Health under Award Number K01HL135466.

Institutional Review Board Statement: Not applicable.

Informed Consent Statement: Not applicable.

Data Availability Statement: Not applicable.

Conflicts of Interest: O.A.O. received an honorarium from Sanofi and D.R.T. served on an advisory board for Sanofi. All other authors declare no competing interests. The funders had no role in the design of the study; in the collection, analyses, or interpretation of data; in the writing of the manuscript; or in the decision to publish the results.

References

1. Joly, B.S.; Coppo, P.; Veyradier, A. An Update on Pathogenesis and Diagnosis of Thrombotic Thrombocytopenic Purpura. *Expert. Rev. Hematol.* **2019**, *12*, 383–395. [CrossRef] [PubMed]
2. Lewis, Q.F.; Lanneau, M.S.; Mathias, S.D.; Terrell, D.R.; Vesely, S.K.; George, J.N. Long-Term Deficits in Health-Related Quality of Life after Recovery from Thrombotic Thrombocytopenic Purpura. *Transfusion* **2009**, *49*, 118–124. [CrossRef] [PubMed]
3. Cuker, A.; Cataland, S.R.; Coppo, P.; de la Rubia, J.; Friedman, K.D.; George, J.N.; Knoebl, P.N.; Kremer Hovinga, J.A.; Lämmle, B.; Matsumoto, M.; et al. Redefining Outcomes in Immune TTP: An International Working Group Consensus Report. *Blood* **2021**, *137*, 1855–1861. [CrossRef]
4. Deford, C.C.; Reese, J.A.; Schwartz, L.H.; Perdue, J.J.; Kremer Hovinga, J.A.; Lämmle, B.; Terrell, D.R.; Vesely, S.K.; George, J.N. Multiple Major Morbidities and Increased Mortality during Long-Term Follow-up after Recovery from Thrombotic Thrombocytopenic Purpura. *Blood* **2013**, *122*, 2023–2029. [CrossRef] [PubMed]
5. Holmes, S.; Podger, L.; Bottomley, C.; Rzepa, E.; Bailey, K.M.A.; Chandler, F. Survival after Acute Episodes of Immune-Mediated Thrombotic Thrombocytopenic Purpura (ITTP)—Cognitive Functioning and Health-Related Quality of Life Impact: A Descriptive Cross-Sectional Survey of Adults Living with ITTP in the United Kingdom. *Hematology* **2021**, *26*, 465–472. [CrossRef]
6. Terrell, D.; Cataland, S.; Beebe, L.; Keller, S.; Panepinto, J.; Vesely, S.K.; George, J.; Kelley, R.A.; Cheney, M. Impact of Residual Effects and Complications of Thrombotic Thrombocytopenic Purpura (TTP) on Daily Living: A Qualitative Study. *Blood* **2019**, *134*, 931. [CrossRef]

7. Han, B.; Page, E.E.; Stewart, L.M.; Deford, C.C.; Scott, J.G.; Schwartz, L.H.; Perdue, J.J.; Terrell, D.R.; Vesely, S.K.; George, J.N. Depression and Cognitive Impairment Following Recovery from Thrombotic Thrombocytopenic Purpura: Depression and Cognitive Impairment Following TTP. *Am. J. Hematol.* **2015**, *90*, 709–714. [CrossRef]
8. Saultz, J.N.; Wu, H.M.; Cataland, S. Headache Prevalence Following Recovery from TTP and AHUS. *Ann. Hematol.* **2015**, *94*, 1473–1476. [CrossRef]
9. Falter, T.; Schmitt, V.; Herold, S.; Weyer, V.; von Auer, C.; Wagner, S.; Hefner, G.; Beutel, M.; Lackner, K.; Lämmle, B.; et al. Depression and Cognitive Deficits as Long-Term Consequences of Thrombotic Thrombocytopenic Purpura: Depression and cognitive deficits in TTP. *Transfusion* **2017**, *57*, 1152–1162. [CrossRef]
10. FDA-NIH Biomarker Working Group. BEST (Biomarkers, EndpointS, and Other Tools) Resource [Internet]. Silver Spring (MD): Food and Drug Administration (US); 2016-. Glossary. 2016 Jan 28 [Updated 2021 Nov 29]. Co-Published by National Institutes of Health (US), Bethesda (MD). Available online: https://www.ncbi.nlm.nih.gov/books/NBK326791/ (accessed on 14 December 2022).
11. Crego, N.; Masese, R.; Bonnabeau, E.; Douglas, C.; Rains, G.; Shah, N.; Tanabe, P. Patient Perspectives of Sickle Cell Management in the Emergency Department. *Crit. Care Nurs. Q.* **2021**, *44*, 160–174. [CrossRef]
12. Kinahan, J.Y.; Graham, J.M.I.; Hébert, Y.V.; Sampson, M.; O'Hearn, K.; Klaassen, R.J. Patient-Reported Outcome Measures in Pediatric Non-Malignant Hematology: A Systematic Review. *J. Pediatr. Hematol. Oncol.* **2021**, *43*, 121–134. [CrossRef] [PubMed]
13. Scully, M.; de la Rubia, J.; Pavenski, K.; Metjian, A.; Knöbl, P.; Peyvandi, F.; Cataland, S.; Coppo, P.; Kremer Hovinga, J.A.; Minkue Mi Edou, J.; et al. Long-term Follow-up of Patients Treated with Caplacizumab and Safety and Efficacy of Repeat Caplacizumab Use: Post-HERCULES Study. *J. Thromb. Haemost.* **2022**, *20*, 2810–2822. [CrossRef] [PubMed]
14. Patient-Reported Outcome Measures: Use in Medical Product Development to Support Labeling Claims: Guidance for Industry. Available online: https://www.fda.gov/regulatory-information/search-fda-guidance-documents/patient-reported-outcome-measures-use-medical-product-development-support-labeling-claims (accessed on 11 November 2022).
15. Moher, D.; Liberati, A.; Tetzlaff, J.; Altman, D.G. The PRISMA Group Preferred Reporting Items for Systematic Reviews and Meta-Analyses: The PRISMA Statement. *PLoS Med.* **2009**, *6*, e1000097. [CrossRef]
16. Page, M.J.; Shamseer, L.; Tricco, A.C. Registration of Systematic Reviews in PROSPERO: 30,000 Records and Counting. *Syst. Rev.* **2018**, *7*, 32. [CrossRef] [PubMed]
17. Covidence. *Covidence Systematic Review Software*; Veritas Health Innovation: Melbourne, Australia, 2022. Available online: https://www.covidence.org/ (accessed on 23 July 2022).
18. Joanna Briggs Institute Checklists for Case Reports and Case Series. Available online: https://jbi.global/critical-appraisal-tools (accessed on 17 April 2023).
19. Cataland, S.R.; Scully, M.A.; Paskavitz, J.; Maruff, P.; Witkoff, L.; Jin, M.; Uva, N.; Gilbert, J.C.; Wu, H.M. Evidence of Persistent Neurologic Injury Following Thrombotic Thrombocytopenic Purpura. *Am. J. Hematol.* **2011**, *86*, 87–89. [CrossRef]
20. Riva, S.; Mancini, I.; Maino, A.; Ferrari, B.; Artoni, A.; Agosti, P.; Peyvandi, F. Long-Term Neuropsychological Sequelae, Emotional Wellbeing and Quality of Life in Patients with Acquired Thrombotic Thrombocytopenic Purpura. *Haematologica* **2020**, *105*, 1957–1962. [CrossRef]
21. Alwan, F.; Mahdi, D.; Tayabali, S.; Cipolotti, L.; Lakey, G.; Hyare, H.; Scully, M. Cerebral MRI Findings Predict the Risk of Cognitive Impairment in Thrombotic Thrombocytopenic Purpura. *Br. J. Haematol.* **2020**, *191*, 868–874. [CrossRef] [PubMed]
22. Greenberg, D.B.; Carey, R.W. The Cost of Surviving Thrombotic Thrombocytopenic Purpura: Case Report. *J. Clin. Psychiatry* **1984**, *45*, 477–479.
23. Kennedy, A.S.; Lewis, Q.F.; Scott, J.G.; Kremer Hovinga, J.A.; Lämmle, B.; Terrell, D.R.; Vesely, S.K.; George, J.N. Cognitive Deficits after Recovery from Thrombotic Thrombocytopenic Purpura. *Transfusion* **2009**, *49*, 1092–1101. [CrossRef]
24. Clinical Outcome Study of ARC1779 Injection in Patients with Thrombotic Microangiopathy. Available online: https://clinicaltrials.gov/Ct2/Show/Study/NCT00726544 (accessed on 12 November 2022).
25. Study to Assess Efficacy and Safety of Anti-von Willebrand Factor (VWF) Nanobody in Patients with Acquired Thrombotic Thrombocytopenic Purpura (ATTP) (TITAN). Available online: https://classic.clinicaltrials.gov/ct2/show/NCT01151423 (accessed on 11 November 2022).
26. The ConNeCT Study: Neurological Complications of TTP. Available online: https://classic.clinicaltrials.gov/ct2/show/NCT04981028 (accessed on 9 September 2022).
27. Efficacy of a Personalized Caplacizumab Regimen Based on ADAMTS13 Activity Monitoring in Adult ATTP (CAPLAVIE). Available online: https://classic.clinicaltrials.gov/ct2/show/NCT04720261 (accessed on 9 September 2022).
28. Dahlan, R.; McCormick, B.B.; Alkhattabi, M.; Gallo, K.; Clark, W.F.; Rock, G. Patients' Quality of Life after Stopping Plasma Exchange: A Pilot Study. *Transfus. Apher. Sci.* **2014**, *51*, 137–140. [CrossRef]
29. Alesci, S.R.; Schwan, V.; Miesbach, W.; Seifried, E.; Klinger, D. Rare Bleeding Disorders Are Associated with Depression and Anxiety. *Hamostaseologie* **2013**, *33* (Suppl. S1), S64–S68. [PubMed]
30. Lins, L.; Carvalho, F.M. SF-36 Total Score as a Single Measure of Health-Related Quality of Life: Scoping Review. *SAGE Open Med.* **2016**, *4*, 205031211667172. [CrossRef] [PubMed]
31. Husson, O.; de Rooij, B.H.; Kieffer, J.; Oerlemans, S.; Mols, F.; Aaronson, N.K.; van der Graaf, W.T.A.; van de Poll-Franse, L.V. The EORTC QLQ-C30 Summary Score as Prognostic Factor for Survival of Patients with Cancer in the "Real-World": Results from the Population-Based PROFILES Registry. *Oncologist* **2020**, *25*, e722–e732. [CrossRef] [PubMed]

32. Schwarz, R.; Hinz, A. Reference Data for the Quality of Life Questionnaire EORTC QLQ-C30 in the General German Population. *Eur. J. Cancer* **2001**, *37*, 1345–1351. [CrossRef]
33. Aaronson, N.K.; Ahmedzai, S.; Bergman, B.; Bullinger, M.; Cull, A.; Duez, N.J.; Filiberti, A.; Flechtner, H.; Fleishman, S.B.; Haes, J.C.J.M.d.; et al. The European Organization for Research and Treatment of Cancer QLQ-C30: A Quality-of-Life Instrument for Use in International Clinical Trials in Oncology. *JNCI J. Natl. Cancer Inst.* **1993**, *85*, 365–376. [CrossRef] [PubMed]
34. Mystakidou, K.; Tsilika, E.; Parpa, E.; Kalaidopoulou, O.; Smyrniotis, V.; Vlahos, L. The EORTC Core Quality of Life Questionnaire (QLQ-C30, Version 3.0) in Terminally Ill Cancer Patients under Palliative Care: Validity and Reliability in a Hellenic Sample. *Int. J. Cancer* **2001**, *94*, 135–139. [CrossRef]
35. Yang, M.; Rendas-Baum, R.; Varon, S.F.; Kosinski, M. Validation of the Headache Impact Test (HIT-6™) across Episodic and Chronic Migraine. *Cephalalgia* **2011**, *31*, 357–367. [CrossRef]
36. Kosinski, M.; Bayliss, M.S.; Bjorner, J.B.; Ware, J.E., Jr.; Garber, W.H.; Batenhorst, A.; Cady, R.; Dahlöf, C.G.H.; Dowson, A.; Tepper, S. A Six-Item Short-Form Survey for Measuring Headache Impact: The HIT-6. *Qual. Life Res.* **2003**, *12*, 963–974. [CrossRef]
37. Kroenke, K.; Spitzer, R.L.; Williams, J.B.W. The PHQ-9: Validity of a Brief Depression Severity Measure. *J. Gen. Intern. Med.* **2001**, *16*, 606–613. [CrossRef]
38. Plemmons, G. Depression and Suicide Screening. In *Adolescent Health Screening: An Update in the Age of Big Data*; Elsevier: Amsterdam, The Netherlands, 2019; pp. 135–149. ISBN 978-0-323-66130-0.
39. Kroenke, K.; Strine, T.W.; Spitzer, R.L.; Williams, J.B.W.; Berry, J.T.; Mokdad, A.H. The PHQ-8 as a Measure of Current Depression in the General Population. *J. Affect. Disord.* **2009**, *114*, 163–173. [CrossRef]
40. Strine, T.W.; Kroenke, K.; Dhingra, S.; Balluz, L.S.; Gonzalez, O.; Berry, J.T.; Mokdad, A.H. The Associations Between Depression, Health-Related Quality of Life, Social Support, Life Satisfaction, and Disability in Community-Dwelling US Adults. *J. Nerv. Ment. Dis.* **2009**, *197*, 61–64. [CrossRef] [PubMed]
41. Beck, A.T.; Steer, R.A.; Carbin, M.G. Psychometric Properties of the Beck Depression Inventory: Twenty-Five Years of Evaluation. *Clin. Psychol. Rev.* **1988**, *8*, 77–100. [CrossRef]
42. Reeves, G.M.; Rohan, K.J.; Langenberg, P.; Snitker, S.; Postolache, T.T. Calibration of Response and Remission Cut-Points on the Beck Depression Inventory-Second Edition for Monitoring Seasonal Affective Disorder Treatment Outcomes. *J. Affect. Disord.* **2012**, *138*, 123–127. [CrossRef] [PubMed]
43. Spitzer, R.L.; Kroenke, K.; Williams, J.B.W.; Löwe, B. A Brief Measure for Assessing Generalized Anxiety Disorder: The GAD-7. *Arch. Intern. Med.* **2006**, *166*, 1092. [CrossRef] [PubMed]
44. Generalised Anxiety Disorder Assessment (GAD-7). Available online: https://www.corc.uk.net/Outcome-Experience-Measures/Generalised-Anxiety-Disorder-Assessment-Gad-7/#:~:Text=The%20GAD%2D7%20is%20a,1%2D2%20minutes%20to%20complete (accessed on 31 May 2023).
45. Zigmond, A.S.; Snaith, R.P. The Hospital Anxiety and Depression Scale. *Acta Psychiatr. Scand.* **1983**, *67*, 361–370. [CrossRef]
46. John Rush, A.; Giles, D.E.; Schlesser, M.A.; Fulton, C.L.; Weissenburger, J.; Burns, C. The Inventory for Depressive Symptomatology (IDS): Preliminary Findings. *Psychiatry Res.* **1986**, *18*, 65–87. [CrossRef]
47. Rush, A.J.; Gullion, C.M.; Basco, M.R.; Jarrett, R.B.; Trivedi, M.H. The Inventory of Depressive Symptomatology (IDS): Psychometric Properties. *Psychol. Med.* **1996**, *26*, 477–486. [CrossRef]
48. Cerimele, J.M.; Goldberg, S.B.; Miller, C.J.; Gabrielson, S.W.; Fortney, J.C. Systematic Review of Symptom Assessment Measures for Use in Measurement-Based Care of Bipolar Disorders. *Psychiatr. Serv.* **2019**, *70*, 396–408. [CrossRef]
49. Brown, E.S.; Murray, M.; Carmody, T.J.; Kennard, B.D.; Hughes, C.W.; Khan, D.A.; Rush, A.J. The Quick Inventory of Depressive Symptomatology-Self-Report: A Psychometric Evaluation in Patients with Asthma and Major Depressive Disorder. *Ann. Allergy Asthma Immunol.* **2008**, *100*, 433–438. [CrossRef]
50. Lovibond, P.F.; Lovibond, S.H. The Structure of Negative Emotional States: Comparison of the Depression Anxiety Stress Scales (DASS) with the Beck Depression and Anxiety Inventories. *Behav. Res. Ther.* **1995**, *33*, 335–343. [CrossRef]
51. Parkitny, L.; McAuley, J. The Depression Anxiety Stress Scale (DASS). *J. Physiother.* **2010**, *56*, 204. [CrossRef]
52. Chaturvedi, S.; Oluwole, O.; Cataland, S.; McCrae, K.R. Post-Traumatic Stress Disorder and Depression in Survivors of Thrombotic Thrombocytopenic Purpura. *Thromb. Res.* **2017**, *151*, 51–56. [CrossRef]
53. Blevins, C.A.; Weathers, F.W.; Davis, M.T.; Witte, T.K.; Domino, J.L. The Posttraumatic Stress Disorder Checklist for *DSM-5* (PCL-5): Development and Initial Psychometric Evaluation: Posttraumatic Stress Disorder Checklist for *DSM-5*. *J. Trauma. Stress* **2015**, *28*, 489–498. [CrossRef]
54. PTSD Checklist for DSM-5 (PCL-5). Available online: https://www.ptsd.va.gov/Professional/Assessment/Adult-Sr/Ptsd-Checklist.Asp (accessed on 31 May 2023).
55. Cella, D.; Riley, W.; Stone, A.; Rothrock, N.; Reeve, B.; Yount, S.; Amtmann, D.; Bode, R.; Buysse, D.; Choi, S.; et al. The Patient-Reported Outcomes Measurement Information System (PROMIS) Developed and Tested Its First Wave of Adult Self-Reported Health Outcome Item Banks: 2005–2008. *J. Clin. Epidemiol.* **2010**, *63*, 1179–1194. [CrossRef] [PubMed]
56. Mücke, F.J.; Hendriks, M.P.; Bien, C.G.; Grewe, P. Discrepancy between Subjective and Objective Memory Change after Epilepsy Surgery: Relation with Seizure Outcome and Depressive Symptoms. *Front. Neurol.* **2022**, *13*, 855664. [CrossRef] [PubMed]
57. Beblo, T.; Kunz, M.; Brokate, B.; Scheurich, A.; Weber, B.; Albert, A.; Richter, P.; Lautenbacher, S. Entwicklung eines Fragebogens zur subjektiven Einschätzung der geistigen Leistungsfähigkeit (FLei) bei Patienten mit psychischen Störungen. *Z. Neuropsychol.* **2010**, *21*, 143–151. [CrossRef]

58. Falter, T.; Böschen, S.; Schepers, M.; Beutel, M.; Lackner, K.; Scharrer, I.; Lämmle, B. Influence of Personality, Resilience and Life Conditions on Depression and Anxiety in 104 Patients Having Survived Acute Autoimmune Thrombotic Thrombocytopenic Purpura. *J. Clin. Med.* **2021**, *10*, 365. [CrossRef] [PubMed]
59. FLEI. Available online: https://marketplace.schuhfried.com/En/FLEI (accessed on 31 May 2023).
60. von Eisenhart Rothe, A.; Zenger, M.; Lacruz, M.E.; Emeny, R.; Baumert, J.; Haefner, S.; Ladwig, K.-H. Validation and Development of a Shorter Version of the Resilience Scale RS-11: Results from the Population-Based KORA-Age Study. *BMC Psychol.* **2013**, *1*, 25. [CrossRef]
61. Wagnild, G.M.; Young, H.M. Development and Psychometric Evaluation of the Resilience Scale. *J. Nurs. Meas.* **1993**, *1*, 165–178.
62. Scheier, M.F.; Carver, C.S.; Bridges, M.W. Distinguishing Optimism from Neuroticism (and Trait Anxiety, Self-Mastery, and Self-Esteem): A Reevaluation of the Life Orientation Test. *J. Personal. Soc. Psychol.* **1994**, *67*, 1063–1078. [CrossRef]
63. Revised Life Orientation Test (LOT-R). Available online: https://sparqtools.org/Mobility-Measure/Revised-Life-Orientation-Test-Lotr/ (accessed on 31 May 2023).
64. Reilly, M.C.; Zbrozek, A.S.; Dukes, E.M. The Validity and Reproducibility of a Work Productivity and Activity Impairment Instrument. *PharmacoEconomics* **1993**, *4*, 353–365. [CrossRef]
65. Tillett, W.; Lin, C.-Y.; Zbrozek, A.; Sprabery, A.T.; Birt, J. A Threshold of Meaning for Work Disability Improvement in Psoriatic Arthritis Measured by the Work Productivity and Activity Impairment Questionnaire. *Rheumatol. Ther.* **2019**, *6*, 379–391. [CrossRef]
66. Page, E.E.; Jiang, Y.; Terrell, D.R.; Vesely, S.K.; George, J.N. Long-Term Outcomes of Health-Related Quality of Life Following Diverse Thrombotic Microangiopathy Syndromes: HRQOL Following Recovery from TMA. *Am. J. Hematol.* **2016**, *91*, E278–E279. [CrossRef] [PubMed]
67. Terrell, D.R.; Tolma, E.L.; Stewart, L.M.; Shirley, E.A. Thrombotic Thrombocytopenic Purpura Patients' Attitudes toward Depression Management: A Qualitative Study. *Health Sci. Rep.* **2019**, *2*, e136. [CrossRef]
68. Kelley, R.A.; Cheney, M.K.; Martin, C.M.; Cataland, S.R.; Quick, L.B.; Keller, S.; Vesely, S.K.; Llaneza, A.J.; Khawandanah, M.; Journeycake, J.; et al. Health Following Recovery from Immune Thrombotic Thrombocytopenic Purpura: The Patient's Perspective. *Blood Adv.* **2022**, *7*, 1813–1822. [CrossRef]
69. Oladapo, A.; Ito, D.; Hibbard, C.; Hare, T.; Krupnick, R.; Ewenstein, B. Development of a Patient-Reported Outcome (PRO) Instrument for Patients with Acquired Thrombotic Thrombocytopenic Purpura. *Value Health* **2018**, *21*, S257. [CrossRef]
70. Oladapo, A.; Ito, D.; Hibbard, C.; Bean, S.; Krupnick, R.; Ewenstein, B. 22nd International Abstracts Book, PSY92 patient-reported outcome (PRO) instrument development for congenital thrombotic thrombocytopenic purpura (cTTP, upshaw-schulman syndrome [USS], hereditary thrombotic thrombocytopenic purpura, hTTP). *Value Health* **2017**, *20*, A225. [CrossRef]
71. Kluzek, S.; Dean, B.; Wartolowska, K.A. Patient-Reported Outcome Measures (PROMs) as Proof of Treatment Efficacy. *BMJ EBM* **2022**, *27*, 153–155. [CrossRef]
72. Churruca, K.; Pomare, C.; Ellis, L.A.; Long, J.C.; Henderson, S.B.; Murphy, L.E.D.; Leahy, C.J.; Braithwaite, J. Patient-reported Outcome Measures (PROMs): A Review of Generic and Condition-specific Measures and a Discussion of Trends and Issues. *Health Expect.* **2021**, *24*, 1015–1024. [CrossRef]
73. Bele, S.; Mohamed, B.; Chugh, A.; Haverman, L.; Santana, M.-J. Impact of Using Patient-Reported Outcome Measures in Routine Clinical Care of Paediatric Patients with Chronic Conditions: A Systematic Review Protocol. *BMJ Open* **2019**, *9*, e027354. [CrossRef]
74. Field, J.; Holmes, M.M.; Newell, D. PROMs Data: Can It Be Used to Make Decisions for Individual Patients? A Narrative Review. *Patient Relat. Outcome Meas.* **2019**, *10*, 233–241. [CrossRef]
75. Thestrup Hansen, S.; Kjerholt, M.; Friis Christensen, S.; Brodersen, J.; Hølge-Hazelton, B. User Experiences on Implementation of Patient Reported Outcome Measures (PROMs) in a Haematological Outpatient Clinic. *J. Patient Rep. Outcomes* **2020**, *4*, 87. [CrossRef] [PubMed]
76. Willik, E.M.; Terwee, C.B.; Bos, W.J.W.; Hemmelder, M.H.; Jager, K.J.; Zoccali, C.; Dekker, F.W.; Meuleman, Y. Patient-reported Outcome Measures (PROMs): Making Sense of Individual PROM Scores and Changes in PROM Scores over Time. *Nephrology* **2021**, *26*, 391–399. [CrossRef] [PubMed]
77. Lordon, R.J.; Mikles, S.P.; Kneale, L.; Evans, H.L.; Munson, S.A.; Backonja, U.; Lober, W.B. How Patient-Generated Health Data and Patient-Reported Outcomes Affect Patient–Clinician Relationships: A Systematic Review. *Health Inform. J.* **2020**, *26*, 2689–2706. [CrossRef]
78. Antunes, B.; Harding, R.; Higginson, I.J.; on behalf of EUROIMPACT. Implementing Patient-Reported Outcome Measures in Palliative Care Clinical Practice: A Systematic Review of Facilitators and Barriers. *Palliat. Med.* **2014**, *28*, 158–175. [CrossRef] [PubMed]
79. Marker, A.M.; Patton, S.R.; McDonough, R.J.; Feingold, H.; Simon, L.; Clements, M.A. Implementing Clinic-wide Depression Screening for Pediatric Diabetes: An Initiative to Improve Healthcare Processes. *Pediatr. Diabetes* **2019**, *20*, 964–973. [CrossRef] [PubMed]
80. Health Measures—Transforming How Health Is Measures. Available online: https://www.healthmeasures.net/Explore-Measurement-Systems/Promis (accessed on 9 June 2023).
81. Singh, S.A.; Bakshi, N.; Mahajan, P.; Morris, C.R. What Is the Future of Patient-Reported Outcomes in Sickle-Cell Disease? *Expert. Rev. Hematol.* **2020**, *13*, 1165–1173. [CrossRef]

82. Meadows, K.A. Patient-Reported Outcome Measures: An Overview. *Br. J. Community Nurs.* **2011**, *16*, 146–151. [CrossRef]
83. Kilgour, J.M.; Wali, G.; Gibbons, E.; Scherwath, A.; Barata Badiella, A.; Peniket, A.; Schoemans, H.; Matin, R.N. Systematic Review of Patient-Reported Outcome Measures in Graft-versus-Host Disease. *Biol. Blood Marrow Transplant.* **2020**, *26*, e113–e127. [CrossRef]
84. FDA Patient-Focused Drug Development Guidance Series for Enhancing the Incorporation of the Patient's Voice in Medical Product Development and Regulatory Decision Making. Available online: https://www.fda.gov/Drugs/Development-Approval-Process-Drugs/Fda-Patient-Focused-Drug-Development-Guidance-Series-Enhancing-Incorporation-Patients-Voice-Medical (accessed on 30 May 2023).

Disclaimer/Publisher's Note: The statements, opinions and data contained in all publications are solely those of the individual author(s) and contributor(s) and not of MDPI and/or the editor(s). MDPI and/or the editor(s) disclaim responsibility for any injury to people or property resulting from any ideas, methods, instructions or products referred to in the content.

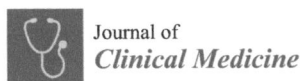

Review

Global Health Resource Utilization and Cost-Effectiveness of Therapeutics and Diagnostics in Immune Thrombotic Thrombocytopenic Purpura (TTP)

Ayesha Butt [1], Cecily Allen [2], Adriana Purcell [3], Satoko Ito [4] and George Goshua [4,*]

1. Department of Internal Medicine, Yale School of Medicine, New Haven, CT 06510, USA
2. Division of Hematology, Department of Medicine, Johns Hopkins University, Baltimore, MD 21218, USA
3. Yale School of Medicine, New Haven, CT 06510, USA
4. Section of Hematology, Department of Internal Medicine, Yale School of Medicine, New Haven, CT 06510, USA
* Correspondence: george.goshua@yale.edu

Abstract: In this review, we examine the current landscape of health resource utilization and cost-effectiveness data in the care of patient populations with immune thrombotic thrombocytopenic purpura. We focus on the therapeutic (therapeutic plasma exchange, glucocorticoids, rituximab, caplacizumab) and diagnostic (ADAMTS13 assay) health technologies employed in the care of patients with this rare disease. Health resource utilization and cost-effectiveness data are limited to the high-income country context. Measurement of TTP-specific utility weights in the high-income country context and collection of health resource utilization data in the low- and middle-income country settings would enable an evaluation of country-specific quality-adjusted life expectancy and cost-effectiveness of these therapeutic and diagnostic health technologies. This quantification of value is one way to mitigate cost concerns where they exist.

Keywords: TTP; thrombotic thrombocytopenic purpura; ADAMTS13; treatment; diagnosis; review; cost; cost-effectiveness; health resource utilization; decision science

1. Introduction

Thrombotic thrombocytopenic purpura (TTP) is a rare and life-threatening thrombotic microangiopathy characterized by a triad of microangiopathic hemolytic anemia, severe thrombocytopenia, and organ ischemia linked to disseminated, microvascular platelet rich-thrombi [1]. Acute episodes of TTP are marked by a severe deficiency of a disintegrin and metalloproteinase with a thrombospondin type 1 motif, member 13 (ADAMTS13), with the standard of care initial diagnosis being defined by enzymatic activity of less than 10% of normal ADAMTS13 in countries where this assay is available [2,3].

Decreased ADAMTS13 activity leads to an accumulation of ultra-large von Willebrand factor multimers, which bind platelets and induce aggregation [1]. Most commonly, a severe deficiency of ADAMTS13 is mediated by the immune-mediated production of autoantibodies to ADAMTS13. In one cross-sectional study of 772 patients with a first episode of thrombotic microangiopathy and ADAMTS13-confirmed diagnosis of TTP, 73% of patients were noted to have positive anti-ADAMTS13 IgG, with an additional 3% being identified beyond the first episode [4]. In this same study, 21% of patients were always anti-ADAMTS13 IgG-negative and 3% had mutation-confirmed (homozygous or compound heterozygous) congenital TTP [1]. The epidemiology of TTP, whether immune-mediated or hereditary, classifies it as a rare disease in every country in the world, being defined, at its most strict, as <650 patients per one million people in Brazil [5]. The estimated annual incidence in different studies is geographic-location-dependent and ranges between 1 and 13 cases per million people, while the prevalence of TTP is 10 per million people [4,6,7].

Citation: Butt, A.; Allen, C.; Purcell, A.; Ito, S.; Goshua, G. Global Health Resource Utilization and Cost-Effectiveness of Therapeutics and Diagnostics in Immune Thrombotic Thrombocytopenic Purpura (TTP). *J. Clin. Med.* **2023**, *12*, 4887. https://doi.org/10.3390/jcm12154887

Academic Editors: Deirdra R. Terrell and Angelo Claudio Molinari

Received: 26 May 2023
Revised: 28 June 2023
Accepted: 21 July 2023
Published: 25 July 2023

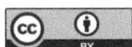

Copyright: © 2023 by the authors. Licensee MDPI, Basel, Switzerland. This article is an open access article distributed under the terms and conditions of the Creative Commons Attribution (CC BY) license (https://creativecommons.org/licenses/by/4.0/).

The first case of what would later be termed "TTP" was reported by Eli Moschcowitz in 1924 [8]. In 1959, the first known documented utilization of whole blood exchange transformed an 11-year old girl's "deep and persistent" coma to the regaining of consciousness and the disappearance of abnormal neurologic signs [9]. In 1977, two patients were reported to recover completely after "intensive plasmapheresis" [10], paving the way for treatment transformation in 1991 through a clinical trial of therapeutic plasma exchange versus plasma infusion that spanned the 1980s [11]. In 1982, the presence of ultra-large von Willebrand Factor (VWF) multimers in four patients with chronic, relapsing TTP suggested a defect in the processing of these multimers after secretion [12]. In 1985, large amounts of VWF (when compared with fibrinogen) were found within the visceral platelet microthrombi via histopathology in a deceased TTP patient [1]. In 1991, the aforementioned clinical trial of therapeutic plasma exchange versus plasma infusion reported an acute survival probability of 96% versus 84%, with 6-month survival holding at 78% and 63%, respectively. These results were a significant increase from a mortality of *up to* 90% prior to plasma infusion or exchange [1,11]. A novel metalloprotease (VWF cleaving-protease) that specifically cleaved VWF was purified from human plasma in 1996, and two years later, a severe functional deficiency of the VWF cleaving-protease was shown to cause TTP [13,14]. Finally, this cleaving-protease was identified as ADAMTS13 in 2001, setting the stage for a biomarker-based diagnostic assay [15].

The treatment of immune TTP is anchored around therapeutic plasma exchange, which serves to remove autoantibodies and ultra-large von Willebrand factor multimers, and to replenish ADAMTS13 [11]. Autoantibody formation is targeted by using immunosuppression with a foundation of glucocorticoids and rituximab [16]. In 2019, caplacizumab, an anti–von Willebrand factor humanized single-variable-domain immunoglobulin (Nanobody, Ablynx) that targets the A1 domain of von Willebrand factor, obtained Food and Drug Administration approval for the management of TTP based on a primary endpoint of time to platelet normalization [17]. Standard-of-care treatment in high-income countries revolves around the aforementioned therapeutics, noting that the addition of glucocorticoids to therapeutic plasma exchange is a strong recommendation and that the addition of rituximab and caplacizumab are conditional recommendations in the 2020 International Society on Thrombosis and Haemostasis Treatment Guidelines [18], with a grade IB recommendation against using caplacizumab in unselected patients in the 2022 American Society of Hematology Education Program [19]. Treatment is initiated based on clinical suspicion in patients for evidence of thrombotic microangiopathy on smear and without a more likely etiology, employing either the PLASMIC and/or French scores [20]. In this primer, we examine the current landscape of health resource utilization and cost-effectiveness studies of the therapeutic armamentarium and diagnostic assay for patients with this rare disease. Specifically, we focus on TPE, glucocorticoids, rituximab, caplacizumab, and the ADAMTS13 assay, with a primary focus on health resource utilization and a secondary one on cost-effectiveness.

2. Therapeutic #1: Therapeutic Plasma Exchange (TPE)

TPE is an established anchor of frontline treatment for immune TTP, improving acute and 6-month mortality even when compared to plasma infusion [1,11,21]. TPE should be started as soon as the diagnosis of TTP is suspected [1,3]. Daily TPE removes autoantibodies against ADAMTS13 while replenishing the missing or inhibited ADAMTS13 enzyme [11]. Treatment with TPE is continued daily until the platelet count is greater than $150 \times 10^9/\text{L}$ on two consecutive days, and TPE may be performed more than once daily in severely ill patients [22–24].

Health resource utilization: A 2008 retrospective analysis that used the South East England TTP Registry, spanning a time period from April 2002 through to December 2006 across 176 patients with 236 acute episodes, reported a median of 15.5 plasma exchanges (range 3–93), with a significant difference between the number of exchanges required in the first acute episode of TTP (median 15 (4–40)) compared to that in relapsed acute TTP episodes (median 9.5 (5–57)) [25]. The authors noted a statistically significant secular trend—in this case, a systematic decrease over time, presumably due to increased clinician experience—within their 56-month study period, with median exchange sessions decreasing from 19 to 12 between the first 20 and last 36 months. A 2016 analysis of 2009–2014 data from the Australian TTP/TMA registry reported similar findings, with TPE used in 67/72 (93%) episodes of 57 confirmed TTP patients with a median of 12 (range 1–8) TPE sessions per acute episode [26].

A 2012 study using data from the HealthCore Integrated Research Database (HIRD), explored healthcare utilization of immune TTP patients in a commercially insured population from many different regions of the United States [27]. The study included 151 patients with the mean total healthcare payments for the TTP hospitalization being USD 56,347 (standard deviation [SD] USD 80,230) [27]. During an acute episode of TTP, the mean number of PE was found to be 8.5 (SD 12.9, range 1–116). The mean duration of the PE treatment was 28.2 days (SD 54.0) [27]. Mean payments for TPE services in the month following discharge were USD 9127 (SD USD 20,840) [27].

A 2014 study including results from a survey of physicians from 32 centers in the US sought to delineate current clinical practices of TTP treatment in the US [28]. At all centers, TPE was started as soon as TTP was the most likely diagnosis [28]. TPE was initiated with plasma as replacement fluid (91%) at 1.0 plasma volume (72%) and stopped with a platelet count of 150×10^9/L (66%), and TPE was then tapered off (69%) [28].

In 2021, an American retrospective study utilized administrative claims data between 2010 and 2018 for US Medicare and non-Medicare populations following immune TTP episodes to describe immune TTP-related hospital resource utilization, cost, complications, and overall survival [29]. The study included 2279 patients at a weighted mean age of 58 across four payer types: Medicare Fee-for-Service (FFS; n = 1486), Medicare Advantage (MA; n = 123), commercial (n = 312), and Managed Medicaid (MM; n = 358). The study reported a mean length of hospitalization across payer types ranging between 12 and 16 days and 61% of Medicare FFS patients received ICU-level care. Notably, Medicare FFS patients experienced a mean of 3 days from admission to TPE initiation, as compared to all other payers for whom TPE initiation occurred less than 1 day from admission. [29] Mean total direct healthcare expenditures for index hospitalization varied by payer (Medicare FFS: USD 29,024; MA: USD 12,860; commercial: USD 9996; MM: USD 10,470) [29]. The FFS cohort had mortality rates of 15.7% and 21% during initial hospitalization and within the first 30 days, respectively [29].

Cost-effectiveness: At this time, there are no cost-effectiveness studies regarding TPE in immune TTP.

3. Therapeutic #2: Steroids

Steroids have long been considered an important therapeutic option for immune TTP, owing to the autoimmune nature of the disease. Although no longer treated with corticosteroids alone, at one point in the pre-ADAMST13 time period, corticosteroids alone were reported to lead to remission in patients with milder cases [30,31]. While there is a paucity of randomized controlled trials exploring the use of steroids in immune TTP, several studies have reported favorable outcomes leading to its use as part of standard of care for TTP alongside TPE [23].

Health resource utilization: In a 2006 Italian randomized open-label trial of 60 TTP patients running from 2000 through 2006, high-dose methylprednisolone (10 mg/kg/day for 3 days followed by 2.5 mg/kg/day) induced a higher complete remission rate by a pre-specified day 23 compared to standard-dose methylprednisolone (1 mg/kg/day) (76.6% vs. 46.6%, respectively) [32]. Costs of care between these two arms were not reported. Another randomized clinical trial examining the adjunct use of prednisone versus cyclosporine to TPE was halted after interim analysis (22 total evaluable patients) showed an increase in exacerbations with the latter strategy during acute immune TTP treatment, in addition to prednisone significantly improving ADAMTS13 activity at weeks 3 and 4 and lowering anti-ADAMTS13 IgG at weeks 2–4 compared to cyclosporine [33]. The 2008 retrospective analysis from the South East England TTP Registry showed that in 80% of all acute episodes, TTP patients received steroids. Most patients received three days of pulsed therapy between 500 mg and 1 g per day of methylprednisolone for up to 3 days [25]. Data from the Australian TTP/TMA registry similarly showed that steroids were used in 71% (51/72) acute TTP episodes with a median steroid exposure being 19.5 days (range 2–108 days) [26]. A 2014 study including results from a survey of physicians from 32 centers in the US reported the standard use of prednisone for TTP treatment in 26/32 centers (81%) [28].

Cost-effectiveness: At this time, there are no cost-effectiveness studies on corticosteroid use in immune TTP.

4. Therapeutic #3: Rituximab

Rituximab is a chimeric monoclonal antibody directed against the CD20 antigen present on B lymphocytes. It is used in the management of diseases like lymphoma and rheumatoid arthritis, where it clears B lymphocytes responsible for antibody production via complement-dependent cytotoxicity, antibody-dependent cellular cytotoxicity, or directly by inducing apoptosis [34]. The role of rituximab in treating patients with TTP emerged first in the refractory or relapsed setting in the 2000s [35–38].

Health resource utilization: A 2009 randomized clinical trial to evaluate the addition of upfront rituximab to TPE and steroids was stopped due to low enrolment [39]. A prospective, non-randomized, single-arm, phase 2 trial reported in 2011 by the South East England TTP study group examined the benefit of upfront rituximab with steroids and TPE versus historical control patients treated without rituximab and with steroids and TPE. The investigators reported a reduction in relapse rates from 57% at a median 18 months in the historical controls to 10% at a median 27 months in 40 trial patients with the use of weekly rituximab at lymphoma-based dosing (375 mg/m^2 weekly for 4 weeks, up to 8 infusions allowed), administered within three days of admission in the acute TTP setting [40]. Across 34 total patients classified as de novo TTP, the authors noted the following three ethnicity categories and their respective, descriptive median number of TPE treatments and range: Afro-Caribbean (24, range: 6–34), White 11.5 (range 4–30), and Indian/Asian 23 (range, 6–34). They then collapsed ethnicity into a binary variable of white versus nonwhite, reporting the number of TPE sessions to be significantly decreased at 14 versus 21, respectively [40]. A study using the United States Thrombotic Microangiopathies Consortium iTTP Registry explored the correlation of race with mortality and relapse-free survival (RFS) in immune TTP in the United States from 1995 to 2020. Black race was associated with shorter RFS (hazard ratio [HR], 1.60; 95% CI, 1.16–2.21), while the addition of rituximab to corticosteroids improved RFS in White (HR, 0.37; 95% CI, 0.18–0.73) but not Black patients (HR, 0.96; 95% CI, 0.71–1.31) [41].

Subsequent to the 2009 study, a 2012 retrospective study from the United Kingdom TTP Study Registry reported the administration of rituximab within 3 days from admission in 54 patients with acute de novo TTP versus rituximab administration more than 3 days from admission in 32 patients with acute de novo TTP over a 2004–2011 time period [42]. In this context, the former strategy yielded earlier remission (12 versus 20 days), fewer TPE sessions (16 versus 24) and a shorter length of hospital admission (16 versus 23 days) [42]. In 2012, the expert-based guidelines from the United Kingdom recommended the utilization of upfront rituximab alongside TPE and steroids for patients with relapsed TTP and suggested consideration for upfront rituximab in the de novo context [43]. Data from the first 5 years of the Australian TTP/TMA microangiopathy registry reported rituximab use in 28/72 (39%) acute TTP episodes spanning the 2009–2014 time period. The authors noted the first registry-documented use of rituximab in Australia in 2010, with its use occurring in 21/52 (40%) and 7/20 (35%) of de novo and relapsed TTP episodes in this time period [26]. A 2019 systematic review and meta-analysis reported on a total of 570 patients across nine included studies dating from 2011 through to 2018 [44]. The odds ratio for the pooled relapse rates as an effect of rituximab administration in the acute phase was 0.40 (95% confidence interval (CI) 0.19–0.85, I^2 = 43%) with an OR of 0.41 ([95% CI 0.18–0.91],

$I^2 = 0\%$) from the six and eight studies, respectively, where these data were reported [44]. A 2014 study including results from a survey of physicians from 32 centers in the US reported heterogeneity in the use of rituximab: 4 centers (13%) did not use rituximab, while 28 centers (88%) used it routinely [28]. Of the 28 centers that used rituximab, 5 (18%) routinely used the drug during the first presentation of TTP, while the remaining 23 centers (82%) use it in relapsed/refractory cases [28]. Rituximab was used concurrently with TPE in 27/28 centers (96%) [28].

In the United States, one major hurdle to adding rituximab into inpatient treatment paradigms for immune TTP is the expense of the medication [45], particularly in the context of a payer system that delineates fixed payments per pre-specified diagnosis-related group and thus incentivizes cost-containment in the inpatient setting. To examine this question, a retrospective single-center study of 27 patients with de novo immune TTP across all relapses over a median follow-up time of 56 months reported on preventable TPE sessions, inpatient hospital days, and cost savings that would have accrued for patients who responded to the addition of incident rituximab therapy to TPE and steroids after subsequent relapses [46]. First in the initial cohort, rituximab use during initial hospitalization was projected to avert 185 inpatient admission days and 137 TPE sessions at cost savings to hospitals of USD 900,000 [46]. Second in the relapse cohort, rituximab use during any earlier relapse was projected to avert 86 inpatient admission days and 64 TPE sessions at cost savings to hospitals of USD 420,000 [46]. This study delineated that, despite financial inpatient formulary concerns, the inpatient use of rituximab in the management of TTP can lead to cost savings (~USD 30,000 per patient with TTP initiated on rituximab inpatient). This supported the practice change to an automatic formulary approval for inpatient rituximab use for all patients with immune TTP in the same hospital health system [46].

Cost-effectiveness: At this time, there are no cost-effectiveness studies on rituximab use in immune TTP.

5. Therapeutic #4: Caplacizumab

Caplacizumab is a humanized monoclonal antibody that binds to vWF, inhibits its interaction with platelet glycoprotein Ib-IX-V, yields rapid suppression of vWF-ristocetin cofactor activity, and prevents platelet adhesion [47]. In 2018 and 2019, caplacizumab was approved by the European Medicines Agency and the Food and Drug Administration based on the time to platelet normalization for the treatment of immune TTP in conjunction with TPE and immunosuppression [47]. In 2020, the International Society on Thrombosis and Haemostasis (ISTH) guidelines for the management of immune TTP noted a conditional recommendation for the use of caplacizumab in the frontline treatment of immune TTP [18].

Health resource utilization: Healthcare utilization with the addition of caplacizumab use to TPE and immunosuppression versus without caplacizumab was descriptively reported in a phase 3, randomized, two-arm clinical trial of patients. Here, with caplacizumab use, the patients (1) received a median of 5 days (range 1–35) of plasma exchange (without: 7.0; range 3–46), (2) underwent a median of 18 L (range 5–102) plasma exchanged (without: 27; range 4–254), (3) had a median 9-day (range 2–37) length hospital of stay (without: 12; range 4–53), with (4) a median 3-day (range 1–10) stay in the intensive care unit (without: 5; range 1–47). The median number of TPE sessions and hospital length of stay observed with caplacizumab use in real-world data from Germany, France, England, and Spain are 9 (range 2–41) and 18 (range 5–79), 5 (IQR 4–7) and 13 (IQR 9–19), 7 (IQR 5–14) and 12 (IQR 8–24), and 8.5 (IQR 6–12.5) and 12 (IQR 9–15), respectively [16,19,48–50]. Of note, healthcare utilization data from trials and real-world data of caplacizumab do not apply to immune TTP patients deemed to be high bleeding risk patients, as these individuals are noted to be excluded in all studies to date. A 2022 systematic review and meta-analysis of caplacizumab use examined data from 632 patients across phase 2 and phase 3 clinical trials, two observational studies with historical controls (total n = 175 treated with caplacizumab with n = 219 historical controls), and one observational study with a concurrent control (total n = 18), with all three observational studies reported as having a high risk of bias [51].

The work had a literature search censor date through July 2021. Noting caveats regarding an inability to adjust for secular trends and confounding as a limitation of historical control arms and the exclusion of high-risk bleeding patients, the authors noted that caplacizumab added to the standard of care versus the following standard of care alone yielded relative risks: (1) RR 1.37 ([CI 1.06, 1.77]) and (RR 7.10 [CI 0.90, 56.14]) for all bleed risk in clinical trial and observational data, respectively; and (2) RR 0.21 [CI 0.05, 1.74]) and 0.62 [CI 0.07, 4.41] for death in clinical trial and observational data, respectively. Focusing on the International Society on Thrombosis and Haemostasis major bleed rate, while again noting the exclusion of patients deemed at high risk of bleeding from receiving caplacizumab, the lowest cumulative per-patient-treated real-world data estimate for ISTH major bleeding with caplacizumab use is 2.4% (Table 1). Included within this, with caplacizumab use through to December 2022, there were 4 intracranial hemorrhages that occurred in 272 immune TTP episodes over a median follow-up of 80 days across English, Spanish, and Austrian experiences [49,50,52]. In contrast, there were 0 intracranial hemorrhages across 219 patients over a median follow-up of 618 days and 0 intracranial hemorrhages over a median follow-up of 2336 days in consecutively treated patients with immune TTP in the Harvard TTP Collaborative and Oklahoma TTP Registry, respectively [53,54].

Table 1. ISTH major bleeding reported in real-world data (RWD), with and without caplacizumab, for patients with immune TTP [55].

Parameter	Caplacizumab RWD (Knöbl et al. [52])	Caplacizumab RWD (Pascual Izquierdo et al. [50])	Caplacizumab RWD (Coppo et al. [16])	Caplacizumab RWD (Dutt et al. [49])	Caplacizumab RWD (Volker et al. [48])
Sample size	20	77	90	85	60
ISTH Major Bleed # (%)	1 (5%)	Not reported	2 (2.2%)	5 (5.9%)	Not reported
Parameter	*Without* Caplacizumab RWD (Harvard Collaborative [53])		*Without* Caplacizumab RWD (Dutt et al. [49])		*Without* Caplacizumab RWD (Page et al. [54])
Sample size	219		39		68
ISTH Major Bleed # (%)	0		0		1 (1.5%) (CVC line placement)

A Sanofi-funded cost analysis (note: not cost-effectiveness) projected healthcare utilization expected with caplacizumab use in US hospital setting based on the phase 3 trial and peer-reviewed literature, with a payer mix of 20% Medicare Fee-for-Service (FFS), 8% Medicare Advantage, 10% Medicaid, and 62% commercial [56]. Specifically, the authors reported a per-patient cost of the standard of care as USD 23,000 versus USD 70,000 for caplacizumab added to the standard of care, with these values being inclusive of projected savings of USD 8000 and USD 15,000 for length of stay and TPE cost-savings, respectively, and yielding an incremental per-patient cost of USD 47,000 with caplacizumab use. The authors note that when considering patients cared for under the Medicare Fee-for-Service model specifically, the incremental per-patient cost with caplacizumab would decrease to USD 5000 when the 2020 Medicare new technology add-on payment (NTAP) for caplacizumab is applied. This is an important consideration in the short run that also does not address the long-term perspective given the 3-year expiration of indication-specific NTAPs in the Medicare Fee-for-Service context.

Cost concerns are also noted in France, where caplacizumab is approved for use in immune TTP [57]. The authors note that the addition caplacizumab per immune TTP patient, at an assumed per-11mg caplacizumab dose cost of EUR 4400, would increase costs three-fold per immune TTP episode treated from a historic baseline of EUR 75,000. With a per-11 mg caplacizumab dose cost of USD 8800, the authors also postulate a 4-fold increase in the United States for the same [57].

Cost-effectiveness: Cost is one concern with the use of caplacizumab, which has been examined in several cost-effectiveness analyses [58–60]. In December 2020, after initial rejection, a series of meetings and re-appraisal of Sanofi's modeling at their fourth meeting, the National Institute for Health and Care Excellence (NICE) officially recommended caplacizumab use with TPE and immunosuppression for patients with immune TTP [58]. Specifically, NICE noted that Sanofi's new modeling reported an ICER of just under GBP

30,000 per quality-adjusted life year (QALY) for caplacizumab use, an upper threshold (the typical is GBP 20,000 per QALY) NICE can employ when considering contextual factors such as innovation. This led to their recommendation of caplacizumab as a cost-effective option for treating immune TTP, paving the way for its use in the National Health Service [58]. Concerns about input parameters and assumptions employed by Sanofi in their final model have now been documented [61]. In no specific order, these include the following: (1) the use of an acute mortality relative risk of 0.5; (2) unsupported utility values—values which reflect quality of life—such as a lifelong 34% quality of life reduction in living in remission if a patient achieved remission without caplacizumab use as compared to the same remission with caplacizumab use; (3) an underestimated annual relapse rate that over a lifetime time-horizon would propagate a significant artificial decrease in the ICER for their drug [61].

A 2020 American cost-effectiveness analysis presented the results of two decision tree models, one for each clinical trial, and a third Markov model with a 5-year time-horizon conducted from the US health system perspective and at a willingness-to-pay threshold of 195,000 USD/QALY [60]. The analysis eschewed the consideration of bleeding—increased with caplacizumab use—and employed utilities preset to minimize the incremental cost-effectiveness ratio for caplacizumab added to the standard of care versus standard of care alone. At a 5-year time-horizon the incremental cost for caplacizumab was USD 400,000 with an incremental QALY of 0.27, resulting in an ICER of USD 1.5 million, far exceeding the willingness-to-pay threshold. In the American context, caplacizumab was reported to be cost-ineffective in 100% of 10,000 iterations in a probabilistic sensitivity analysis with deterministic sensitivity analysis identifying drug price as the one parameter that could significantly decrease the ICER, beginning at a price reduction of at least 80% [60,61].

A 2021 Italian health technology assessment conducted a cost-effectiveness analysis of capalcizumab added to the standard of care versus the standard of care at a lifetime time-horizon, an Italian hospital perspective and at a willingness-to-pay threshold of 60,000 EUR/QALY previously suggested in Italy [59]. The authors reported an expected increase in 3.27 life years and 3.06 quality-adjusted life years with caplacizumab use at an incremental cost-effectiveness ratio of 44,600 EUR/QALY. These results are accrued in the context of acute mortality probabilities of 0.0% with caplacizumab use and 13.2% without caplacizumab use per each immune TTP across a lifetime time-horizon. Deterministic sensitivity analysis did not evaluate a non-0% probability of acute mortality with caplacizumab use and the probabilistic sensitivity analysis reported the probability of caplacizumab being cost-effective at 82.4% without discounts for 10-mg caplacizumab per-vial pricing at EUR 3900 in the Italian setting.

In the context of a 2022 open-label single-arm phase 3 trial (MAYARI, NCT 05468320) to examine the use of caplacizumab without frontline TPE in immune TTP with a planned 1-year follow-up, a cost-effectiveness analysis examined the efficacy threshold of a 1-year relapse-free survival this single-arm trial would need to meet for caplacizumab to be a cost-effective replacement of the standard of care [62]. The analysis employed clinical trial data, assuming caplacizumab without TPE is exactly as effective as caplacizumab with TPE and with all inpatient costs eliminated. A relapse-free survival of 100% at 1-year would not meet any accepted US willingness-to-pay threshold. This analysis also entirely ignored bleeding complications, assumed no drop-off in efficacy from opting for no TPE therapy and reported that a minimum 78% price decrease in caplacizumab would be needed. TPE-based care was the cost-effective strategy in 100% of 10,000 iterations in a probabilistic sensitivity analysis [62].

A sample state transition diagram for model-based cost-effectiveness analysis is shown in Figure 1.

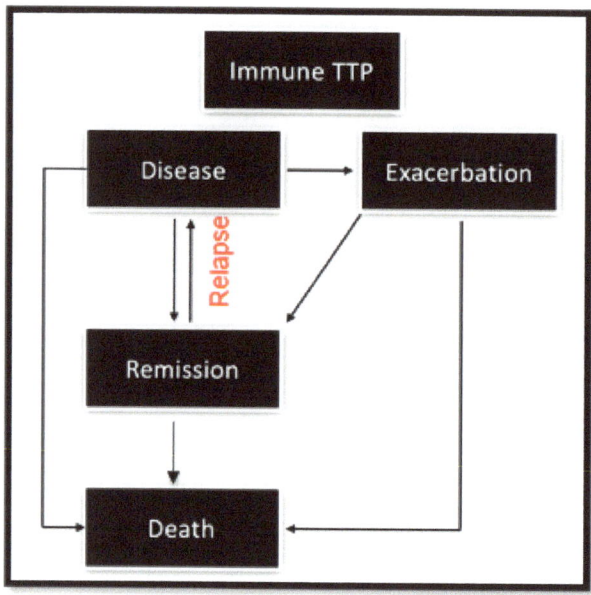

Figure 1. Sample state transition diagram for modeling treatment decisions in immune TTP [62]. Shown are the various health states possible for patients with TTP, which include the disease state (i.e., active TTP necessitating treatment), the remission state (no active TTP), exacerbation state and death. In this sample, relapse is a transitory event. All patients start in the disease state, with possibility of exacerbation, remission, and relapse back to disease. At all disease states, patients accrue background mortality risk, in addition to mortality specific to a given disease state.

A comparative summary of the costs, advantages, disadvantages, and side effects for the four therapeutics can be found in Table 2. Of note, costs vary greatly across and within countries; thus, we largely focus on the largest payer in the United States, the Centers for Medicare and Medicaid Services (Table 2).

Table 2. Comparative summary of selected costs, advantages, disadvantages, and side effects of the therapeutic plasma exchange, steroids, rituximab, and caplacizumab. Legend: CMS = Centers for Medicare and Medicaid Services; mg = milligram.

Therapies	Therapeutic Plasma Exchange (TPE)	Steroids	Rituximab	Caplacizumab
Cost per CMS unit	Average cost per 1 TPE session: USD 4900 Cost range: USD 3000–USD 6600 [56,60,63,64]	USD 0.02/mg of prednisone [65] USD 5.95/125 mg of methylprednisone [65]	USD 81.75 per 10 mg [65]	USD 718.64 per mg [65]
Advantages	Total of 30 years of data, Lifesaving [11]	Globally available, low cost	Total of 20 years of data; associated with increased time to relapse [66] in the short-run; can be cost-saving to hospitals in the long-run [46]	Easy administration, associated with decreased exacerbations [3]
Disadvantages	Requires logistical coordination; not available at all hospitals	Need to minimize unnecessary patient steroid exposure (i.e., overly prolonged tapers)	Recent observational study reporting differential effect of the social construct of race on relapse-free survival [41]	Associated with longer time to ADAMTS13 recovery [67], increased relapses [3], increased major bleeding [19], high cost [19]
Side Effects	Fever, urticaria, and hypocalcemic symptoms [68]	Immunosuppression leading to increased risk of infections; osteoporosis, myopathy, increase in blood glucose levels, weight gain, hypertension, arrhythmias, skin atrophy, acne, mild hirsutism, stria, impaired wound healing [69]	Immunosuppression leading to increased risk of infections; rituximab hypersensitivity; serum sickness and exacerbation of cardiac symptoms [42]	Bleeding (Table 1) [19]

6. Diagnostics

Testing for ADAMTS13 activity requires laboratory skill and time, making in-house and same-day assay output challenging. Clinical scoring systems are free of charge and include the French and PLASMIC scores. Neither score has perfect test characteristics and this worsens with older age [70]. Due to these limitations, there is a demand for rapid diagnostic testing and, given the associated costs, a need for cost-effectiveness analyses to convince hospital stakeholders that investment is worthwhile.

Health resource utilization: ADAMTS13 activity assay availability was limited in the early 2000s and the options included immunoradiometric, collagen-binding, and ristocetin-cofactor assays [71–74]. The availability of testing has since expanded, with some simplification achieved in testing complexity. Most current assays for ADAMTS13 utilize fluorescence resonance energy transfer (FRET) to detect proteolysis of vWF [75], improving the turnaround time of results in the context of reduced testing complexity observed with other assays [76]. Calls for further testing simplification led to the development of fully automated assays. The HemosIL AcuStar ADAMTS13 activity assay is a fully automated, chemiluminescent assay that takes 33 min for analysis output [77]. Studies comparing the HemosIL chemiluminescent immunoassay to chromogenic ELISA and FRET-based assays revealed high concordance in results [77–81]. The HemosIL Acustar ADAMTS13 activity assay may then decrease the burden placed on laboratories to run skill- and time-intensive assays and increase the turnaround time of ADAMTS13 testing. The latter would help decrease unnecessary risk exposure of patients suspected to have immune TTP to TTP-specific therapeutic modalities that each have associated risks. A cost analysis (note: not cost-effectiveness) compared what the theoretical costs in 2019 would have been at a single center if an AcuStar was used instead of the ELISA-based Technozym ADAMTS13 [82]. From ELISA-based testing of 165 patient plasma samples across 93 patients received in that year for ADAMTS13 activity testing, 9 patients underwent unnecessary TPEs. The authors reported this corresponded to 18 TPE sessions and 227 units of fresh frozen plasma with a total cost of EUR 41,700. While the counterfactual clinical outcome cannot be known and the authors did not employ a measure of effectiveness, there is an implied clinical benefit of avoiding unnecessary patient risk exposure to TPE. Compared to the 2019 analysis year, in this 2022 study, the availability of caplacizumab and its attendant bleeding risk puts patients at unnecessary increased risk exposure for bleeding when diagnostic assay turnaround times are prolonged.

Cost-effectiveness: Two cost-effectiveness analyses conducted by the same group have examined the comparative value of in-house versus send-out FRET-based ADAMTS13 activity (Table 3) [64,83]. The first in 2017 reported on four competing testing strategies for a patient suspected of having immune TTP: (1) send-out ADAMTS13 activity versus (2) in-house ADAMTS13 activity versus (3) PLASMIC clinical score application followed by send-out ADAMTS13 testing for intermediate-to-high risk PLASMIC-scoring patients versus (4) PLASMIC clinical score application followed by in-house ADAMTS13 testing for intermediate-to-high risk PLASMIC-scoring patients [83]. The respective 3-day costs and deaths averted (the effectiveness outcome the authors employed) were USD 15,600 and 0.98, USD 4900 and 0.91, USD 9400 and 0.95, and USD 4700 and 0.91, respectively. Judged at a threshold of <USD 50,000 per death averted, the authors noted strategy #2 was the cost-effective strategy at an ICER of 49,600 per death averted. In a 2020 cost-effectiveness analysis, the authors examined the impact of delayed FRET-based ADAMTS13 activity testing over a 6-day time-horizon with a focus on the number of days delayed [64]. They reported an incremental cost to the health system ranging from USD 4200 to USD 5100 for every 1-day delay in obtaining ADAMTS13 activity assay results, with life days, their metric of effectiveness, decreasing from 5.89 with a 1-day delay to 5.85 with a 5-day delay.

Table 3. ADAMTS13 cost-effectiveness analyses with noted effectiveness metrics, time-horizon, and thresholds [64,83].

Effectiveness Metric and Time-Horizon	Strategies and/or Comparators	Effectiveness I Cost	Cost-Effective Strategy I at Threshold
Deaths averted and 3-day time-horizon [64]	Send-out vs. In-house vs. PLASMIC → send-out vs. PLAMSIC → in-house	0.98 I USD 15,600 0.91 I USD 4900 0.95 I USD 9400 0.91 I USD 4700	In-house (USD 49,600 per death averted), at threshold: <USD 50,000 per death averted
Life days and 6-day time-horizon [83]	Delay to ADAMTS13 results: day x vs. day x + 1, where x = 1 − 4	1 Day Delay: 5.89 I USD 27,500 5 Day Delay: 5.85 I USD 46,500	Not applicable

7. Conclusions

In 2023, health resource utilization data and cost-effectiveness evaluation of therapeutics and diagnostics in the care of patients with immune TTP are preferentially available in high-income country settings. Despite this, in high-income countries, the measurement of quality-adjusted life expectancy and cost-effectiveness evaluation is limited by the lack of TTP-specific utility weights. In low- and middle-income countries, these limitations are compounded by the lack of health resource utilization data, impaired access to the standard of care therapeutics, and the lack of ADAMTS13 assay availability due to cost concerns [84,85]. Although health technology assessments in country-specific contexts would quantify the value of each therapeutic and diagnostic in the care of patients with immune TTP, the measurement of input parameters and their uncertainty is needed for such quantification. For this reason, we believe the pressing research needs include the direct measurement of TTP-specific utility weights for high-income country settings and the collection of health resource utilization data in low- and middle-income country settings.

Author Contributions: A.B., C.A., A.P., S.I. and G.G. wrote and edited the manuscript. All authors have read and agreed to the published version of the manuscript.

Funding: GG is supported by the American Society of Hematology RTAF, Yale Bunker Endowment, and The Frederick A. DeLuca Foundation. The funding sources had no role in the study design; collection, analysis, or interpretation of the data; writing of the manuscript; or the decision to submit the manuscript for publication.

Institutional Review Board Statement: Not applicable.

Informed Consent Statement: Not applicable.

Data Availability Statement: Not applicable.

Conflicts of Interest: The authors declare no conflict of interest.

References

1. Joly, B.S.; Coppo, P.; Veyradier, A. Thrombotic thrombocytopenic purpura. *Blood* **2017**, *129*, 2836–2846. [CrossRef] [PubMed]
2. Sadler, J.E. What's new in the diagnosis and pathophysiology of thrombotic thrombocytopenic purpura. *Hematol. Am. Soc. Hematol. Educ. Program* **2015**, *2015*, 631–636. [CrossRef] [PubMed]
3. Zheng, X.L.; Vesely, S.K.; Cataland, S.R.; Coppo, P.; Geldziler, B.; Iorio, A.; Matsumoto, M.; Mustafa, R.A.; Pai, M.; Rock, G.; et al. ISTH guidelines for the diagnosis of thrombotic thrombocytopenic purpura. *J. Thromb. Haemost.* **2020**, *18*, 2486–2495. [CrossRef] [PubMed]
4. Mariotte, E.; Azoulay, E.; Galicier, L.; Rondeau, E.; Zouiti, F.; Boisseau, P.; Poullin, P.; de Maistre, E.; Provôt, F.; Delmas, Y.; et al. Epidemiology and pathophysiology of adulthood-onset thrombotic microangiopathy with severe ADAMTS13 deficiency (thrombotic thrombocytopenic purpura): A cross-sectional analysis of the French national registry for thrombotic microangiopathy. *Lancet Haematol.* **2016**, *3*, e237–e245. [CrossRef] [PubMed]
5. Wainstock, D.; Katz, A. Advancing rare disease policy in Latin America: A call to action. *Lancet Reg. Health* **2023**, *18*, 100434. [CrossRef]

6. George, J.N.; Al-Nouri, Z.L. Diagnostic and therapeutic challenges in the thrombotic thrombocytopenic purpura and hemolytic uremic syndromes. *Hematol. Am. Soc. Hematol. Educ. Program* **2012**, *2012*, 604–609. [CrossRef]
7. Stanley, M.; Killeen, R.B.; Michalski, J.M. Thrombotic Thrombocytopenic Purpura. In *StatPearls*; StatPearls Publishing: Treasure Island, FL, USA, 2023. Available online: https://www.ncbi.nlm.nih.gov/books/NBK430721/ (accessed on 2 April 2023).
8. Moschcowitz, E. Hyaline thrombosis of the terminal arterioles and capillaries: A hitherto undescribed disease. *Proc. N. Y. Pathol. Soc.* **1924**, *24*, 21–24.
9. Rubinstein, M.; Kagan, B.; Macgillviray, M.; Merliss, R.; Sacks, H. Unusual remission in a case of thrombotic thrombocytopenic purpura syndrome following fresh blood exchange transfusions. *Ann. Intern. Med.* **1959**, *51*, 1409–1419. [CrossRef]
10. Bukowski, R.M.; King, J.W.; Hewlett, J.S. Plasmapheresis in the treatment of thrombotic thrombocytopenic purpura. *Blood* **1977**, *50*, 413–417. [CrossRef]
11. Rock, G.A.; Shumak, K.H.; Buskard, N.A.; Blanchette, V.S.; Kelton, J.G.; Nair, R.C.; Spasoff, R.A.; Canadian Apheresis Study Group. Comparison of plasma exchange with plasma infusion in the treatment of thrombotic thrombocytopenic purpura. *N. Engl. J. Med.* **1991**, *325*, 393–397. [CrossRef]
12. Moake, J.L.; Rudy, C.K.; Troll, J.H.; Weinstein, M.J.; Colannino, N.M.; Azocar, J.; Seder, R.H.; Hong, S.L.; Deykin, D. Unusually large plasma factor VIII:von Willebrand factor multimers in chronic relapsing thrombotic thrombocytopenic purpura. *N. Engl. J. Med.* **1982**, *307*, 1432–1435. [CrossRef] [PubMed]
13. Furlan, M.; Robles, R.; Galbusera, M.; Remuzzi, G.; Kyrle, P.A.; Brenner, B.; Krause, M.; Scharrer, I.; Aumann, V.; Mittler, U.; et al. von Willebrand factor-cleaving protease in thrombotic thrombocytopenic purpura and the hemolytic-uremic syndrome. *N. Engl. J. Med.* **1998**, *339*, 1578–1584. [CrossRef] [PubMed]
14. Tsai, H.M.; Lian, E.C. Antibodies to von Willebrand factor-cleaving protease in acute thrombotic thrombocytopenic purpura. *N. Engl. J. Med.* **1998**, *339*, 1585–1594. [CrossRef] [PubMed]
15. Soejima, K.; Mimura, N.; Hirashima, M.; Maeda, H.; Hamamoto, T.; Nakagaki, T.; Nozaki, C. A novel human metalloprotease synthesized in the liver and secreted into the blood: Possibly, the von Willebrand factor-cleaving protease? *J. Biochem.* **2001**, *130*, 475–480. [CrossRef]
16. Coppo, P.; Bubenheim, M.; Azoulay, E.; Galicier, L.; Malot, S.; Bigé, N.; Poullin, P.; Provôt, F.; Martis, N.; Presne, C.; et al. A regimen with caplacizumab, immunosuppression, and plasma exchange prevents unfavorable outcomes in immune-mediated TTP. *Blood* **2021**, *137*, 733–742. [CrossRef]
17. Scully, M.; Cataland, S.R.; Peyvandi, F.; Coppo, P.; Knöbl, P.; Kremer Hovinga, J.A.; Metjian, A.; de la Rubia, J.; Pavenski, K.; Callewaert, F.; et al. Caplacizumab Treatment for Acquired Thrombotic Thrombocytopenic Purpura. *N. Engl. J. Med.* **2019**, *380*, 335–346. [CrossRef]
18. Zheng, X.L.; Vesely, S.K.; Cataland, S.R.; Coppo, P.; Geldziler, B.; Iorio, A.; Matsumoto, M.; Mustafa, R.A.; Pai, M.; Rock, G.; et al. ISTH guidelines for treatment of thrombotic thrombocytopenic purpura. *J. Thromb. Haemost.* **2020**, *18*, 2496–2502. [CrossRef]
19. Goshua, G.; Bendapudi, P.K. Evidence-Based Minireview: Should caplacizumab be used routinely in unselected patients with immune thrombotic thrombocytopenic purpura? *Hematol. Am. Soc. Hematol. Educ. Program* **2022**, *2022*, 491–494. [CrossRef]
20. Bendapudi, P.K.; Hurwitz, S.; Fry, A.; Marques, M.B.; Waldo, S.W.; Li, A.; Sun, L.; Upadhyay, V.; Hamdan, A.; Brunner, A.M.; et al. Derivation and external validation of the PLASMIC score for rapid assessment of adults with thrombotic microangiopathies: A cohort study. *Lancet Haematol.* **2017**, *4*, e157–e164. [CrossRef]
21. Picod, A.; Provôt, F.; Coppo, P. Therapeutic plasma exchange in thrombotic thrombocytopenic purpura. *Presse Med.* **2019**, *48*, 319–327. [CrossRef]
22. Soucemarianadin, M.; Benhamou, Y.; Delmas, Y.; Pichereau, C.; Maury, E.; Pène, F.; Halimi, J.M.; Presne, C.; Thouret, J.M.; Veyradier, A.; et al. Twice-daily therapeutical plasma exchange-based salvage therapy in severe autoimmune thrombotic thrombocytopenic purpura: The French TMA reference center experience. *Eur. J. Haematol.* **2016**, *97*, 183–191. [CrossRef]
23. Subhan, M.; Scully, M. Advances in the management of TTP. *Blood Rev.* **2022**, *55*, 100945. [CrossRef] [PubMed]
24. Nguyen, L.; Li, X.; Duvall, D.; Terrell, D.R.; Vesely, S.K.; George, J.N. Twice-daily plasma exchange for patients with refractory thrombotic thrombocytopenic purpura: The experience of the Oklahoma Registry, 1989 through 2006. *Transfusion* **2008**, *48*, 349–357. [CrossRef] [PubMed]
25. Scully, M.; Yarranton, H.; Liesner, R.; Cavenagh, J.; Hunt, B.; Benjamin, S.; Bevan, D.; Mackie, I.; Machin, S. Regional UK TTP registry: Correlation with laboratory ADAMTS 13 analysis and clinical features. *Br. J. Haematol.* **2008**, *142*, 819–826. [CrossRef] [PubMed]
26. Blombery, P.; Kivivali, L.; Pepperell, D.; McQuilten, Z.; Engelbrecht, S.; Polizzotto, M.N.; Phillips, L.E.; Wood, E.; Cohney, S.; TTP registry steering committee. Diagnosis and management of thrombotic thrombocytopenic purpura (TTP) in Australia: Findings from the first 5 years of the Australian TTP/thrombotic microangiopathy registry. *Intern. Med. J.* **2016**, *46*, 71–79. [CrossRef]
27. Wahl, P.M.; Bohn, R.L.; Terrell, D.R.; George, J.N.; Ewenstein, B. Health care utilization of patients diagnosed with idiopathic thrombotic thrombocytopenic purpura in a commercially insured population in the United States. *Transfusion* **2012**, *52*, 1614–1621. [CrossRef]
28. Mazepa, M.A.; Raval, J.S.; Brecher, M.E.; Park, Y.A. Treatment of acquired Thrombotic Thrombocytopenic Purpura in the U.S. remains heterogeneous: Current and future points of clinical equipoise. *J. Clin. Apher.* **2018**, *33*, 291–296. [CrossRef]
29. Pollissard, L.; Shah, A.; Punekar, R.S.; Petrilla, A.; Pham, H.P. Burden of illness among Medicare and non-Medicare US populations with acquired thrombotic thrombocytopenic purpura. *J. Med. Econ.* **2021**, *24*, 706–716. [CrossRef]

30. Bell, W.R.; Braine, H.G.; Ness, P.M.; Kickler, T.S. Improved survival in thrombotic thrombocytopenic purpura-hemolytic uremic syndrome. Clinical experience in 108 patients. *N. Engl. J. Med.* **1991**, *325*, 398–403. [CrossRef]
31. Petitt, R.M. Thrombotic thrombocytopenic purpura: A thirty year review. *Semin. Thromb. Hemost.* **1980**, *6*, 350–355. [CrossRef]
32. Balduini, C.L.; Gugliotta, L.; Luppi, M.; Laurenti, L.; Klersy, C.; Pieresca, C.; Quintini, G.; Iuliano, F.; Re, R.; Spedini, P.; et al. High versus standard dose methylprednisolone in the acute phase of idiopathic thrombotic thrombocytopenic purpura: A randomized study. *Ann. Hematol.* **2010**, *89*, 591–596. [CrossRef]
33. Cataland, S.R.; Kourlas, P.J.; Yang, S.; Geyer, S.; Witkoff, L.; Wu, H.; Masias, C.; George, J.N.; Wu, H.M. Cyclosporine or steroids as an adjunct to plasma exchange in the treatment of immune-mediated thrombotic thrombocytopenic purpura. *Blood Adv.* **2017**, *1*, 2075–2082. [CrossRef] [PubMed]
34. Garvey, B. Rituximab in the treatment of autoimmune haematological disorders. *Br. J. Haematol. Rev.* **2008**, *141*, 149–169. [CrossRef]
35. Arnold, D.M.; Dentali, F.; Crowther, M.A.; Meyer, R.M.; Cook, R.J.; Sigouin, C.; Fraser, G.A.; Lim, W.; Kelton, J.G. Systematic review: Efficacy and safety of rituximab for adults with idiopathic thrombocytopenic purpura. *Ann. Intern. Med.* **2007**, *146*, 25–33. [CrossRef] [PubMed]
36. Caramazza, D.; Quintini, G.; Abbene, I.; Coco, L.L.; Malato, A.; Di Trapani, R.; Saccullo, G.; Pizzo, G.; Palazzolo, R.; Barone, R.; et al. Rituximab for managing relapsing or refractory patients with idiopathic thrombotic thrombocytopenic purpura--haemolytic uraemic syndrome. *Blood Transfus.* **2010**, *8*, 203–210. [CrossRef] [PubMed]
37. de la Rubia, J.; Moscardó, F.; Gómez, M.J.; Guardia, R.; Rodríguez, P.; Sebrango, A.; Zamora, C.; Debén, G.; Goterris, R.; López, R.; et al. Efficacy and safety of rituximab in adult patients with idiopathic relapsing or refractory thrombotic thrombocytopenic purpura: Results of a Spanish multicenter study. *Transfus. Apher. Sci.* **2010**, *43*, 299–303. [CrossRef]
38. Rüfer, A.; Brodmann, D.; Gregor, M.; Kremer Hovinga, J.A.; Lämmle, B.; Wuillemin, W.A. Rituximab for acute plasma-refractory thrombotic thrombocytopenic purpura. A case report and concise review of the literature. *Swiss Med. Wkly.* **2007**, *137*, 518–524.
39. Uhl, L.; Kiss, J.E.; Malynn, E.; Terrell, D.R.; Vesely, S.K.; George, J.N. Rituximab for thrombotic thrombocytopenic purpura: Lessons from the STAR trial. *Transfusion* **2017**, *57*, 2532–2538. [CrossRef]
40. Scully, M.; McDonald, V.; Cavenagh, J.; Hunt, B.J.; Longair, I.; Cohen, H.; Machin, S.J. A phase 2 study of the safety and efficacy of rituximab with plasma exchange in acute acquired thrombotic thrombocytopenic purpura. *Blood* **2011**, *118*, 1746–1753. [CrossRef]
41. Chaturvedi, S.; Antun, A.G.; Farland, A.M.; Woods, R.; Metjian, A.; Park, Y.A.; de Ridder, G.; Gibson, B.; Kasthuri, R.S.; Liles, D.K.; et al. Race, rituximab, and relapse in TTP. *Blood* **2022**, *140*, 1335–1344. [CrossRef]
42. Westwood, J.-P.; Webster, H.; McGuckin, S.; McDonald, V.; Machin, S.J.; Scully, M. Rituximab for thrombotic thrombocytopenic purpura: Benefit of early administration during acute episodes and use of prophylaxis to prevent relapse. *J. Thromb. Haemost.* **2013**, *11*, 481–490. [CrossRef] [PubMed]
43. Scully, M.; Hunt, B.J.; Benjamin, S.; Liesner, R.; Rose, P.; Peyvandi, F.; Cheung, B.; Machin, S.J. British Committee for Standards in Haematology. Guidelines on the diagnosis and management of thrombotic thrombocytopenic purpura and other thrombotic microangiopathies. *Br. J. Haematol.* **2012**, *158*, 323–335. [CrossRef]
44. Owattanapanich, W.; Wongprasert, C.; Rotchanapanya, W.; Owattanapanich, N.; Ruchutrakool, T. Comparison of the long-term remission of rituximab and conventional treatment for acquired thrombotic thrombocytopenic Purpura: A systematic review and meta-analysis. *Clin. Appl. Thromb. Hemost.* **2019**, *25*, 1076029618825309. [CrossRef] [PubMed]
45. Westwood, J.P.; Thomas, M.; Alwan, F.; McDonald, V.; Benjamin, S.; Lester, W.A.; Lowe, G.C.; Dutt, T.; Hill, Q.A.; Scully, M. Rituximab prophylaxis to prevent thrombotic thrombocytopenic purpura relapse: Outcome and evaluation of dosing regimens. *Blood Adv.* **2017**, *1*, 1159–1166. [CrossRef] [PubMed]
46. Goshua, G.; Gokhale, A.; Hendrickson, J.E.; Tormey, C.; Lee, A.I. Cost savings to hospital of rituximab use in severe autoimmune acquired thrombotic thrombocytopenic purpura. *Blood Adv.* **2020**, *4*, 539–545. [CrossRef] [PubMed]
47. Duggan, S. Caplacizumab: First Global Approval. *Drugs* **2018**, *78*, 1639–1642, Erratum in *Drugs* **2018**, *78*, 1955. [CrossRef]
48. Völker, L.A.; Kaufeld, J.; Miesbach, W.; Brähler, S.; Reinhardt, M.; Kühne, L.; Mühlfeld, A.; Schreiber, A.; Gaedeke, J.; Tölle, M.; et al. Real-world data confirm the effectiveness of caplacizumab in acquired thrombotic thrombocytopenic purpura. *Blood Adv.* **2020**, *4*, 3085–3092. [CrossRef]
49. Dutt, T.; Shaw, R.J.; Stubbs, M.; Yong, J.; Bailiff, B.; Cranfield, T.; Crowley, M.P.; Desborough, M.; Eyre, T.A.; Gooding, R.; et al. Real-world experience with caplacizumab in the management of acute TTP. *Blood* **2021**, *137*, 1731–1740. [CrossRef]
50. Izquierdo, C.P.; Mingot-Castellano, M.E.; Fuentes, A.E.K.; García-Arroba Peinado, J.; Cid, J.; Jimenez, M.M.; Valcarcel, D.; Gómez-Seguí, I.; de la Rubia, J.; Martin, P.; et al. Real-world effectiveness of caplacizumab vs the standard of care in immune thrombotic thrombocytopenic purpura. *Blood Adv.* **2022**, *6*, 6219–6227. [CrossRef]
51. Djulbegovic, M.; Tong, J.; Xu, A.; Yang, J.; Chen, Y.; Cuker, A.; Pishko, A. Adding caplacizumab to standard of care in thrombotic thrombocytopenic purpura: A systematic review and meta-analysis. *Blood Adv.* **2023**, *7*, 2132–2142. [CrossRef]
52. Knöbl, P.E.K.; Buxhofer-Ausch, V.; Thaler, J.; Gleixner, K.; Sperr, W. Management of thrombotic thrombocytopenic purpura (TTP) without plasma exchange: An update on the Austrian experience. In Proceedings of the ISTH Congress 2022, London, UK, 9–13 July 2022.
53. Colling, M.; Sun, L.; Upadhyay, V.; Ryu, J.; Li, A.; Uhl, L.; Kaufman, R.M.; Stowell, C.P.; Dzik, W.H.; Makar, R.S.; et al. Deaths and complications associated with the management of acute immune thrombotic thrombocytopenic purpura. *Transfusion* **2020**, *60*, 841–846. [CrossRef] [PubMed]

54. Page, E.E.; Kremer Hovinga, J.A.; Terrell, D.R.; Vesely, S.K.; George, J.N. Thrombotic thrombocytopenic purpura: Diagnostic criteria, clinical features, and long-term outcomes from 1995 through 2015. *Blood Adv.* **2017**, *1*, 590–600. [CrossRef] [PubMed]
55. Goshua, G. Debate: Most/All Patients with Acquired (Immune) Thrombotic Thrombocytopenia Purpura Receive Caplacizumab. Education Spotlight. In Proceedings of the 64th Annual American Society of Hematology Meeting, New Orleans, LA, USA, 10–13 December 2022.
56. Pollissard, L.; Leinwand, B.I.; Fournier, M.; Pham, H.P. Cost analysis of the impact of caplacizumab in the treatment of acquired thrombotic thrombocytopenic purpura from a US hospital perspective. *J. Med. Econ.* **2021**, *24*, 1178–1184. [CrossRef] [PubMed]
57. Picod, A.; Veyradier, A.; Coppo, P. Should all patients with immune-mediated thrombotic thrombocytopenic purpura receive caplacizumab? *J. Thromb. Haemost.* **2021**, *19*, 58–67. [CrossRef] [PubMed]
58. National Institute for Health and Care Excellence. Final Appraisal Document: Caplacizumab with Plasma Exchange and Immunosuppression for Treating Acute Acquired Thrombotic Thrombocytopenic Purpura. Available online: https://www.nice.org.uk/guidance/ta667/documents/final-appraisal-determination-document (accessed on 18 October 2022).
59. Di Minno, G.; Ravasio, R. Cost-effectiveness analysis of caplacizumab in the new standard of care for immune Thrombotic Thrombocytopenic Purpura in Italy. *Grhta* **2021**, *8*, 43–52. Available online: https://journals.aboutscience.eu/index.php/grhta/article/view/2191 (accessed on 2 April 2023). [CrossRef]
60. Goshua, G.; Sinha, P.; Hendrickson, J.E.; Tormey, C.; Bendapudi, P.K.; Lee, A.I. Cost effectiveness of caplacizumab in acquired thrombotic thrombocytopenic purpura. *Blood* **2021**, *137*, 969–976. [CrossRef]
61. Goshua, G.; Prasad, V.; Lee, A.I.; Bendapudi, P.K. Accurate accounting of caplacizumab cost effectiveness. *Lett. Lancet Haematol.* **2021**, *8*, e315. [CrossRef]
62. Butt, A.; Lee, A.I.; Goshua, G. Cost-Effectiveness of Caplacizumab without First-Line Therapeutic Plasma Exchange vs. Standard-of-Care for Patients with Immune Thrombotic Thrombocytopenic Purpura: Setting Future Clinical Trial Thresholds. *Blood* **2022**, *140* (Suppl. S1), 1621–1622. [CrossRef]
63. Heatwole, C.; Johnson, N.; Holloway, R.; Noyes, K. Plasma exchange versus intravenous immunoglobulin for myasthenia gravis crisis: An acute hospital cost comparison study. *J. Clin. Neuromuscul. Dis.* **2011**, *13*, 85–94. [CrossRef]
64. Kim, C.H.; Simmons, S.C.; Wattar, S.F.; Azad, A.; Pham, H.P. Potential impact of a delayed ADAMTS13 result in the treatment of thrombotic microangiopathy: An economic analysis. *Vox Sang* **2020**, *115*, 433–442. [CrossRef]
65. Centers for Medicare & Medicaid Services. 2022 ASP Drug Pricing Files. Available online: https://www.cms.gov/medicare/medicare-part-b-drug-average-sales-price/2022-asp-drug-pricing-files (accessed on 2 April 2023).
66. Anderson, D.; Ali, K.; Blanchette, V.; Brouwers, M.; Couban, S.; Radmoor, P.; Huebsch, L.; Hume, H.; McLeod, A.; Meyer, R.; et al. Guidelines on the Use of Intravenous Immune Globulin for Hematologic Conditions. Article. *Transfus. Med. Rev.* **2007**, *21* (Suppl. S1), S9–S56. [CrossRef] [PubMed]
67. Prasannan, N.; Thomas, M.; Stubbs, M.; Westwood, J.P.; de Groot, R.; Singh, D.; Scully, M. Delayed normalization of ADAMTS13 activity in acute thrombotic thrombocytopenic purpura in the caplacizumab era. *Blood* **2023**, *141*, 2206–2213. [CrossRef] [PubMed]
68. Shemin, D.; Briggs, D.; Greenan, M. Complications of therapeutic plasma exchange: A prospective study of 1727 procedures. *J. Clin. Apher.* **2007**, *22*, 270–276. [CrossRef] [PubMed]
69. Yasir, M.; Goyal, A.; Sonthalia, S. Corticosteroid Adverse Effects. In *StatPearls*; StatPearls Publishing: Treasure Island, FL, USA, 2023. Available online: https://www.ncbi.nlm.nih.gov/books/NBK531462/ (accessed on 2 April 2023).
70. Liu, A.; Dhaliwal, N.; Upreti, H.; Kasmani, J.; Dane, K.; Moliterno, A.; Braunstein, E.; Brodsky, R.; Chaturvedi, S. Reduced sensitivity of PLASMIC and French scores for the diagnosis of thrombotic thrombocytopenic purpura in older individuals. *Transfusion* **2021**, *61*, 266–273. [CrossRef] [PubMed]
71. Studt, J.D.; Böhm, M.; Budde, U.; Girma, J.P.; Varadi, K.; Lämmle, B. Measurement of von Willebrand factor-cleaving protease (ADAMTS-13) activity in plasma: A multicenter comparison of different assay methods. *J. Thromb. Haemost.* **2003**, *1*, 1882–1887. [CrossRef] [PubMed]
72. Böhm, M.; Vigh, T.; Scharrer, I. Evaluation and clinical application of a new method for measuring activity of von Willebrand factor-cleaving metalloprotease (ADAMTS13). *Ann. Hematol.* **2002**, *81*, 430–435. [CrossRef]
73. Gerritsen, H.E.; Turecek, P.L.; Schwarz, H.P.; Lämmle, B.; Furlan, M. Assay of von Willebrand factor (vWF)-cleaving protease based on decreased collagen binding affinity of degraded vWF: A tool for the diagnosis of thrombotic thrombocytopenic purpura (TTP). *Thromb. Haemost.* **1999**, *82*, 1386–1389. [CrossRef]
74. Obert, B.; Tout, H.; Veyradier, A.; Fressinaud, E.; Meyer, D.; Girma, J.P. Estimation of the von Willebrand factor-cleaving protease in plasma using monoclonal antibodies to VWF. *Thromb. Haemost.* **1999**, *82*, 1382–1385. [CrossRef]
75. Kokame, K.; Nobe, Y.; Kokubo, Y.; Okayama, A.; Miyata, T. FRETS-VWF73, a first fluorogenic substrate for ADAMTS13 assay. *Br. J. Haematol.* **2005**, *129*, 93–100. [CrossRef]
76. Kremer Hovinga, J.A.; Mottini, M.; Lämmle, B. Measurement of ADAMTS-13 activity in plasma by the FRETS-VWF73 assay: Comparison with other assay methods. *J. Thromb. Haemost.* **2006**, *4*, 1146–1148. [CrossRef]
77. Valsecchi, C.; Mirabet, M.; Mancini, I.; Biganzoli, M.; Schiavone, L.; Faraudo, S.; Mane-Padros, D.; Giles, D.; Serra-Domenech, J.; Blanch, S.; et al. Evaluation of a New, Rapid, Fully Automated Assay for the Measurement of ADAMTS13 Activity. *Thromb. Haemost.* **2019**, *119*, 1767–1772. [CrossRef]
78. Stratmann, J.; Ward, J.N.; Miesbach, W. Evaluation of a rapid turn-over, fully-automated ADAMTS13 activity assay: A method comparison study. *J. Thromb. Thrombolysis* **2020**, *50*, 628–631. [CrossRef]

79. Beranger, N.; Benghezal, S.; Joly, B.S.; Capdenat, S.; Delton, A.; Stepanian, A.; Coppo, P.; Veyradier, A. Diagnosis and follow-up of thrombotic thrombocytopenic purpura with an automated chemiluminescent ADAMTS13 activity immunoassay. *Res. Pract. Thromb. Haemost.* **2021**, *5*, 81–93. [CrossRef] [PubMed]
80. Favaloro, E.J.; Mohammed, S.; Chapman, K.; Swanepoel, P.; Zebeljan, D.; Sefhore, O.; Malan, E.; Clifford, J.; Yuen, A.; Donikian, D.; et al. A multicenter laboratory assessment of a new automated chemiluminescent assay for ADAMTS13 activity. *J. Thromb. Haemost.* **2021**, *19*, 417–428. [CrossRef]
81. Pascual, C.; Nieto, J.M.; Fidalgo, T.; Seguí, I.G.; Díaz-Ricart, M.; Docampo, M.F.; Del Rio, J.; Salinas, R. Multicentric evaluation of the new HemosIL Acustar® chemiluminescence ADAMTS13 activity assay. *Int. J. Lab. Hematol.* **2021**, *43*, 485–493. [CrossRef]
82. Jousselme, E.; Sobas, F.; Guerre, P.; Simon, M.; Nougier, C. Cost-effectiveness of thrombotic thrombocytopenic purpura diagnosis: A retrospective analysis in the University Hospital Center of Lyon (France). *Blood Coagul. Fibrinolysis* **2022**, *33*, 119–123. [CrossRef]
83. Kim, C.H.; Simmons, S.C.; Williams, L.A., III; Staley, E.M.; Zheng, X.L.; Pham, H.P. ADAMTS13 test and/or PLASMIC clinical score in management of acquired thrombotic thrombocytopenic purpura: A cost-effective analysis. *Transfusion* **2017**, *57*, 2609–2618. [CrossRef] [PubMed]
84. Kirui, N.; Sokwala, A. A case of refractory thrombotic thrombocytopenic purpura treated with plasmapheresis and rituximab. *S. Afr. Med. J.* **2016**, *106*, 689–691. [CrossRef] [PubMed]
85. Chaurasiya, P.S.; Khatri, A.; Gurung, S.; Karki, S.; Shahi, S.; Aryal, L. Rituximab for acute plasma-refractory thrombotic thrombocytopenic purpura: A case report. *Ann. Med. Surg.* **2022**, *82*, 104789. [CrossRef] [PubMed]

Disclaimer/Publisher's Note: The statements, opinions and data contained in all publications are solely those of the individual author(s) and contributor(s) and not of MDPI and/or the editor(s). MDPI and/or the editor(s) disclaim responsibility for any injury to people or property resulting from any ideas, methods, instructions or products referred to in the content.

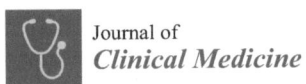
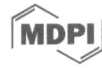

Review

Clinical Manifestations, Current and Future Therapy, and Long-Term Outcomes in Congenital Thrombotic Thrombocytopenic Purpura

Kazuya Sakai [1] and Masanori Matsumoto [1,2,*]

[1] Department of Blood Transfusion Medicine, Nara Medical University, Kashihara 634-8522, Japan; ks13122@naramed-u.ac.jp
[2] Department of Hematology, Nara Medical University, Kashihara 634-8521, Japan
* Correspondence: mmatsumo@naramed-u.ac.jp; Tel.: +81-744-22-3051

Abstract: Congenital thrombotic thrombocytopenic purpura (cTTP) is an extremely rare disease characterized by the severe deficiency of a disintegrin and metalloproteinase with thrombospondin type 1 motifs 13 (ADAMTS13), caused by *ADAMTS13* mutations. While ADAMTS13 supplementation by fresh frozen plasma (FFP) infusion immediately corrects platelet consumption and resolves thrombotic symptoms in acute episodes, FFP treatment can lead to intolerant allergic reactions and frequent hospital visits. Up to 70% of patients depend on regular FFP infusions to normalize their platelet counts and avoid systemic symptoms, including headache, fatigue, and weakness. The remaining patients do not receive regular FFP infusions, mainly because their platelet counts are maintained within the normal range or because they are symptom-free without FFP infusions. However, the target peak and trough levels of ADAMTS13 to prevent long-term comorbidity with prophylactic FFP and the necessity of treating FFP-independent patients in terms of long-term clinical outcomes are yet to be determined. Our recent study suggests that the current volumes of FFP infusions are insufficient to prevent frequent thrombotic events and long-term ischemic organ damage. This review focuses on the current management of cTTP and its associated issues, followed by the importance of upcoming recombinant ADAMTS13 therapy.

Keywords: congenital thrombotic thrombocytopenic purpura; ADAMTS13; fresh frozen plasma; prophylaxis; quality of life

Citation: Sakai, K.; Matsumoto, M. Clinical Manifestations, Current and Future Therapy, and Long-Term Outcomes in Congenital Thrombotic Thrombocytopenic Purpura. *J. Clin. Med.* 2023, *12*, 3365. https://doi.org/10.3390/jcm12103365

Academic Editors: Ilaria Mancini and Andrea Artoni

Received: 28 February 2023
Revised: 5 May 2023
Accepted: 8 May 2023
Published: 9 May 2023

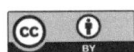

Copyright: © 2023 by the authors. Licensee MDPI, Basel, Switzerland. This article is an open access article distributed under the terms and conditions of the Creative Commons Attribution (CC BY) license (https://creativecommons.org/licenses/by/4.0/).

1. Introduction

Thrombotic thrombocytopenic purpura (TTP) is an extremely rare disease clinically characterized by severe thrombocytopenia, hemolytic anemia, and ischemic organ damage [1–3]. The estimated incidence of TTP is 2–6 per million persons [4]. In patients with TTP, the levels of the von Willebrand factor (VWF)-cleaving protease ADAMTS13 are severely decreased. This leads to secreted VWF remaining as an uncleaved large multimetric form called an ultra-large VWF multimer (UL-VWFM), which captures circulating platelets under high shear force via interactions between the VWF A1 domain and the GpIb domain of platelets [5,6]. As a result, VWF/platelet-rich thrombi occlude the systemic microvasculature, leading to life-threatening ischemic organ crises such as stroke and myocardial infarction [7,8]. Either autoantibodies against ADAMTS13 or causative *ADAMTS13* mutations in a homozygous or compound heterozygous state cause severe ADAMTS13 depletion in patients with TTP, which can be classified into immune-mediated TTP (iTTP) [9,10] or congenital TTP (cTTP) [11,12], also known as Upshaw–Schulman syndrome (USS), respectively. cTTP accounts for <5% of all TTP cases [13].

In 1960, Schulman et al. first described the condition of an 8-year-old girl with persistent thrombocytopenia (<100 × 10^9/L) and repeated bleeding symptoms as "chronic thrombocytopenia". Her platelet count responded to 6 mL/kg of fresh frozen plasma (FFP)

infusions but decreased after 12 days [14]. Subsequently, Upshaw also reported an identical case of a 29-year-old woman who frequently developed high fever, petechial rash, and severe thrombocytopenia triggered by acute viral or bacterial infections. FFP infusion dramatically improved severe thrombocytopenia and normalized platelet counts. While this patient showed similar laboratory findings to typical TTP, the clinical presentation did not fulfill the five classic pentads of iTTP [15]. At that time, this disease, named after these two researchers, was not considered typical TTP, in which the disease mortality exceeded 90% without effective treatment [16,17]. Levy et al. successfully found several *ADAMTS13* mutations among USS families, leading to the recognition of USS as cTTP [11]. In the mid-2000s, causative *ADAMTS13* mutations were identified over the ADAMTS13 domains without a specific hot spot [18–21]. ADAMTS13 supply through FFP infusion is sufficient to resolve acute episodes in patients with cTTP [14,15,22], while patients with iTTP require intensive plasma exchange with FFP and immunosuppressors to survive.

Several TTP reference centers have established nationwide or international cTTP cohorts to clarify demographic characteristics, variations in causative *ADAMTS13* mutations, current ADAMTS13 replenishment, and TTP-related organ damage [18–21]. So far, more than 200 *ADAMTS13* mutations have been reported to cause cTTP. Furthermore, the anti-thrombotic effect of ADAMTS13 has been reported in experimental thrombotic mice, and the imbalanced VWF-ADAMTS13 axis has gained more attention in diverse areas of research.

The ultra-rarity of cTTP has prevented the full characterization of the clinical manifestations and optimal patient care. Since >90–95% of patients with TTP are diagnosed with iTTP, many physicians may assume that the following points are true for "all" TTP patients: (i) severe thrombocytopenia, hemolytic anemia, and ischemic organ damage occur when ADAMTS13 levels fall <10%; (ii) without suitable therapeutic interventions, >90% of cases lead to a fatal outcome; (iii) all acute and recurrent cases must be treated in the hospital, sometimes in an intensive care unit; and (iv) treatment options are expanding and there are relatively well-established treatment protocols. These four points are recognized in the field of iTTP [1–3]. However, although severe ADAMTS13 deficiency is present in both iTTP and cTTP, the aforementioned clinical features may vary for patients with cTTP. This review discusses cTTP-specific clinical features in comparison with those of iTTP.

Hence, we must investigate the appropriate treatment and management for better long-term outcomes, likely through enriched international cohort studies and clinical trials of novel therapies.

2. Diagnostic Flow for cTTP

Among patients with severe thrombocytopenia and hemolytic anemia of unknown cause, the reduction in ADAMTS13 levels to <10% of normal values confirms a diagnosis of TTP [23]. Two assays developed in Japan are commonly used to measure ADAMTS13 activity. The first is the chromogenic ADAMTS13 act-enzyme-linked immunosorbent assay (ELISA), in which the N10 monoclonal antibody directly detects the cleavage site of a synthetic 73-amino-acid peptide, VWF73 [24,25]. The second, the fluorescence resonance energy transfer (FRET)-VWF73 assay, detects increased fluorescence generated by the FRET-VWF73 substrate cleaved by ADAMTS13 in the plasma [26]. Recently, a fully automated assay, the HemosIL AcuStar ADAMTS13 activity assay, became available, which helps to more rapidly measure ADAMTS13 activity (33 min) [27]. However, measuring ADAMTS13 activity with the FRET-VWF73 assay requires careful attention as extremely high levels of serum bilirubin (>100 μmol/L, 5.85 mg/dL) can interfere with fluorescence evolution by acting as a quencher at an emission wavelength of 450 nm [28].

The detection of autoantibodies against ADAMTS13 using the Bethesda assay or anti-ADAMTS13 IgG ELISA is required to distinguish between iTTP and cTTP [29]. In cases of negative results, the assay must be repeated on samples drawn at different time points because patients at presentation of the acute TTP event sometimes do not present autoantibodies, probably due to immunocomplexes with ADAMTS13 and autoantibodies in circulation [30]. Measuring ADAMTS13 activity in the parents of affected individuals to confirm mild–moderate ADAMTS13 depletion, usually seen in individuals with heterozygous ADAMTS13 mutations [31], is also useful for cTTP diagnosis.

A diagnosis of cTTP is confirmed through genetic analysis and identification of causative *ADAMTS13* mutations (homozygous or compound heterozygous). Polymerase chain reaction (PCR) direct sequencing, also known as Sanger's method, is used to analyze the 29 exons [32]. Genetic confirmation is straightforward when the detected *ADAMTS13* mutations have been proven to be causative or pathogenic variants based on in vitro ADAMTS13 expression studies. In the Japanese registry data, 67 clinically diagnosed patients underwent genetic analysis, which identified 68 different mutations in 60 families as of May 2022; these mutations included missense mutations, nonsense mutations, insertions/deletions, structural variants, and aberrant splicing [31]. Comprehensive genomic quantitative PCR can compensate for the limitations of direct PCR sequencing [33]. Some complex cases may also show variants including copy number variants, deep-intronic splice site variants, repeat expansions, structural variants, or mobile element insertions. In addition, a recent in silico study showed that some synonymous single nucleotide variants (sSNVs) in *ADAMTS13* change mRNA folding energy/stability, disrupt mRNA splicing, disturb microRNA-binding sites, and alter synonymous codon or codon pair usage [34].

3. Current Treatments for Patients with cTTP

In most cases, cTTP diagnosis is not confirmed when patients experience their first episode of severe TTP because autoantibody detection via ELISA sometimes fails to distinguish between iTTP and cTTP [23]. FFP infusion is typically sufficient to achieve clinical remission [22]. However, these initial cases are generally treated with therapeutic plasma exchange (TPE), the standard therapy for iTTP. Based on previous experiences, acute TTP episodes in confirmed cTTP can be treated with several FFP infusions [22]. The exact amount of ADAMTS13 required to resolve acute TTP episodes has not been determined; however, sole FFP infusions can successfully adjust the unbalanced ADAMTS13-VWF axis in patients with cTTP compared to that in patients with iTTP with numerous neutralizing autoantibodies against ADAMTS13. The recent International Society on Thrombosis and Haemostasis (ISTH) TTP guidelines suggest daily plasma infusions for symptomatic patients until the symptoms resolve and platelet counts reach the normal range [35,36]. If the underlying trigger is treatable (e.g., bacterial or influenza virus infection), suitable medication should be administered in parallel to prevent further VWF secretion by the endothelial cells. However, the level of ADAMTS13 activity required to overcome acute TTP episodes remains unknown.

As maintenance therapy, the ISTH TTP guidelines recommend treating cTTP with FFP (10–15 mL/kg) every 1–3 weeks to prevent further acute episodes [35,36]. In the international hereditary TTP registry, 83 patients (70% of the total) received regular treatment, with a median interval of regular infusions of 14.0 days (range: 2–75 days) [19]. Another report on the annual incidence of TTP episodes reported a mean plasma volume dose of <15 mL/kg every 2 weeks in 79% (60 out of 76) of patients with available information [37]. In the UK registry, 67% of the patients received regular prophylactic therapy, 12% received on-demand therapy, and 21% had never received therapy since the initial diagnosis of cTTP. The interval between infusions was determined in a stepwise manner until once weekly. The single dosage of replacement therapy per body weight was not available [20]. In Japan, 240–480 mL of prophylactic FFP infusion every 2 weeks has been recommended over the past two decades based on our experience [38].

The decision to administer regular FFP is based on the opinion of the attending physician, with the aim of maintaining a sufficient platelet count. As mentioned above, large cohort studies revealed that not all patients receive prophylactic FFP infusions, and that up to 30% of patients require FFP infusions only if they develop thrombocytopenia due to triggers such as infection, trauma, or pregnancy (on-demand FFP infusions) [19,20,39]. For instance, some children do not receive FFP infusions because of the difficulty in finding suitable venous access. Patients also tend to reject prophylactic FFP infusion if they are not FFP-dependent (e.g., normal platelet count, no hemolytic anemia, and no recurrence of TTP episodes).

In patients requiring ADAMTS13 supplementation, prophylactic FFP infusion is often burdensome in multiple ways (Figure 1). First, FFP infusions are performed only in a hospital setting, frequently (once every 1–3 weeks). Patients outside urban areas may have to move closer to the city to continue receiving ADAMTS13 replacement therapy. Moreover, FFP administration takes several hours of infusion due to its high volume. Care is usually taken to avoid volume overload in patients with impaired cardiac or renal function. Second, FFP contains not only the ADAMTS13 protein but also other proteins that may cause allergic reactions and can potentially transmit pathogens to patients [39]. Allergic reactions can range from hives to life-threatening anaphylactic shock and are more apparent in patients receiving prophylactic FFP compared to those receiving on-demand FFP. Our registry data showed that 58% of patients receiving prophylactic FFP infusion required premedication against allergic reactions before each FFP infusion, including steroids (hydrocortisone, prednisolone, and betamethasone), antihistamine agents (d-chlorpheniramine maleate and hydroxyzine), and anti-allergic medicines (fexofenadine and epinastine) [39]. A UK group has demonstrated the efficacy of two plasma-derived factor VIII/VWF concentrates as a source of ADAMTS13 (Koate-DVI and BPL 8Y). Since these agents have smaller volume and fewer other plasma proteins than FFP, they can be helpful for small children or patients requiring desensitization because of intolerant hypersensitivity to FFP [40,41]. Notably, ISTH TTP guidelines do not recommend the use of FVIII concentrate for most patients with cTTP in remission because of lacking clear evidence about the variability of ADAMTS13 concentrations across various FVIII concentrate products with intermediate purity [35]. Solvent–detergent-inactivated and amotosalen-UVA pathogen-inactivated FFP can reduce severe allergic reactions [42–44]. However, these manipulated plasma products are not available in some countries.

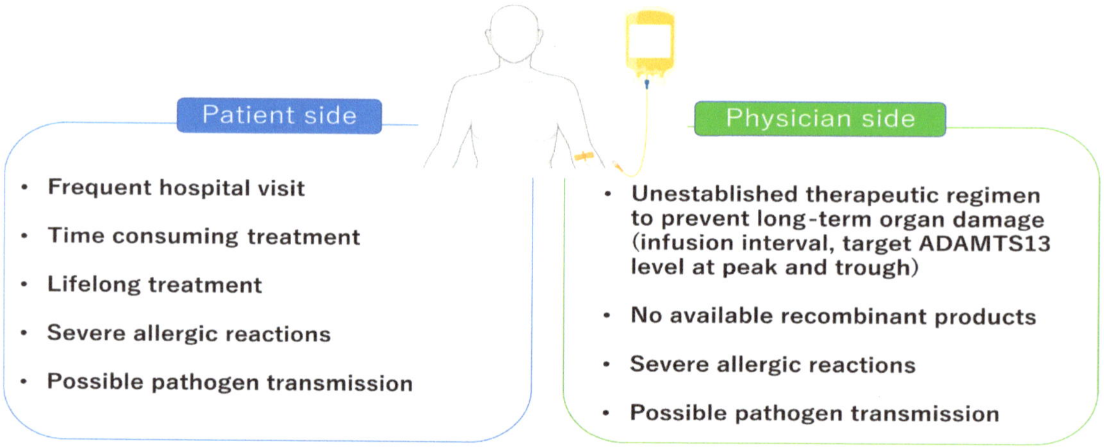

Patient side
- Frequent hospital visit
- Time consuming treatment
- Lifelong treatment
- Severe allergic reactions
- Possible pathogen transmission

Physician side
- Unestablished therapeutic regimen to prevent long-term organ damage (infusion interval, target ADAMTS13 level at peak and trough)
- No available recombinant products
- Severe allergic reactions
- Possible pathogen transmission

Figure 1. Current issues related to the use of prophylactic fresh frozen plasma infusion in patients with cTTP. Patients and physicians are concerned about several limitations of this treatment, which can decrease patients' quality of life.

In addition, a recent case report showed that a single dose of caplacizumab plus FFP infusion reduced the required FFP volume and hospital stay in refractory cTTP relapse [45]. Caplacizumab is a humanized nanobody that inhibits the interaction between VWF multimers and platelet glycoprotein 1b, and it has been approved for acute iTTP [46]. The treatment experience for cTTP is limited; however, it may benefit patients with refractory cTTP, sustained ischemic organ damage, and FFP intolerance due to allergic reactions. Moreover, caplacizumab has not yet been approved for cTTP as of March 2023.

4. Long-Term Organ Damage and Mortality in Patients with cTTP

The therapeutic regimen proposed in the ISTH guidelines mainly focuses on avoiding acute TTP episodes, including severe thrombocytopenia and ischemic organ damage. The most frequent acute TTP episodes during follow-up are of mild severity and are caused by acute infection [37]. However, the long-term organ damage in cTTP impacting the quality of life (QOL) of patients remains unclear (Figure 1). To clarify this risk among patients with cTTP, we conducted a questionnaire study in a Japanese cTTP cohort and analyzed the data from 55 eligible patients [39]. Forty-one patients received prophylactic FFP infusions (prophylactic FFP group), 14 of whom were included in the on-demand FFP group. In the prophylactic FFP group, the median dose of FFP infusion was 13.2 mL/kg/month, which was lower than that suggested in the ISTH guidelines (roughly 20–30 mL/kg/month). The trough levels of ADAMTS13 activity were available for 24 of 41 patients in the prophylactic FFP group, while 16 of these cases had levels below the detection limit (<1%). Laboratory findings immediately before FFP infusion revealed mild-to-moderate thrombocytopenia (median 138×10^9/L). A total of sixteen patients developed organ damage. Chronic kidney disease (CKD) was observed in 13 patients; five had end-stage renal failure and required renal replacement therapy, four required hemodialysis, and one underwent renal transplantation from his father. Six patients developed cerebral infarction and one patient developed cardiac hypofunction, during follow-up. Another study showed that all 25 enrolled patients reported the presence of more than two neuropsychiatric symptoms including headaches, difficulty in concentration, and depression. Headaches with aura (presumed to be migraines), vision changes, forgetfulness, fatigue, neuropathy, dysarthria, loss of vision, seizures, transient weakness, falls, and dysphagia were also reported [47]. Notably, 17 of the 25 patients developed strokes as they aged, and 11 had stroke-related sequelae. Stroke can occur in two different ways: during acute TTP episodes or from a gradual occlusion of cerebral vessels by latent microthrombi; however, which mechanism occurs more commonly in cTTP is not known. In another literature review, 202 patients identified between 2001 and 2020 were analyzed for their morbidities. Among those over 40 years of age, 20 (51%) had a major comorbidity, and 11 (28%) patients experienced a recurrence of a major morbidity after starting prophylactic FFP [48].

In contrast, in our previous study, none of the 14 patients with asymptomatic cTTP, who maintained platelet count within the normal range without regular FFP infusions, developed the kind of organ damage described above [39]. Indeed, the median serum creatinine level in this group was significantly lower than that among FFP-dependent patients (0.58 mg/mL vs. 0.71 mg/mL, $p = 0.009$). The trough levels of ADAMTS13 activity were available for only seven patients, and three cases were below the detection limit (<1%). Thus, these asymptomatic patients did not show relatively higher levels of ADAMTS13 activity, although previous studies showed that residual ADAMTS13 activity prevented more acute TTP episodes. These findings are summarized in Table 1.

Table 1. Long-term consequences reported in follow-up studies on congenital thrombotic thrombocytopenic purpura (cTTP).

Summary	Reference
The prophylactic FFP group received a lower FFP dose than suggested in the ISTH guidelines (13.2 mL/kg/month vs. 20–30 mL/kg/month). These patients showed mild thrombocytopenia immediately before FFP infusions (median 138×10^9/L). Chronic kidney disease was the most prevalent organ damage among these patients (32%), followed by cerebral infarction (15%) and cardiac hypofunction (2%) during follow-up.	Japanese registry [39]

Table 1. *Cont.*

Summary	Reference
Sixty-eight percent of patients developed strokes as they aged and 44% had stroke-related sequelae.	Oklahoma registry [47]
Among patients over 40 years of age, 51% had a major comorbidity, and 28% of patients experienced a major morbidity recurrence after initiating prophylactic FFP.	Literature review [48]
The FFP on-demand group maintained platelet counts within a normal range without regular treatment and did not develop long-term organ damage during follow-up.	Japanese registry [39]

As of May 2022, 10 of the 68 patients in the Japanese cTTP registry had died during follow-up. A young female patient who had received prophylactic FFP infusions after her first TTP episode during pregnancy committed suicide. Except for this case, the 10-year overall survival rate after the clinical diagnosis was 91.1% [31]. The causes of death are summarized in Table 2. The median patient age at the time of death was 44 years (IQR: 41–52 years). Two patients died due to thrombosis-related events. Five other patients died suddenly, suggesting abrupt cardiopulmonary dysfunction such as fatal arrhythmia or heart failure due to myocardial infarction. Three of the sudden death cases (60%) were in renal replacement. Previous studies on non-cTTP patients undergoing dialysis revealed a 2.2-fold higher mortality in patients with elevated VWF antigen levels compared to patients without elevated antigen levels [49]. Up to one-quarter of non-cTTP patients undergoing hemodialysis died of sudden cardiac death, suggesting that hemodialysis is associated with ventricular arrhythmia and dynamic electrocardiographic changes [50,51]. In patients with cTTP, more chronic glomerular sclerotic changes with C4d deposits were identified in the histopathological findings of renal biopsies with progressive renal impairment compared to controls, suggesting that C4d immunostaining provides evidence for complement-mediated glomerular damage in patients with cTTP [52]. The follow-up data from the international hTTP registry also showed that 4 of 87 patients died during prospective follow-up due to large cerebral infarction, heart failure, lethal arrhythmia with asystole during sepsis, and death from an unknown cause, respectively [37].

Table 2. Causes of death among patients in the Japanese cohort with congenital thrombotic thrombocytopenic purpura (cTTP).

Code	Age at Death (Years)	Sex	Follow-Up (Years)	Cause of Death	Renal Impairment	Complications/ Backgrounds	Prophylactic FFP Infusion
C3	38	M	30	Unknown *	ESRD (HD)		Yes
H3	52	M	1	Uremia	ESRD (HD)	GIH	No
R5	37	F	14	Suicide			Yes
X5	44	F	4	Unknown *		SLE	No
2G2	79	M	3	Cerebral infarction			Yes
2N4	23	F	0	Unknown *		Pregnancy	No
2O	41	M	2	Unknown *	ESRD (HD)		No
2P4	44	F	17	Status epilepticus, NOMI		Paralysis after stroke	Yes
2R	48	M	14	Unknown *	ESRD (HD)		Yes
2T	66	M	1	Sepsis	ESRD (HD)		Yes

* Sudden death, suggesting sudden cardiac death. Abbreviations: NOMI, non-occlusive mesenteric ischemia; ESRD, end-stage renal disease; HD, hemodialysis; GIH, gastrointestinal hemorrhage; SLE, systemic lupus erythematosus; FFP, fresh frozen plasma.

Considering this limited information, stroke and progressive renal failure during long-term follow-up substantially affect patients' QOL. Although the amount and frequency of ADAMTS13 supplementation needed to prevent long-term organ damage in patients with FFP-dependent cTTP is not well known, further investigations based on the clinical use of recombinant ADAMTS13 products and large-scale cTTP cohorts are needed to address this unmet medical need. In addition, we must determine whether asymptomatic patients with cTTP can be followed up without ADAMTS13 replenishment.

5. Determinants of FFP-Dependent or Asymptomatic Phenotypes in cTTP

Intriguingly, some patients with cTTP require regular FFP infusions to avoid severe thrombocytopenia and ischemic organ damage due to TTP episodes, whereas others seem to be free from TTP episodes unless a triggering factor is present. Schulman et al. reported a case of a 9-year-old patient who could not maintain platelet counts within the normal range without FFP [14], and Upshaw et al. described a 29-year-old patient who developed thrombocytopenia and petechial rash only when she had an infection [15]. These patients were classified as having FFP-dependent cTTP and asymptomatic cTTP, respectively. As acute TTP episodes triggered by infection [37] or pregnancy [53,54] have received increasing attention, there are few observations regarding FFP dependency after recovery from acute TTP episodes.

To clarify the determinants of FFP-dependent or asymptomatic phenotypes in cTTP, we hypothesized that the clinical presentation is derived from different genotypes (*ADAMTS13* mutations). As mentioned above, cTTP causative mutations are distributed throughout the ADAMTS13 sequence, predominantly R193W in the metalloprotease domain and C908Y in the TSP5 domain [31]. However, the presence of these mutations has not been shown as evidence of FFP dependency. c.4143_4144dupA (p.E1382Rfs*6) and p.R1060W are commonly observed in patients in Western countries [19,20], and a recent report from the international hTTP registry indicated that 12 of 87 patients who were compound heterozygous carriers of p.R1060W mutations had a residual ADAMTS13 activity of 1–9% and had a low incidence rate of acute episodes [37].

We sometimes encounter siblings with the same ADAMTS13 mutations presenting with different clinical pictures, suggesting that the cTTP severity might be determined not only by the type of ADAMTS13 mutation but also by other underlying factors [37,39].

6. Emerging Novel Therapies Will Improve the QOL and Long-Term Outcomes of Patients with cTTP

Current FFP dosages vary widely depending on patient characteristics and physician preferences, suggesting that it is difficult to establish an equal standard of care for all patients. Recombinant ADAMTS13 concentrate (r-ADAMTS13; codename: TAK-755) was developed in the early 2010s. The efficacy of r-ADAMTS13 was proven in cTTP mice, in which acute TTP was induced using a VWF concentrate. r-ADAMTS13 prevented severe thrombocytopenia and microthrombi in systemic tissues [55]. In the phase I first-in-human clinical trial, the pharmacokinetic (PK) profiling of r-ADAMTS13 was similar to that of FFP in a dose-dependent manner [56]. Its safety, immunogenicity, and tolerability were also demonstrated in the participants. Notably, patients were free from the physical burden and intolerant allergic reactions compared to regular FFP treatments [57]. Similar to hemophilia therapy, r-ADAMTS13 home infusion will become more common in patients with cTTP, regardless of generation. A phase III international multicenter clinical trial is currently underway to identify the side effects of long-term treatment with r-ADAMTS13 (https://www.clinicaltrials.gov/ct2/show/NCT04683003, accessed on 1 February 2023). Very recently, two important papers from a phase III trial described the efficacy and safety of r-ADAMTS13 in severe neonatal and pregnancy cases [58,59]. r-ADAMTS13 will soon be approved for clinical use and enable more patients with cTTP to easily maintain much higher ADAMTS13 activity at peak and trough levels. Meanwhile, additional clinical information on prophylactic r-ADAMTS13 will supply more robust evidence of long-term preventable effects against recurrent acute TTP episodes and progressive organ damage.

ADAMTS13 was also shown to down-regulate platelet adhesion to the exposed subendothelium and thrombus formation in injured arterioles [60] and reduce ischemic brain injury in experimental stroke [61,62]. Moreover, recombinant ADAMTS13 reduced oxidative stress by cleaving VWF in ischemia/reperfusion-induced acute kidney injury [63]. Even in healthy individuals, a slight decrease in ADAMTS13 activity (<70%) is a risk for stroke [64]. The anti-thrombotic effects of ADAMTS13 have also been described in myocardial infarction [65], chronic thrombotic pulmonary hypertension [66], and inflammatory bowel disease [67]. Hence, prophylactic r-ADAMTS13 infusion can benefit asymptomatic patients with cTTP, although data from our Japanese cohort showed no long-term organ damage in this group.

Regarding the progress of treatments for patients with hemophilia A and B, longer-acting recombinant factor concentrates have become widely available, and therapeutic intervals have been extended to maintain suitable factor levels since mid-2010. In November 2022, the U.S. Food and Drug Administration (FDA) approved Hemgenix (etranacogene dezaparvovec), an adeno-associated virus (AAV) vector-based gene therapy for the treatment of adults with HB who currently use Factor IX prophylaxis therapy or have a history of life-threatening hemorrhage, or have repeated, severe spontaneous bleeding events [68]. Although gene therapy has been thought of as a costly treatment, a recent study reported that a single use of gene therapy could compensate for lifelong consecutive factor prophylaxis [69]. Hence, gene therapy could also overcome the limitation of short-term ADAMTS13 replacement because the ADAMTS13 transgene would allow the long-term expression of ADAMTS13 and free cTTP patients from lifelong replacement therapy [70]. Some research groups have already shown promising long-term ADAMTS13 or MDTCS expression in *ADAMTS13* knock-out mice via different applications, including hematopoietic progenitor-cell transgene, in utero gene transfer of the lentiviral vector, adenoviral vector-mediated transgene, AAV-mediated transgene, and sleeping-beauty transposon-mediated gene transfer [71–75]. Therefore, gene therapy for cTTP may be a reasonable therapeutic option once its long-term efficiency and safety have been established.

7. Conclusions

This review discussed in detail the clinical manifestations of the very rare congenital TTP condition, the challenges with current plasma therapy, and the long-term prognosis based on the latest reports. Physicians treating patients with FFP often use platelet counts as a basis because the link between the peak/trough levels of ADAMTS13 activity and long-term organ damage has not been well investigated. Collecting data from cTTP registries could offer greater insights into morbidity and mortality during long-term follow-up. The emerging novel r-ADAMTS13 product has the potential to keep ADAMTS13 activity higher than conventional FFP infusions and improve the QOL. Further investigations are necessary to determine if r-ADAMTS13 could improve long-term outcomes in patients with cTTP.

Author Contributions: Conceptualization, K.S. and M.M.; writing—original draft preparation, K.S.; writing—review and editing, M.M. All authors have read and agreed to the published version of the manuscript.

Funding: This study was financially supported by research grants from the Ministry of Health, Labour, and Welfare of Japan (20FC1024 to M.M.).

Institutional Review Board Statement: Not applicable.

Informed Consent Statement: Not applicable.

Data Availability Statement: Not applicable.

Acknowledgments: The authors thank Emeritus Yoshihiro Fujimura for his contribution to the cTTP registry in Japan and all physicians for sending the data and samples of Japanese patients with cTTP.

Conflicts of Interest: M.M. is a member of the advisory board of Takeda Yakuhin and Sanofi. He is also an inventor of the ADAMTS13 actELISA.

References

1. Sadler, J.E. Pathophysiology of thrombotic thrombocytopenic purpura. *Blood* **2017**, *130*, 1181–1188. [CrossRef] [PubMed]
2. Kremer Hovinga, J.A.; Coppo, P.; Lammle, B.; Moake, J.L.; Miyata, T.; Vanhoorelbeke, K. Thrombotic thrombocytopenic purpura. *Nat. Rev. Dis. Primers* **2017**, *3*, 17020. [CrossRef] [PubMed]
3. Joly, B.S.; Coppo, P.; Veyradier, A. Thrombotic thrombocytopenic purpura. *Blood* **2017**, *129*, 2836–2846. [CrossRef] [PubMed]
4. Zheng, X.L.; Vesely, S.K.; Cataland, S.R.; Coppo, P.; Geldziler, B.; Iorio, A.; Matsumoto, M.; Mustafa, R.A.; Pai, M.; Rock, G.; et al. ISTH guidelines for the diagnosis of thrombotic thrombocytopenic purpura. *J. Thromb. Haemost.* **2020**, *18*, 2486–2495. [CrossRef] [PubMed]
5. South, K.; Lane, D.A. ADAMTS-13 and von Willebrand factor: A dynamic duo. *J. Thromb. Haemost.* **2018**, *16*, 6–18. [CrossRef]
6. Sarig, G. ADAMTS-13 in the diagnosis and management of thrombotic microangiopathies. *Rambam. Maimonides. Med. J.* **2014**, *5*, e0026. [CrossRef]
7. Patschan, D.; Witzke, O.; Dührsen, U.; Erbel, R.; Philipp, T.; Herget-Rosenthal, S. Acute myocardial infarction in thrombotic microangiopathies—Clinical characteristics, risk factors and outcome. *Nephrol. Dial. Transplant* **2006**, *21*, 1549–1554. [CrossRef]
8. Nichols, L.; Berg, A.; Rollins-Raval, M.A.; Raval, J.S. Cardiac injury is a common postmortem finding in thrombotic thrombocytopenic purpura patients: Is empiric cardiac monitoring and protection needed? *Ther. Apher. Dial.* **2015**, *19*, 87–92. [CrossRef]
9. Furlan, M.; Robles, R.; Galbusera, M.; Remuzzi, G.; Kyrle, P.A.; Brenner, B.; Krause, M.; Scharrer, I.; Aumann, V.; Mittler, U.; et al. von Willebrand factor-cleaving protease in thrombotic thrombocytopenic purpura and the hemolytic-uremic syndrome. *N. Engl. J. Med.* **1998**, *339*, 1578–1584. [CrossRef]
10. Tsai, H.M.; Lian, E.C. Antibodies to von Willebrand factor-cleaving protease in acute thrombotic thrombocytopenic purpura. *N. Engl. J. Med.* **1998**, *339*, 1585–1594. [CrossRef]
11. Levy, G.G.; Nichols, W.C.; Lian, E.C.; Foroud, T.; McClintick, J.N.; McGee, B.M.; Yang, A.Y.; Siemieniak, D.R.; Stark, K.R.; Gruppo, R.; et al. Mutations in a member of the ADAMTS gene family cause thrombotic thrombocytopenic purpura. *Nature* **2001**, *413*, 488–494. [CrossRef] [PubMed]
12. Zheng, X.; Chung, D.; Takayama, T.K.; Majerus, E.M.; Sadler, J.E.; Fujikawa, K. Structure of von Willebrand factor-cleaving protease (ADAMTS13), a metalloprotease involved in thrombotic thrombocytopenic purpura. *J. Biol. Chem.* **2001**, *276*, 41059–41063. [CrossRef] [PubMed]
13. Kremer Hovinga, J.A.; George, J.N. Hereditary thrombotic thrombocytopenic purpura. *N. Engl. J. Med.* **2019**, *381*, 1653–1662. [CrossRef] [PubMed]
14. Schulman, I.; Pierce, M.; Lukens, A.; Currimbhoy, Z. Studies on thrombopoiesis. I. A factor in normal human plasma required for platelet production; chronic thrombocytopenia due to its deficiency. *Blood* **1960**, *16*, 943–957. [CrossRef]
15. Upshaw, J.D., Jr. Congenital deficiency of a factor in normal plasma that reverses microangiopathic hemolysis and thrombocytopenia. *N. Engl. J. Med.* **1978**, *298*, 1350–1352. [CrossRef] [PubMed]
16. Rock, G.A.; Shumak, K.H.; Buskard, N.A.; Blanchette, V.S.; Kelton, J.G.; Nair, R.C.; Spasoff, R.A. Comparison of plasma exchange with plasma infusion in the treatment of thrombotic thrombocytopenic purpura. Canadian Apheresis Study Group. *N. Engl. J. Med.* **1991**, *325*, 393–397. [CrossRef]
17. Bell, W.R.; Braine, H.G.; Ness, P.M.; Kickler, T.S. Improved survival in thrombotic thrombocytopenic purpura-hemolytic uremic syndrome. Clinical experience in 108 patients. *N. Engl. J. Med.* **1991**, *325*, 398–403. [CrossRef]
18. Fujimura, Y.; Matsumoto, M.; Isonishi, A.; Yagi, H.; Kokame, K.; Soejima, K.; Murata, M.; Miyata, T. Natural history of Upshaw-Schulman syndrome based on ADAMTS13 gene analysis in Japan. *J. Thromb. Haemost.* **2011**, *9* (Suppl. 1), 283–301. [CrossRef]
19. Van Dorland, H.A.; Taleghani, M.M.; Sakai, K.; Friedman, K.D.; George, J.N.; Hrachovinova, I.; Knobl, P.N.; von Krogh, A.S.; Schneppenheim, R.; Aebi-Huber, I.; et al. The international hereditary thrombotic thrombocytopenic purpura registry: Key findings at enrollment until 2017. *Haematologica* **2019**, *104*, 2107–2115. [CrossRef]
20. Alwan, F.; Vendramin, C.; Liesner, R.; Clark, A.; Lester, W.; Dutt, T.; Thomas, W.; Gooding, R.; Biss, T.; Watson, H.G.; et al. Characterization and treatment of congenital thrombotic thrombocytopenic purpura. *Blood* **2019**, *133*, 1644–1651. [CrossRef]
21. Joly, B.S.; Boisseau, P.; Roose, E.; Stepanian, A.; Biebuyck, N.; Hogan, J.; Provot, F.; Delmas, Y.; Garrec, C.; Vanhoorelbeke, K.; et al. ADAMTS13 gene mutations influence ADAMTS13 conformation and disease age-onset in the French cohort of upshaw-Schulman syndrome. *Thromb. Haemost.* **2018**, *118*, 1902–1917. [CrossRef] [PubMed]
22. Byrnes, J.J.; Khurana, M. Treatment of thrombotic thrombocytopenic purpura with plasma. *N. Engl. J. Med.* **1977**, *297*, 1386–1389. [CrossRef] [PubMed]
23. Matsumoto, M.; Fujimura, Y.; Wada, H.; Kokame, K.; Miyakawa, Y.; Ueda, Y.; Higasa, S.; Moriki, T.; Yagi, H.; Miyata, T.; et al. Diagnostic and treatment guidelines for thrombotic thrombocytopenic purpura (TTP) 2017 in Japan. *Int. J. Hematol.* **2017**, *106*, 3–15. [CrossRef] [PubMed]
24. Kato, S.; Matsumoto, M.; Matsuyama, T.; Isonishi, A.; Hiura, H.; Fujimura, Y. Novel monoclonal antibody-based enzyme immunoassay for determining plasma levels of ADAMTS13 activity. *Transfusion* **2006**, *46*, 1444–1452. [CrossRef] [PubMed]
25. Kokame, K.; Matsumoto, M.; Fujimura, Y.; Miyata, T. VWF73, a region from D1596 to R1668 of von Willebrand factor, provides a minimal substrate for ADAMTS-13. *Blood* **2004**, *103*, 607–612. [CrossRef]
26. Kokame, K.; Nobe, Y.; Kokubo, Y.; Okayama, A.; Miyata, T. FRETS-VWF73, a first fluorogenic substrate for ADAMTS13 assay. *Br. J. Haematol.* **2005**, *129*, 93–100. [CrossRef]

27. Valsecchi, C.; Mirabet, M.; Mancini, I.; Biganzoli, M.; Schiavone, L.; Faraudo, S.; Mane-Padros, D.; Giles, D.; Serra-Domenech, J.; Blanch, S.; et al. Evaluation of a new, rapid, fully automated assay for the measurement of ADAMTS13 activity. *Thromb. Haemost.* **2019**, *119*, 1767–1772. [CrossRef]
28. Meyer, S.C.; Sulzer, I.; Lämmle, B.; Kremer Hovinga, J.A. Hyperbilirubinemia interferes with ADAMTS-13 activity measurement by FRETS-VWF73 assay: Diagnostic relevance in patients suffering from acute thrombotic microangiopathies. *J. Thromb. Haemost.* **2007**, *5*, 866–867. [CrossRef]
29. Scully, M.; Cataland, S.; Coppo, P.; de la Rubia, J.; Friedman, K.D.; Kremer Hovinga, J.; Lammle, B.; Matsumoto, M.; Pavenski, K.; Sadler, E.; et al. Consensus on the standardization of terminology in thrombotic thrombocytopenic purpura and related thrombotic microangiopathies. *J. Thromb. Haemost.* **2017**, *15*, 312–322. [CrossRef]
30. Lotta, L.A.; Valsecchi, C.; Pontiggia, S.; Mancini, I.; Cannavò, A.; Artoni, A.; Mikovic, D.; Meloni, G.; Peyvandi, F. Measurement and prevalence of circulating ADAMTS13-specific immune complexes in autoimmune thrombotic thrombocytopenic purpura. *J. Thromb. Haemost.* **2014**, *12*, 329–336. [CrossRef]
31. Sakai, K.; Hamada, E.; Kokame, K.; Matsumoto, M. Congenital thrombotic thrombocytopenic purpura: Genetics and emerging therapies. *Ann. Blood*, 2022; 1–14, in press.
32. Kokame, K.; Matsumoto, M.; Soejima, K.; Yagi, H.; Ishizashi, H.; Funato, M.; Tamai, H.; Konno, M.; Kamide, K.; Kawano, Y.; et al. Mutations and common polymorphisms in ADAMTS13 gene responsible for von Willebrand factor-cleaving protease activity. *Proc. Natl. Acad. Sci. USA* **2002**, *99*, 11902–11907. [CrossRef] [PubMed]
33. Eura, Y.; Kokame, K.; Takafuta, T.; Tanaka, R.; Kobayashi, H.; Ishida, F.; Hisanaga, S.; Matsumoto, M.; Fujimura, Y.; Miyata, T. Candidate gene analysis using genomic quantitative PCR: Identification of ADAMTS13 large deletions in two patients with Upshaw-Schulman syndrome. *Mol. Genet. Genomic. Med.* **2014**, *2*, 240–244. [CrossRef] [PubMed]
34. Jankowska, K.I.; Meyer, D.; Holcomb, D.D.; Kames, J.; Hamasaki-Katagiri, N.; Katneni, U.K.; Hunt, R.C.; Ibla, J.C.; Kimchi-Sarfaty, C. Synonymous ADAMTS13 variants impact molecular characteristics and contribute to variability in active protein abundance. *Blood. Adv.* **2022**, *6*, 5364–5378. [CrossRef]
35. Zheng, X.L.; Vesely, S.K.; Cataland, S.R.; Coppo, P.; Geldziler, B.; Iorio, A.; Matsumoto, M.; Mustafa, R.A.; Pai, M.; Rock, G.; et al. ISTH guidelines for treatment of thrombotic thrombocytopenic purpura. *J. Thromb. Haemost.* **2020**, *18*, 2496–2502. [CrossRef]
36. Zheng, X.L.; Vesely, S.K.; Cataland, S.R.; Coppo, P.; Geldziler, B.; Iorio, A.; Matsumoto, M.; Mustafa, R.A.; Pai, M.; Rock, G.; et al. Good practice statements (GPS) for the clinical care of patients with thrombotic thrombocytopenic purpura. *J. Thromb. Haemost.* **2020**, *18*, 2503–2512. [CrossRef] [PubMed]
37. Tarasco, E.; Butikofer, L.; Friedman, K.D.; George, J.N.; Hrachovinova, I.; Knobl, P.N.; Matsumoto, M.; von Krogh, A.S.; Aebi-Huber, I.; Cermakova, Z.; et al. Annual incidence and severity of acute episodes in hereditary thrombotic thrombocytopenic purpura. *Blood* **2021**, *137*, 3563–3575. [CrossRef] [PubMed]
38. Kinoshita, S.; Yoshioka, A.; Park, Y.D.; Ishizashi, H.; Konno, M.; Funato, M.; Matsui, T.; Titani, K.; Yagi, H.; Matsumoto, M.; et al. Upshaw-Schulman syndrome revisited: A concept of congenital thrombotic thrombocytopenic purpura. *Int. J. Hematol.* **2001**, *74*, 101–108. [CrossRef] [PubMed]
39. Sakai, K.; Fujimura, Y.; Miyata, T.; Isonishi, A.; Kokame, K.; Matsumoto, M. Current prophylactic plasma infusion protocols do not adequately prevent long-term cumulative organ damage in the Japanese congenital thrombotic thrombocytopenic purpura cohort. *Br. J. Haematol.* **2021**, *194*, 444–452. [CrossRef] [PubMed]
40. Naik, S.; Mahoney, D.H. Successful treatment of congenital TTP with a novel approach using plasma-derived factor VIII. *J. Pediatr. Hematol. Oncol.* **2013**, *35*, 551–553. [CrossRef]
41. Scully, M.; Gattens, M.; Khair, K.; Liesner, R. The use of intermediate purity factor VIII concentrate BPL 8Y as prophylaxis and treatment in congenital thrombotic thrombocytopenic purpura. *Br. J. Haematol.* **2006**, *135*, 101–104. [CrossRef]
42. McGonigle, A.M.; Patel, E.U.; Waters, K.M.; Moliterno, A.R.; Thoman, S.K.; Vozniak, S.O.; Ness, P.M.; King, K.E.; Tobian, A.A.R.; Lokhandwala, P.M. Solvent detergent treated pooled plasma and reduction of allergic transfusion reactions. *Transfusion* **2020**, *60*, 54–61. [CrossRef] [PubMed]
43. Sidhu, D.; Snyder, E.L.; Tormey, C.A. Two approaches to the clinical dilemma of treating TTP with therapeutic plasma exchange in patients with a history of anaphylactic reactions to plasma. *J. Clin. Apher.* **2017**, *32*, 158–162. [CrossRef] [PubMed]
44. Garraud, O.; Malot, S.; Herbrecht, R.; Ojeda-Uribe, M.; Lin, J.S.; Veyradier, A.; Payrat, J.M.; Liu, K.; Corash, L.; Coppo, P. Amotosalen-inactivated fresh frozen plasma is comparable to solvent-detergent inactivated plasma to treat thrombotic thrombocytopenic purpura. *Transfus. Apher. Sci.* **2019**, *58*, 102665. [CrossRef] [PubMed]
45. Boothby, A.; Mazepa, M. Caplacizumab for congenital thrombotic thrombocytopenic purpura. *Am. J. Hematol.* **2022**, *97*, e420–e421. [CrossRef] [PubMed]
46. Scully, M.; Cataland, S.R.; Peyvandi, F.; Coppo, P.; Knobl, P.; Kremer Hovinga, J.A.; Metjian, A.; de la Rubia, J.; Pavenski, K.; Callewaert, F.; et al. Caplacizumab treatment for acquired thrombotic thrombocytopenic purpura. *N. Engl. J. Med.* **2019**, *380*, 335–346. [CrossRef]
47. Borogovac, A.; Tarasco, E.; Kremer Hovinga, J.A.; Friedman, K.D.; Asch, A.S.; Vesely, S.K.; Prodan, C.; Terrell, D.R.; George, J.N. Prevalence of neuropsychiatric symptoms and stroke in patients with hereditary thrombotic thrombocytopenic purpura. *Blood* **2022**, *140*, 785–789. [CrossRef]
48. Borogovac, A.; Reese, J.A.; Gupta, S.; George, J.N. Morbidities and mortality in patients with hereditary thrombotic thrombocytopenic purpura. *Blood Adv.* **2022**, *6*, 750–759. [CrossRef]

49. Ocak, G.; Roest, M.; Verhaar, M.C.; Rookmaaker, M.B.; Blankestijn, P.J.; Bos, W.J.W.; Fijnheer, R.; Péquériaux, N.C.; Dekker, F.W. Von Willebrand factor, ADAMTS13 and mortality in dialysis patients. *BMC Nephrol.* **2021**, *22*, 222. [CrossRef]
50. Green, D.; Roberts, P.R.; New, D.I.; Kalra, P.A. Sudden cardiac death in hemodialysis patients: An in-depth review. *Am. J. Kidney Dis. Off. J. Natl. Kidney Found.* **2011**, *57*, 921–929. [CrossRef]
51. Makar, M.S.; Pun, P.H. Sudden cardiac death among hemodialysis patients. *Am. J. Kidney Dis. Off. J. Natl. Kidney Found.* **2017**, *69*, 684–695. [CrossRef]
52. Itami, H.; Hara, S.; Matsumoto, M.; Imamura, H.; Kanai, R.; Nishiyama, K.; Ishimura, M.; Ohga, S.; Yoshida, M.; Tanaka, R.; et al. Complement activation associated with ADAMTS13 deficiency may contribute to the characteristic glomerular manifestations in Upshaw-Schulman syndrome. *Thromb. Res.* **2018**, *170*, 148–155. [CrossRef] [PubMed]
53. Sakai, K.; Fujimura, Y.; Nagata, Y.; Higasa, S.; Moriyama, M.; Isonishi, A.; Konno, M.; Kajiwara, M.; Ogawa, Y.; Kaburagi, S.; et al. Success and limitations of plasma treatment in pregnant women with congenital thrombotic thrombocytopenic purpura. *J. Thromb. Haemost.* **2020**, *18*, 2929–2941. [CrossRef] [PubMed]
54. Von Krogh, A.S.; Kremer Hovinga, J.A.; Tjonnfjord, G.E.; Ringen, I.M.; Lammle, B.; Waage, A.; Quist-Paulsen, P. The impact of congenital thrombotic thrombocytopenic purpura on pregnancy complications. *Thromb. Haemost.* **2014**, *111*, 1180–1183. [CrossRef]
55. Schiviz, A.; Wuersch, K.; Piskernik, C.; Dietrich, B.; Hoellriegl, W.; Rottensteiner, H.; Scheiflinger, F.; Schwarz, H.P.; Muchitsch, E.M. A new mouse model mimicking thrombotic thrombocytopenic purpura: Correction of symptoms by recombinant human ADAMTS13. *Blood* **2012**, *119*, 6128–6135. [CrossRef] [PubMed]
56. Scully, M.; Knobl, P.; Kentouche, K.; Rice, L.; Windyga, J.; Schneppenheim, R.; Kremer Hovinga, J.A.; Kajiwara, M.; Fujimura, Y.; Maggiore, C.; et al. Recombinant ADAMTS-13: First-in-human pharmacokinetics and safety in congenital thrombotic thrombocytopenic purpura. *Blood* **2017**, *130*, 2055–2063. [CrossRef] [PubMed]
57. Sarode, R. Recombinant ADAMTS-13: Goodbye, allergic reactions! *Blood* **2017**, *130*, 2045–2046. [CrossRef] [PubMed]
58. Asmis, L.M.; Serra, A.; Krafft, A.; Licht, A.; Leisinger, E.; Henschkowski-Serra, J.; Ganter, M.T.; Hauptmann, S.; Tinguely, M.; Kremer Hovinga, J.A. Recombinant ADAMTS13 for hereditary thrombotic thrombocytopenic purpura. *N. Engl. J. Med.* **2022**, *387*, 2356–2361. [CrossRef]
59. Stubbs, M.J.; Kendall, G.; Scully, M. Recombinant ADAMTS13 in severe neonatal thrombotic thrombocytopenic purpura. *N. Engl. J. Med.* **2022**, *387*, 2391–2392. [CrossRef]
60. Chauhan, A.K.; Motto, D.G.; Lamb, C.B.; Bergmeier, W.; Dockal, M.; Plaimauer, B.; Scheiflinger, F.; Ginsburg, D.; Wagner, D.D. Systemic antithrombotic effects of ADAMTS13. *J. Exp. Med.* **2006**, *203*, 767–776. [CrossRef]
61. Xu, H.; Cao, Y.; Yang, X.; Cai, P.; Kang, L.; Zhu, X.; Luo, H.; Lu, L.; Wei, L.; Bai, X.; et al. ADAMTS13 controls vascular remodeling by modifying VWF reactivity during stroke recovery. *Blood* **2017**, *130*, 11–22. [CrossRef]
62. South, K.; Saleh, O.; Lemarchand, E.; Coutts, G.; Smith, C.J.; Schiessl, I.; Allan, S.M. Robust thrombolytic and anti-inflammatory action of a constitutively active ADAMTS13 variant in murine stroke models. *Blood* **2022**, *139*, 1575–1587. [CrossRef]
63. Zhou, S.; Guo, J.; Liao, X.; Zhou, Q.; Qiu, X.; Jiang, S.; Xu, N.; Wang, X.; Zhao, L.; Hu, W.; et al. rhADAMTS13 reduces oxidative stress by cleaving VWF in ischaemia/reperfusion-induced acute kidney injury. *Acta Physiol.* **2022**, *234*, e13778. [CrossRef] [PubMed]
64. Sonneveld, M.A.; de Maat, M.P.; Portegies, M.L.; Kavousi, M.; Hofman, A.; Turecek, P.L.; Rottensteiner, H.; Scheiflinger, F.; Koudstaal, P.J.; Ikram, M.A.; et al. Low ADAMTS13 activity is associated with an increased risk of ischemic stroke. *Blood* **2015**, *126*, 2739–2746. [CrossRef] [PubMed]
65. Witsch, T.; Martinod, K.; Sorvillo, N.; Portier, I.; De Meyer, S.F.; Wagner, D.D. Recombinant human ADAMTS13 treatment improves myocardial remodeling and functionality after pressure overload injury in mice. *J. Am. Heart Assoc.* **2018**, *7*, e007004. [CrossRef] [PubMed]
66. Newnham, M.; South, K.; Bleda, M.; Auger, W.R.; Barberà, J.A.; Bogaard, H.; Bunclark, K.; Cannon, J.E.; Delcroix, M.; Hadinnapola, C.; et al. The ADAMTS13-VWF axis is dysregulated in chronic thromboembolic pulmonary hypertension. *Eur. Respir. J.* **2019**, *53*, 1801805. [CrossRef] [PubMed]
67. Zitomersky, N.L.; Demers, M.; Martinod, K.; Gallant, M.; Cifuni, S.M.; Biswas, A.; Snapper, S.; Wagner, D.D. ADAMTS13 deficiency worsens colitis and exogenous ADAMTS13 administration decreases colitis severity in mice. *TH Open* **2017**, *1*, e11–e23. [CrossRef] [PubMed]
68. Pipe, S.W.; Leebeek, F.W.G.; Recht, M.; Key, N.S.; Castaman, G.; Miesbach, W.; Lattimore, S.; Peerlinck, K.; Van der Valk, P.; Coppens, M.; et al. Gene therapy with etranacogene dezaparvovec for hemophilia B. *N. Engl. J. Med.* **2023**, *388*, 706–718. [CrossRef]
69. Cook, K.; Forbes, S.P.; Adamski, K.; Ma, J.J.; Chawla, A.; Garrison, L.P., Jr. Assessing the potential cost-effectiveness of a gene therapy for the treatment of hemophilia A. *J. Med. Econ.* **2020**, *23*, 501–512. [CrossRef]
70. Dekimpe, C.; Roose, E.; Sakai, K.; Tersteeg, C.; De Meyer, S.F.; Vanhoorelbeke, K. Toward gene therapy for congenital thrombotic thrombocytopenic purpura. *J. Thromb. Haemost.* **2022**, *21*, 1090–1099. [CrossRef]
71. Laje, P.; Shang, D.; Cao, W.; Niiya, M.; Endo, M.; Radu, A.; DeRogatis, N.; Scheiflinger, F.; Zoltick, P.W.; Flake, A.W.; et al. Correction of murine ADAMTS13 deficiency by hematopoietic progenitor cell-mediated gene therapy. *Blood* **2009**, *113*, 2172–2180. [CrossRef]

72. Niiya, M.; Endo, M.; Shang, D.; Zoltick, P.W.; Muvarak, N.E.; Cao, W.; Jin, S.Y.; Skipwith, C.G.; Motto, D.G.; Flake, A.W.; et al. Correction of ADAMTS13 deficiency by in utero gene transfer of lentiviral vector encoding ADAMTS13 genes. *Mol. Ther.* **2009**, *17*, 34–41. [CrossRef] [PubMed]
73. Trionfini, P.; Tomasoni, S.; Galbusera, M.; Motto, D.; Longaretti, L.; Corna, D.; Remuzzi, G.; Benigni, A. Adenoviral-mediated gene transfer restores plasma ADAMTS13 antigen and activity in ADAMTS13 knockout mice. *Gene Ther.* **2009**, *16*, 1373–1379. [CrossRef] [PubMed]
74. Jin, S.Y.; Xiao, J.; Bao, J.; Zhou, S.; Wright, J.F.; Zheng, X.L. AAV-mediated expression of an ADAMTS13 variant prevents shigatoxin-induced thrombotic thrombocytopenic purpura. *Blood* **2013**, *121*, 3825–3829. [CrossRef] [PubMed]
75. Verhenne, S.; Vandeputte, N.; Pareyn, I.; Izsvák, Z.; Rottensteiner, H.; Deckmyn, H.; De Meyer, S.F.; Vanhoorelbeke, K. Long-Term Prevention of Congenital Thrombotic Thrombocytopenic Purpura in ADAMTS13 Knockout Mice by Sleeping Beauty Transposon-Mediated Gene Therapy. *Arterioscler. Thromb. Vasc. Biol.* **2017**, *37*, 836–844. [CrossRef]

Disclaimer/Publisher's Note: The statements, opinions and data contained in all publications are solely those of the individual author(s) and contributor(s) and not of MDPI and/or the editor(s). MDPI and/or the editor(s) disclaim responsibility for any injury to people or property resulting from any ideas, methods, instructions or products referred to in the content.

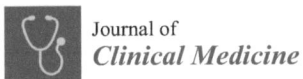

Case Report

Hypercoagulability and Inflammatory Markers in a Case of Congenital Thrombotic Thrombocytopenic Purpura Complicated by Fetal Demise

Leslie Skeith [1], Kelle Hurd [1], Shruti Chaturvedi [2], Lorraine Chow [3], Joshua Nicholas [3], Adrienne Lee [4], Daniel Young [5], Dawn Goodyear [1], Jennifer Soucie [6], Louis Girard [1], Antoine Dufour [7] and Ejaife O. Agbani [7,8,*]

1. Department of Family Medicine, Cumming School of Medicine, University of Calgary, Calgary, AB T2N 4N1, Canada
2. Department of Medicine, Johns Hopkins University School of Medicine, Baltimore, MD 21205, USA
3. Department of Anaesthesiology, Perioperative and Pain Medicine, Cumming School of Medicine, University of Calgary, Calgary, AB T2N 4N1, Canada
4. Department of Medicine, University of British Columbia, Vancouver, BC V6T 1Z4, Canada
5. McCaig Institute for Bone and Joint Health, University of Calgary, Calgary, AB T2N 4N1, Canada
6. Department of Obstetrics and Gynecology, Cumming School of Medicine, University of Calgary, Calgary, AB T2N 4N1, Canada
7. Department of Physiology & Pharmacology, Cumming School of Medicine, University of Calgary, Calgary, AB T2N 4N1, Canada
8. Libin Cardiovascular Institute, University of Calgary, Calgary, AB T2N 1N4, Canada
* Correspondence: ejaife.agbani@ucalgary.ca

Citation: Skeith, L.; Hurd, K.; Chaturvedi, S.; Chow, L.; Nicholas, J.; Lee, A.; Young, D.; Goodyear, D.; Soucie, J.; Girard, L.; et al. Hypercoagulability and Inflammatory Markers in a Case of Congenital Thrombotic Thrombocytopenic Purpura Complicated by Fetal Demise. *J. Clin. Med.* 2022, 11, 7115. https://doi.org/10.3390/jcm11237115

Academic Editors: Ilaria Mancini and Andrea Artoni

Received: 5 October 2022
Accepted: 29 November 2022
Published: 30 November 2022

Publisher's Note: MDPI stays neutral with regard to jurisdictional claims in published maps and institutional affiliations.

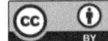

Copyright: © 2022 by the authors. Licensee MDPI, Basel, Switzerland. This article is an open access article distributed under the terms and conditions of the Creative Commons Attribution (CC BY) license (https://creativecommons.org/licenses/by/4.0/).

Abstract: Background: Congenital thrombotic thrombocytopenic purpura (cTTP) is a rare disorder caused by an inherited genetic deficiency of ADAMTS13 and affects less than one per million individuals. Patients who are diagnosed with TTP during pregnancy are at increased risk of maternal and fetal complications including fetal demise. We present a case of a 32-year-old G3P0 (gravida 3, para 0) who presented at 20 weeks gestation with a new diagnosis of congenital TTP (cTTP) and fetal demise. Methods: We describe the pathophysiology of pregnancy complications in a patient with cTTP using platelet procoagulant membrane dynamics analysis and quantitative proteomic studies, compared to four pregnant patients with gestational hypertension, four pregnant patients with preeclampsia, and four healthy pregnant controls. Results: The cTTP patient had increased P-selectin, tissue factor expression, annexin-V binding on platelets and neutrophils, and localized thrombin generation, suggestive of hypercoagulability. Among 15 proteins that were upregulated, S100A8 and S100A9 were distinctly overexpressed. Conclusions: There is platelet-neutrophil activation and interaction, platelet hypercoagulability, and proinflammation in our case of cTTP with fetal demise.

Keywords: platelets; thrombosis; procoagulant membrane dynamics; inflammatory markers; congenital; thrombotic thrombocytopenic purpura; fetal demise

1. Introduction

Patients who are diagnosed with thrombotic thrombocytopenic purpura (TTP) during pregnancy are at increased risk of fetal and maternal complications. There is a high rate of preterm birth, preeclampsia, late fetal demise including stillbirth, and maternal complications such as neurological, renal, or arterial sequelae, and rarely maternal death [1–6]. Thrombotic thrombocytopenic purpura may occur for the first time in pregnancy or the postpartum period and may be acquired (autoimmune) or congenital [7]. Fetal complications are more likely to occur in the first pregnancy and/or when the patient is not receiving prophylactic therapy [1]. Here, we present a case of congenital TTP (cTTP) during pregnancy (ADAMTS13 activity < 10% and *ADAMTS13* gene variants) that was complicated by fetal demise. Congenital TTP is a form of a thrombotic microangiopathy where a severe deficiency of ADAMTS13 due to *ADAMTS13* gene mutations leads to ultra-large VWF multimers accumulating, which binds to endothelial surfaces and platelets to promote microvascular thrombosis [8]. In a small case series of pregnant patients with cTTP who had pregnancy complications, there was macroscopic evidence of fetal and maternal vascular lesions of under perfusion in their placentas, along with intraplacental infarcts, fibrin thrombi, and intervillous fibrin deposition [9]. To understand the pathophysiology further, we evaluated platelets, neutrophils, and inflammatory markers to elucidate the pathophysiology of complications associated with cTTP in pregnancy. Our platelet imaging, immunofluorescence, and proteomics studies identified interactions on a molecular level in a case of cTTP in pregnancy.

2. Case

We report a case of a 32-year-old G3P0 (gravida 3, para 0) who presented at 20 weeks gestational age (GA) with new cTTP and fetal demise. The patient had an elevated body mass index (BMI 38 during pregnancy) with no other medical conditions and had spontaneous abortions at 6 weeks and 9 weeks GA of unknown cause, which included normal cytogenetics of the fetuses. The maternal platelet counts at the time of the earlier pregnancy losses were unknown. In addition to a prenatal vitamin including folate, the patient was started on aspirin 81 mg daily during her most recent pregnancy to prevent placental-mediated complications. She had a normal platelet count in first trimester (338×10^9/L) and normal obstetric ultrasounds (12^5 weeks GA; 19^4 weeks GA). The patient presented at 19^5 weeks GA with epigastric pain and intermittent high blood pressure (range 130/70 to 186/96), with a platelet count 194×10^9/L, LDH 306 U/L (Upper limit of normal, ULN 100 U/L), ALT 41 U/L (ULN 39 U/L), normal urate, creatinine 49 μmol/L, and no proteinuria. She presented to hospital again at 20^3 weeks GA with petechiae, hyperreflexia, a platelet count of 13×10^9/L, microangiopathic hemolytic anemia (hemoglobin 95 g/L, LDH 833 U/L, haptoglobin < 0.15 g/L, reticulocyte count 5.3%, bilirubin 19 μmol/L [ULN 24 μmol/L]), and occasional schistocytes. She also had an elevated ALT 42 U/L, elevated labile blood pressure, creatinine 95 μmol/L (approximately doubled), and new proteinuria of 0.162 g/mmol. Although fetal viability was confirmed upon initial presentation, an intrauterine fetal death occurred during the following twelve hours. The placenta showed marked increased intervillous fibrin scattered with acute intervillositis, decidual necrosis, and hemorrhage. Chromosome microarray analysis and karyotyping of the fetus was normal.

While the working diagnosis was preeclampsia/HELLP (Hemolysis, Elevated Liver Enzymes, Low Platelets) syndrome, the critically low platelets also kept TTP on the differential. Within 24 h of presentation, ADAMTS13 activity testing confirmed TTP. Using ADAMTS13 activity and inhibitor profile tests, a diagnosis of cTTP was made based on severely deficient ADAMTS13 activity of 0.69% (normal 40–130%) and no ADAMTS13 antibodies (<12 units/mL), and two heterozygous *ADAMTS13* variants; with *ADAMTS13* c.578G>A, p.(Arg193Gln), a missense variant previously reported in cTTP [10] and *ADAMTS13* variant c.2420+4_2420+19del (Blueprint Genetics, Seattle, WA, USA). The second variant is in the intronic splice region and has not previously been described. Autoimmune testing including ANA, ENA, ds-DNA, C3, C4, C50, and antiphospholipid antibodies (anticardiolipin antibody, anti-beta-2 glycoprotein antibody, and lupus anticoagulant) were negative.

Once the ADAMTS13 activity result returned, the patient received a plasma infusion and high-dose steroids, followed by an induction of labor and 6 cycles of plasma exchange. Her blood pressure, renal function, platelet count, and hemolytic markers normalized by postpartum day 5 without evidence of recurrent thrombocytopenia or hemolysis, although her anemia took a month to fully resolve. Outside of this episode, her ADAMTS13 activity remained <10% and ADAMTS13 antibody testing remained negative, with results available up to 4 months postpartum.

3. Materials and Methods

We completed platelet procoagulant membrane dynamics analysis and quantitative proteomic studies in a patient with cTTP, as well as control participants. Study participants were screened and enrolled between July and December 2021. Control participants, but not the cTTP participant, were enrolled in a related preeclampsia study [11]. We utilized a detailed fluorescent imaging approach which we previously described [12,13], in platelet-rich-plasma re-constituted to contain neutrophils (PRP+). We derived PRP+ fractions by centrifuging whole blood at 180× g for 17 min, followed by a careful extraction of both the upper plasma-platelet fraction (PRP) and the buffy coat [14]. Citrated PRP+ from study participants were allowed to adhere to bovine serum albumin coated surfaces. Extended focus images at the 45 min timepoint are shown. To visualize homotypical and heterotypical platelet microaggregate or microthrombi in whole plasma (Figure 1B,D), we examined PRP+ fractions. Platelets were labelled with Alexa-fluor® 488 anti-human CD62P (P-Selectin) antibody to detect membrane P-selectin exposure, Alexa-fluor® 568 Annexin-V to monitor phosphatidylserine (PS) externalization, and Alexa-fluor® 405 anti-human tissue factor antibody. In addition, Alexa-fluor® 647 conjugated mouse monoclonal antibody specific for an epitope, mapped between amino acids 331–376 within an internal region of human thrombin, was used to determine platelet membrane thrombin generation. We then conducted plasma quantitative shotgun proteomics analysis as previously reported [11], and compared proteomics and platelet imaging in the described patient with cTTP to 4 healthy pregnant controls (PC), 4 gestational hypertension (GH), and 4 preeclampsia (PE) patients (Research Ethics Board Approval #REB18-1545). The proteomics data of our study are publicly available via ProteomeXchange with identifier PXD037898. The R codes are available upon request. Additional data relating to healthy PCs, GH, and PE participants have been reported elsewhere [11]. Study data were analyzed using GraphPad Prism 9.3 (Dotmatics, San Diego, CA, USA). Statistical significance was determined by 2-way analysis of variance (ANOVA) test, followed by Sidak multiple comparison tests; $p < 0.05$ (*) or $p < 0.01$ (**) were considered significant.

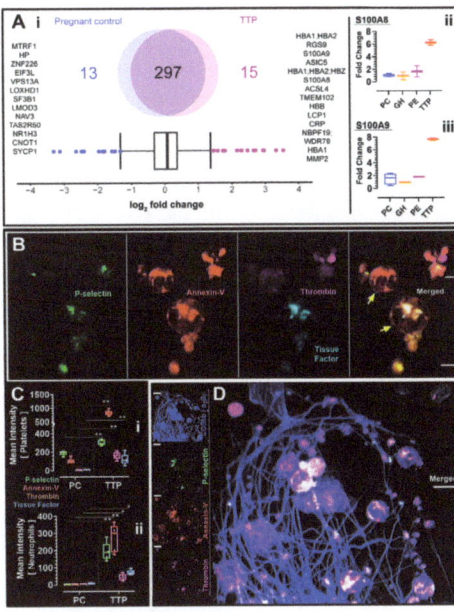

Figure 1. Platelet Proteomics and Procoagulant Membrane Dynamics Study in a Case of Congenital TTP Complicated by Fetal Demise.

4. Results

In addition to a pregnant patient with cTTP, samples were also drawn from four PCs (mean age 32, mean GA 39.4 weeks, range 49–40.2 weeks), four GH (mean age 35, mean GA 35.8 weeks, range 32–40.8 weeks), and four preeclampsia patients (mean age 32, GA 31.4 weeks, range 24.6–36.6 weeks) within a six-month period; all control participants had a normal hemoglobin, platelet count, and creatinine values.

We identified 15 proteins upregulated in TTP (Figure 1(A-i)), and sub-analysis revealed that S100A8 and S100A9 were distinctly overexpressed (6-7-fold increase) in our TTP patient, but not in the controls used in this study with PC, GH, or PE. (Figure 1(A-ii,iii)). High-resolution platelet imaging from our TTP patient showed acquired platelet and neutrophil activation (determined through signals of fluorescent indicators) and classic structures of platelet-neutrophil aggregates [15,16] (Figure 1B). Compared to all other participant groups, our cTTP patient had increased P-selectin (mean $\pm$ SD, PC vs. cTTP: 190.2 $\pm$ 23.5 vs. 299.6 $\pm$ 29.1; p = 0.0033), tissue factor expression (mean $\pm$ SD, PC vs. cTTP: 5.6 $\pm$ 3.5 vs. 116.2 $\pm$ 60.4; p = 0.0029), annexin-V binding (mean $\pm$ SD, PC vs. cTTP: 105.5 $\pm$ 24.9 vs. 819.5 $\pm$ 99.3; p < 0.001), and localized thrombin generation on platelets (mean $\pm$ SD, PC vs. cTTP: 3.5 $\pm$ 3.2 vs. 159.7 $\pm$ 40.1; p < 0.001), suggestive of hypercoagulability (Figure 1(C-i)). Results were similar in neutrophil analysis (Figure 1(C-i)).

We visualised in the plasma sample of the described participant with cTTP, but not in the PC, GH, or PE control samples, loose thrombus consisting of activated and procoagulant platelets and neutrophils trapped within mesh-like structures resembling a fibrin-network, as measured by increased staining of procoagulation markers (Figure 1D). The range of procoagulation signals from the cells of the one cTTP participant is relatively larger compared to measures from control PCs. Likely this is indicative of the relatively quiescent/non active state of platelets and neutrophils in PC compared to cTTP where active procoagulation is progressing at varying degrees in the different cell population analysed in cTTP. This notwithstanding, the minimum, mean, median, and maximum procoagulation values recoded were higher in cTTP, compared to PCs.

Quantification results of plasma proteomics of pregnant controls vs. one patient with thrombotic thrombocytopenic purpura (TTP) as illustrated by Venn Diagrams (Figure 1(A-i)). Interquartile box plot analysis was performed to identify the differently expressed proteins as represented by outliers. "(Figure 1(A-ii)) S100A8 and (Figure 1(A-iii)) S100A9 intensities between pregnant control (PC), gestational hypertension (GH), preeclampsia (PE), and congenital TTP (TTP) as quantified by shotgun proteomics. Data are represented as boxplots. (Figure 1B,D): Images shown in B and D were from the one patient with cTTP. Yellow arrows in B are pointing to procoagulant neutrophils interacting with activated platelets. In (Figure 1C), fluorescent signal intensity data from the 4 PC participants and the one TTP patient (replicates shown) were analyzed using GraphPad Prism 9.3 (Dotmatics, San Diego, CA, USA) and presented as box-and-whiskers plots showing minimum to maximum values, replicate data inclusive. Images were captured at Nyquist using Nikon A1R laser scanning confocal microscope (original objective magnification, $\times$60) and analyzed using Volocity® Software (Quorum Technologies, Laughton, UK). Scale bars: 3 µm (Figure 1B), 7 µm (Figure 1D).

5. Discussion

Thrombocytopenia and microangiopathic hemolytic anemia in pregnancy are manifestations of HELLP syndrome, preeclampsia, TTP, antiphospholipid syndrome, all of which have overlapping clinical and biochemical features that can make it difficult to distinguish between them [17]. Congenital TTP is a rare disorder caused by an inherited genetic deficiency of ADAMTS13 and affects less than one per million individuals, and makes up <5% of all TTP cases [8]. TTP can present for the first time in pregnancy or the postpartum period, and up to 25% of pregnancy-associated TTP cases are from cTTP [1]. In this case, cTTP was confirmed by ADAMTS13 activity < 10%, negative ADAMTS13 antibody testing, and biallelic mutations with at least one mutation previously reported with cTTP [10].

Furthermore, the ADAMTS13 level remained low (<10%) beyond the 3-month postpartum period with no ADAMTS13 antibodies detected, further supporting the diagnosis of cTTP.

There is overlap between TTP and preeclampsia. While TTP has been reported more often in the third trimester and postpartum, fetal loss may be highest in the second trimester [4]. Another observational study identified TTP presentations more commonly occurring in the second trimester and early postpartum [5]. Preeclampsia, typically diagnosed after 20 weeks gestation, is a common feature of pregnancies complicated by TTP, so proteinuria and a clinical overlap may be seen [5,6,18]. This supports the use of low-dose aspirin for preeclampsia prevention in pregnant patients with known TTP. While not specific to this case, ADAMTS13 levels are lower in preeclampsia in the absence of TTP, although are not as severe (defined as <10%) and is an area of future research in preeclampsia and other conditions such as antiphospholipid syndrome [19–21].

While the condition is rare, delays in the diagnosis of TTP in pregnancy can lead to important maternal and fetal complications. In addition to the diagnostic challenge of having clinical overlap with other conditions, the turnaround time of the ADAMTS13 activity testing is variable and is often not available to make immediate decisions. We advocate for pursuing early investigations for TTP, and to initiate empiric therapies while test results are pending, depending on the clinical scenario.

Platelets have a proinflammatory role; using P-selectin and beta(2) and beta(3) integrins (CD11b/CD18, CD41/CD61), platelets can interact with neutrophils to promote the recruitment of neutrophils into inflammatory tissue [22]. Furthermore, platelet–neutrophil interaction has been reported in other prothrombotic conditions such as in severe SARS-Cov-2 infection, thrombosis, atherosclerosis, and tissue injury and repair [23]. Our data are hypothesis generating on the role of platelets and inflammation in the area of cTTP-related pregnancy complications.

There are limitations to this study evaluating platelet, neutrophils, and inflammatory markers. This study is a single case report of cTTP and there are small sample sizes of control participants. We were not able to control for other factors in the control participants, such as age, BMI, gestational age, or prior pregnancy outcomes. Additionally, we are not able to describe temporal changes in a pregnancy with only a single time point drawn. We chose a control group that was at risk of similar placental complications, in hopes to better understand the pathophysiology of placental complications related to cTTP. However, this group was not exactly matched because they did not have low platelets and microangiopathic hemolytic anemia or had an outcome of a fetal demise. The inflammation seen in the participant with cTTP could have been the body's inflammatory response to a fetal demise and not the preceding cause. Lastly, our research testing methods are not available for routine use in practice, so how to implement additional testing into clinical practice deserves further study. Further research is still needed to understand the implications of our findings.

6. Conclusions

This case report highlights the challenging diagnostic overlap with other clinical TTP syndromes like preeclampsia/HELLP syndrome, and that additional laboratory ADAMTS13 testing can be invaluable. Using platelet procoagulant membrane dynamics and proteomics studies, we identified platelet–neutrophil activation and interaction, platelet hypercoagulability, and proinflammation in the case of cTTP with a fetal demise. However, further research is still needed to confirm our findings and the pathophysiology of pregnancy complications of fetal demise and preeclampsia in pregnant patients with TTP.

Author Contributions: Study conceptualization (A.L., L.S. and E.O.A.); patient recruitment (A.L., D.G., J.S., L.G. and L.C.); study/experimental design (A.L. and E.O.A.); study supervision (E.O.A.); experimentation (A.D., D.Y. and E.O.A.); data analysis (E.O.A.); discussion (L.S., K.H., S.C., A.D., J.N., L.C., A.L., D.G., J.S., L.G. and E.O.A.); manuscript preparation (L.S. and E.O.A.), review and revision (L.S., K.H., S.C., A.D., J.N., A.L., L.C., D.G., J.S., L.G. and E.O.A.). All authors have read and agreed to the published version of the manuscript.

Funding: This work was supported by the Anesthesia Academic Council (1210/2021) and the Research Funds of Timothy & Linda Tang, Department of Anaesthesiology, Perioperative and Pain Medicine, Cumming School of Medicine, University of Calgary, Alberta, Canada.

Institutional Review Board Statement: The study was conducted in accordance with the Declaration of Helsinki, and approved by the University of Calgary, Research Ethics Board approval (REB18-1545).

Informed Consent Statement: Informed consent was obtained from all subjects involved in the study.

Data Availability Statement: The proteomics data of our study are publicly available via ProteomeXchange with identifier PXD037898. The R codes are available upon request.

Acknowledgments: This work was supported by the Live Cell Imaging Facility, funded by the Snyder Institute at the University of Calgary and the Microscopy and Imaging Facility (MIF) of the University of Calgary. A.L., L.S. and E.O.A. are members of CanVECTOR, the Canadian Venous Thromboembolism Research Network. E.O.A. is supported by the Cumming School of Medicine and Libin Cardiovascular Institute, University of Calgary, Alberta, Canada.

Conflicts of Interest: The authors declare no conflict of interest.

References

1. Moatti-Cohen, M.; Garrec, C.; Wolf, M.; Boisseau, P.; Galicier, L.; Azoulay, E.; Stepanian, A.; Delmas, Y.; Rondeau, E.; Bezieau, S.; et al. Unexpected frequency of Upshaw-Schulman syndrome in pregnancy-onset thrombotic thrombocytopenic purpura. *Blood* **2012**, *119*, 5888–5897. [CrossRef] [PubMed]
2. Fujimura, Y.; Matsumoto, M.; Kokame, K.; Isonishi, A.; Soejima, K.; Akiyama, N.; Tomiyama, J.; Natori, K.; Kuranishi, Y.; Imamura, Y.; et al. Pregnancy-induced thrombocytopenia and TTP, and the risk of fetal death, in Upshaw-Schulman syndrome: A series of 15 pregnancies in 9 genotyped patients. *Br. J. Haematol.* **2009**, *144*, 742–754. [CrossRef] [PubMed]
3. Alwan, F.; Vendramin, C.; Liesner, R.; Clark, A.; Lester, W.; Dutt, T.; Thomas, W.; Gooding, R.; Biss, T.; Watson, H.G.; et al. Characterization and treatment of congenital thrombotic thrombocytopenic purpura. *Blood* **2019**, *133*, 1644–1651. [CrossRef] [PubMed]
4. Scully, M.; Thomas, M.R.; Underwood, M.; Watson, H.; Langley, K.; Camilleri, R.S.; Clark, A.; Creagh, D.; Rayment, R.; McDonald, V.; et al. Thrombotic thrombocytopenic purpura and pregnancy: Presentation, management, and subsequent pregnancy outcomes. *Blood* **2014**, *124*, 211–219. [CrossRef] [PubMed]
5. Martin, J.N.; Bailey, A.P.; Rehberg, J.F.; Owens, M.T.; Keiser, S.D.; May, W.L. Thrombotic thrombocytopenic purpura in 166 pregnancies: 1955-2006. *Am. J. Obstet. Gynecol.* **2008**, *199*, 98–104. [CrossRef] [PubMed]
6. Brown, J.; Potugari, B.; Mazepa, M.A.; Kohli, R.; Moliterno, A.R.; Brodsky, R.A.; Vaught, J.A.; Burwick, R.; Chaturvedi, S. Maternal and fetal outcomes of pregnancy occurring after a diagnosis of immune-mediated thrombotic thrombocytopenic purpura. *Ann. Hematol.* **2022**, *101*, 2159–2167. [CrossRef] [PubMed]
7. Tarasco, E.; Bütikofer, L.; Friedman, K.D.; George, J.N.; Hrachovinova, I.; Knöbl, P.N.; Matsumoto, M.; von Krogh, A.S.; Aebi-Huber, I.; Cermakova, Z.; et al. Annual incidence and severity of acute episodes in hereditary thrombotic thrombocytopenic purpura. *Blood* **2021**, *137*, 3563–3575. [CrossRef] [PubMed]
8. Kremer Hovinga, J.A.; George, J.N. Hereditary Thrombotic Thrombocytopenic Purpura. *New Engl. J. Med.* **2019**, *381*, 1653–1662. [CrossRef]
9. Miodownik, S.; Pikovsky, O.; Erez, O.; Kezerle, Y.; Lavon, O.; Rabinovich, A. Unfolding the pathophysiology of congenital thrombotic thrombocytopenic purpura in pregnancy: Lessons from a cluster of familial cases. *Am. J. Obstet. Gynecol.* **2021**, *225*, e1–e177. [CrossRef]
10. Lotta, L.A.; Wu, H.M.; Mackie, I.J.; Noris, M.; Veyradier, A.; Scully, M.A.; Remuzzi, G.; Coppo, P.; Liesner, R.; Donadelli, R.; et al. Residual plasmatic activity of ADAMTS13 is correlated with phenotype severity in congenital thrombotic thrombocytopenic purpura. *Blood* **2012**, *120*, 440–448. [CrossRef]
11. de Almeida, L.G.N.; Young, D.; Chow, L.; Nicholas, J.; Lee, A.; Poon, M.C.; Dufour, A.; Agbani, E.O. Proteomics and Metabolomics Profiling of Platelets and Plasma Mediators of Thrombo-Inflammation in Gestational Hypertension and Preeclampsia. *Cells* **2022**, *11*, 1256. [CrossRef] [PubMed]
12. Agbani, E.O.; van den Bosch, M.T.; Brown, E.; Williams, C.M.; Mattheij, N.J.; Cosemans, J.M.; Collins, P.W.; Heemskerk, J.W.; Hers, I.; Poole, A.W. Coordinated membrane ballooning and procoagulant spreading in human platelets. *Circulation* **2015**, *132*, 1414–1424. [CrossRef] [PubMed]
13. Agbani, E.O.; Williams, C.M.; Li, Y.; Bosch, M.V.D.; Moore, S.; Mauroux, A.; Hodgson, L.; Verkman, A.S.; Hers, I.; Poole, A.W. Aquaporin-1 regulates platelet procoagulant membrane dynamics and in vivo thrombosis. *JCI Insight* **2018**, *3*, e99062. [CrossRef] [PubMed]
14. Agbani, E.O.; Mahe, E.; Chaturvedi, S.; Yamaura, L.; Schneider, P.; Barber, M.R.; Choi, M.; Lee, A.; Skeith, L. Platelets and neutrophils co-drive procoagulant potential in second-ary antiphospholipid syndrome during pregnancy. *Thromb. Res.* **2022**, *220*, 141–144. [CrossRef] [PubMed]

15. Finsterbusch, M.; Schrottmaier, W.C.; Kral-Pointner, J.B.; Salzmann, M.; Assinger, A. Measuring and interpreting platelet-leukocyte aggregates. *Platelets* **2018**, *29*, 677–685. [CrossRef]
16. Mauler, M.; Seyfert, J.; Haenel, D.; Seeba, H.; Guenther, J.; Stallmann, D.; Schoenichen, C.; Hilgendorf, I.; Bode, C.; Ahrens, I.; et al. Platelet-neutrophil complex formation-a detailed in vitro analysis of murine and human blood samples. *J. Leukoc. Biol.* **2016**, *99*, 781–789. [CrossRef]
17. George, J.N.; Nester, C.M.; McIntosh, J.J. Syndromes of thrombotic microangiopathy associated with pregnancy. *Hematology* **2015**, *2015*, 644–648. [CrossRef]
18. Dap, M.; Romiti, J.; Dolenc, B.; Morel, O. Thrombotic thrombocytopenic purpura and severe preeclampsia: A clinical overlap during pregnancy and a possible coexistence. *J. Gynecol. Obstet. Human Reprod.* **2022**, *51*, 102422. [CrossRef]
19. Bitsadze, V.; Bouvier, S.; Khizroeva, J.; Cochery-Nouvellon, É.; Mercier, É.; Perez-Martin, A.; Makatsariya, A.; Gris, J.C. Early ADAMTS13 testing associates with pre-eclampsia occurrence in antiphospholipid syndrome. *Thromb. Res.* **2021**, *203*, 101–109. [CrossRef]
20. Neave, L.; Thomas, M.; de Groot, R.; Doyle, A.; David, A.; Maksym, K.; Whitten, M.; Scully, M. Changes in VWF, ADAMTS13, and Complement in Preeclampsia, HELLP syndrome and Other Obstetric Complications: A Single Centre Observational Study. In Proceedings of the ISTH 2022 Congress, London, UK, 9–13 July 2022.
21. Xiao, J.; Feng, Y.; Li, X.; Li, W.; Fan, L.; Liu, J.; Zeng, X.; Chen, K.; Chen, X.; Zhou, X.; et al. Expression of ADAMTS13 in normal and abnormal placentae and its potential role in angiogenesis and placenta development. *Arterioscler. Thromb. Vasc. Biol.* **2017**, *37*, 1748–1756. [CrossRef]
22. Zarbock, A.; Polanowska-Grabowska, R.K.; Ley, K. Platelet-neutrophil-interactions: Linking hemostasis and inflammation. *Blood Rev.* **2007**, *21*, 99–111. [CrossRef] [PubMed]
23. Lisman, T. Platelet–neutrophil interactions as drivers of inflammatory and thrombotic disease. *Cell Tissue Res.* **2018**, *371*, 567–576. [CrossRef] [PubMed]

MDPI AG
Grosspeteranlage 5
4052 Basel
Switzerland
Tel.: +41 61 683 77 34

Journal of Clinical Medicine Editorial Office
E-mail: jcm@mdpi.com
www.mdpi.com/journal/jcm

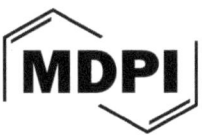

Disclaimer/Publisher's Note: The title and front matter of this reprint are at the discretion of the Guest Editors. The publisher is not responsible for their content or any associated concerns. The statements, opinions and data contained in all individual articles are solely those of the individual Editors and contributors and not of MDPI. MDPI disclaims responsibility for any injury to people or property resulting from any ideas, methods, instructions or products referred to in the content.

www.ingramcontent.com/pod-product-compliance
Lightning Source LLC
LaVergne TN
LVHW070001100526
838202LV00019B/2599